essential guide to
natural home
remedies

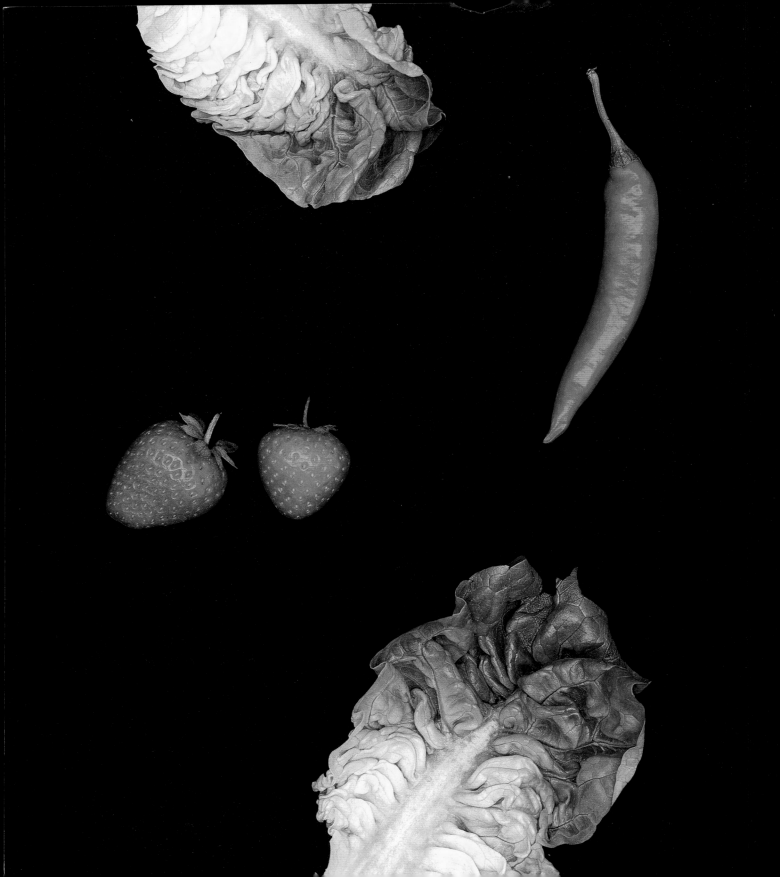

essential guide to

natural
home
remedies

penelope ody

KYLE CATHIE LIMITED

For John Clive, as always

First published in Great Britain in 2002 by
Kyle Cathie Limited
122 Arlington Road
London NW1 7HP
general.enquiries@kyle-cathie.com
www.kylecathie.com

This paperback edition published 2003

ISBN 1 85626 480 7

Editor: Caroline Taggart
Editorial Assistant: Sarah Epton
Designer: Caroline Hillier
Photographer: Laura Hodgson
See also other picture acknowledgements on page 256
Production: Lorraine Baird and Sha Huxtable

Much of the material in this book is taken from
100 Great Natural Remedies by Penelope Ody,
published in 1997.

A CIP catalogue record for this book is available from
the British Library.

Printed and bound in Singapore through Tien-Wah Press

contents

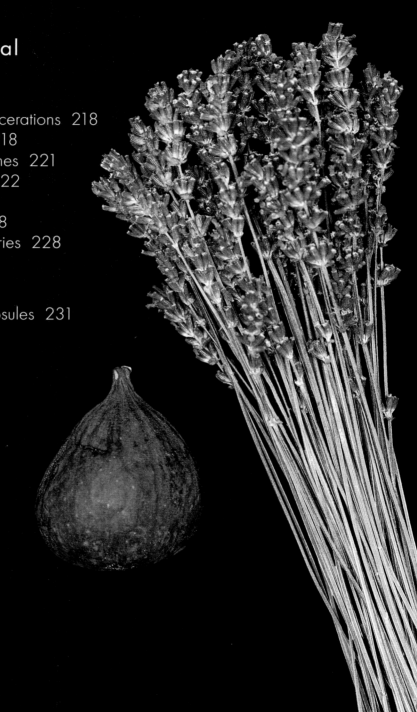

All nature is like one single apothecary's shop, covered only with the roof of heaven; and only One Being works the pestle as far as the world extends. But man has such a shop only in part, not wholly; he possesses something, not everything. For nature's apothecary's shop is greater than man's.

Paracelsus (1493 – 1541)

Author's acknowledgements
Thanks are due to Caroline Taggart and Sarah Epton for their eagle-eyed editing, patience and constant good humour.

Important note
The information and advice contained in this book is intended as a general guide to using plants and is not specific to individuals or their particular circumstances. Many plant substances, whether sold as foods or medicines, and used externally or internally, can cause an allergic reaction in some people. Neither the author nor the publishers can be held responsible for claims arising from the inappropriate use of any remedy or healing regime. Do not attempt self-diagnosis or self-treatment for serious or long-term conditions before consulting a medical professional or qualified practitioner. Do not undertake any self-treatment while taking other prescribed drugs or receiving therapy without first seeking professional guidance. Always seek medical advice if any symptoms persist.

Quantities for making your own remedies are given in metric and imperial measurements. Use one or the other and do not interchange them, as conversions are not always exact equivalents and concentrations need to be consistent for each remedy e.g. 25g of herb to 500ml of water gives the same concentration as 1oz of herb to 1pt of water, but 25g of herb to 1pt of water does not.

introduction

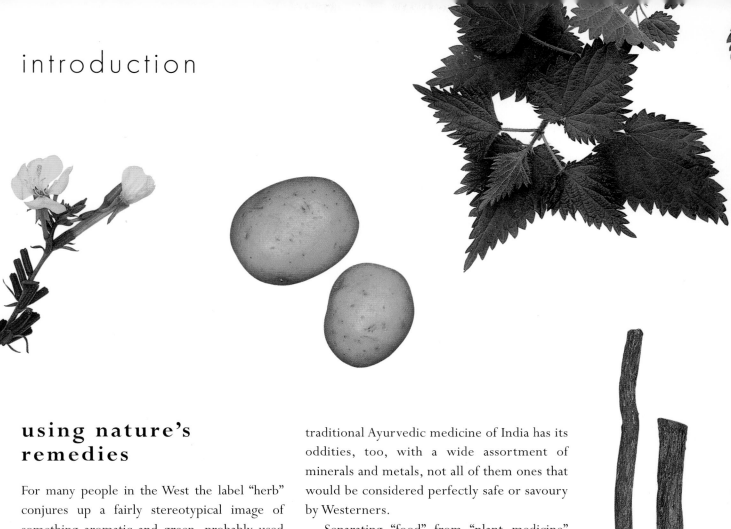

using nature's remedies

For many people in the West the label "herb" conjures up a fairly stereotypical image of something aromatic and green, probably used for flavouring and sometimes displaying medicinal properties. The *Shorter Oxford English Dictionary* confirms the imagery defining herbs as "…plants of which the leaves, or stem and leaves, are used for food or medicine, or for their scent and flavour".

We can, however, put a great many more items into the "natural remedies" category than a few archetypal leaves and stems. Flowers, fruits, roots, barks, seaweeds and fungi all figure in the herbal repertoire, while Chinese medicine is notorious for its use of animal parts and the macabre practices used by suppliers trying to obtain them. The

traditional Ayurvedic medicine of India has its oddities, too, with a wide assortment of minerals and metals, not all of them ones that would be considered perfectly safe or savoury by Westerners.

Separating "food" from "plant medicine" is similarly no easy task: the garlic sold in the supermarket is technically food, but the same cloves could just as easily be prescribed as a heart tonic or used to combat colds and catarrh. Today's increasing appreciation of plant properties has seen a spate of recommendations and media headlines urging us to eat broccoli or carrots to help protect against cancer, to drink wine to combat heart disease or to fight depression with oats. Are we talking here of foods or medicines?

We also live in an age of "magic bullets" where medicine is something powerful, shrink-wrapped, and promises to clear symptoms in hours rather than days; to "bring instant relief" or make us "feel better – faster" as the advertisements usually proclaim. The idea that well-being requires personal effort and involvement is as alien to many people as the concept of using beans, rather than highly processed granules, to make coffee.

Many in modern Western society are also "time poor" – we have too many things to do and too little time in which to do them. The keyword in food shopping nowadays is "convenience" and the recipe writers tell us that life is too short to stuff a mushroom. In such a world it is hardly surprising that gathering herbs, drying them slowly and carefully at home, and then taking the time and trouble to blend them to make healing teas, or spend hours over a hot stove stirring creams and ointments, seems to belong to another age. Yet it is just this sort of involvement that is needed if we are really to heal ourselves.

Until the arrival of low-cost, state-sponsored health care and potent, readily available pharmaceutical drugs, the only medicines available to most people were the ones they made themselves – remedies that could be found in the local wood, meadow or physic garden.

learning lessons from the past

Plant medicines have been in regular, well-documented use for at least 5,000 years and probably much longer: there is evidence that many mammals will seek out and eat particular plants when they feel ill and who is to know whether or not our cave-dwelling ancestors did exactly the same? Traces of medicinal herbs such as yarrow and marshmallow have been found in Neanderthal graves of 65,000 years ago, suggesting at least some contemporary significance for these plants.

Our Western tradition of herbal medicine is largely derived from Greek and Roman practice, with many herbs used today much as they were by Dioscorides – a surgeon with Nero's army who wrote one of our earliest surviving herbals in the first century AD. Greek medicine, as originally described by Hippocrates, the "father of modern medicine" (c. 460–c. 370 BC), was based on the belief that all matter is made up of four elements: earth, air, fire and water. These elements had their own characteristics and qualities: "earth", for example, was regarded as heavy, stable and firm, while "fire" travels upwards, intermingles and permeates all things.

The Greeks applied the concept of elements to the four bodily fluids or "humours" which early physicians had observed coming from the body. These were "blood", associated with air; "phlegm", linked with water; "yellow bile" or the "choleric humour", linked with fire; and "black bile", corresponding to earth. Like the elements, these humours had to be kept in balance and excess was believed to lead to ill health. Those suffering from a surfeit of black bile (described as "melancholic") would have been given strong purgatives as the resulting diarrhoea was visible evidence of the removal of excess black bile from the system. Those with too much blood (sanguine) were good humoured but prone to over-indulgence – hence the habit of "bleeding" patients.

Elements and humours were also defined in terms of cold or hot, dry or damp. Earth and black bile, for example, were both cold and dry, while blood was – understandably – hot and moist. The aim was always to maintain balance between the humours by adjusting diet and lifestyle as need be so that cold conditions would be countered by additional heat or excessive dryness corrected with additional moisture.

Seasonal characteristics were central to the model. Hippocrates, in his famous *Regimen in Health* written around 420 BC, urges that in cold, damp winter one should: "…eat as much as possible and drink as little as possible; drink should be wine as undiluted as possible and food should be bread with all meats roasted; during this season take as few vegetables as possible for so will the body be mostly hot and dry…".

The humoural model was codified by Galen (131–199 AD), so is often termed "Galenic medicine". With the fall of the Roman Empire in the fifth century, this Greek tradition was kept alive by the Arabs and was further refined and developed by such notable physicians as Avicenna al-Hussain (also known as Abdullah Ibn Sina who died in 1037). Today, it survives in the Tibb or Unani medical tradition, which is practised throughout the Islamic world.

Avicenna's work was highly regarded by later European herbalists and was widely quoted by herbal writers until well into the 18th century, when Galenic theories began to be replaced by a more modern approach to medicine.

When it came to identifying plant properties, these early herbalists had largely to depend on trial and error, but to support the guesswork they used a theory known as the "Doctrine of Signatures". This maintained that the appearance of plants provided clues to their properties. Yellow-flowered plants such as dandelion were believed to be good for treating jaundice, for example, while the nodular roots of lesser celandine were said to resemble piles, giving the plant its country name of pilewort. While much of this theory has been discredited by the findings of modern science, both pilewort and dandelion live up to their signatures and are used, respectively, for treating piles and liver disorders today.

While many associated the doctrine with the noted German herbalist Paracelsus (1493–1541), similar theories are found in many cultures. The Chinese, for example, recommend cinnamon twigs to warm the hands and toes, while the tree trunk's bark is more suitable for warming the body.

Like elements and humours, both herbs and foods in Western tradition were also classified as hot or cold, dry or damp, and over the centuries the descriptions became ever more sophisticated with the introduction of several "degrees" of hotness, dampness and so on.

The great Elizabethan herbalist John Gerard, writing in 1597, tells us that horseradish is "hot and dry in the third degree". It would therefore have been used to combat severe problems of cold and damp – excess phlegm – by restoring the balance. In contrast chickweed is "cold and moist and of a waterish substance", so would be helpful with problems of heat and dryness, such as the dry, scaling, irritant eczema for which it is still recommended today.

entering the era of modern medicine

With the coming of the Industrial Revolution to Europe and the population drift from countryside to towns and cities, this sort of knowledge was gradually lost. By the 1850s, the emphasis was firmly on patent remedies, and a new generation of urban poor had little help when it came to illness.

In North America, the early settlers had introduced many of their favourite healing plants from Europe; typical was common plantain which spread so rapidly that the Native Americans called it "white man's foot", as its arrival inevitably followed the pioneers. New World plants were also introduced to the repertoire, with European settlers readily adopting such herbs as echinacea, black cohosh, Virginian skullcap and golden seal.

This blending of traditions can be seen in the "Physiomedical" and "Eclectic" movements founded in 18th-century New England and derived, in part, from the Galenic model combined with Native American traditions of sweat houses and heating remedies. Samuel Thomson, founder of the Physiomedical movement, believed that all disease was caused by cold and he used sweat treatments combined with emetics and purgatives to clear the system of cold and damp phlegm. By the 1830s more than three million Americans had subscribed to Thomson's self-help manuals and were enthusiastically using his remedies.

Thomson's followers, Albert Coffin and Wooster Beech, introduced these new theories to Britain, successfully treating the typhoid and cholera epidemics associated with Victorian slums. Eclectic herbalists continued to practise in Britain until well into the 1930s and many traditional over-the-counter herbal products are still based on their theories. North American plants are important for the British herbal *materia medica* and while these plants remain popular in the UK, there is often little tradition of using them in other parts of Europe where Physiomedicalism never penetrated.

By the 20th century, herbal medicine may have become a minority interest but many of the traditional remedies live on as the basis of newer orthodox drugs: aspirin was extracted from willow bark, heart drugs such as digoxin from foxglove. Today researchers are continuing to discover new cures in our old traditions: yew gives us Taxol, a cancer treatment, while bluebells are being investigated as a possible treatment for AIDS.

looking east

Mainstream herbal medicine has also embraced other new and fashionable influences, as Ayurvedic and traditional Chinese products enter the marketplace. A few years ago it was virtually impossible to buy Chinese herbs in Europe. The intrepid could venture into Soho's Chinatown and similar centres and, if the language problems were not insurmountable, emerge with a bag of miscellaneous brown things which may or may not have been what they wanted. Today, Chinese herbs are being tested in state hospitals and Chinese "doctors" thrive in numerous shops and clinics throughout Europe and North America.

Traditional Chinese medicine is, like Galenic theory, based on a model that links elements with bodily functions. In this case there are five elements (earth, wood, fire, water and metal) related to the five main organs of the body (spleen, liver, heart, kidney and lungs), five emotions (worry, anger, joy, fear and grief), five body fluids (saliva, tears, sweat, urine and mucus), five tastes (sweet, sour, bitter, pungent and salty) and so on. Herbs are defined by taste and temperature, which links them to associated body organs and function. Sweet herbs, for example, are nutritious and toning for the spleen and stomach; salty herbs are associated with fluid balance and kidney function.

As well as the five-element model, the Chinese also believe in the duality of vital energy or *Qi* (sometimes spelt *ch'i*), which has both *yang* and *yin* aspects. *Yang* is associated with the male, light and heat, whereas *yin* is seen as female, dark and cold. Herbs are similarly divided: Korean ginseng, for example, is a *yang* tonic and Siberian ginseng is considered as benefiting *yin* energy.

A number of Chinese herbs are now being included in mainstream herbal products. Ginseng has been available for years, but a newcomer is *Dang Gui* (Chinese angelica), which is defined in Chinese theory as a blood tonic and is widely used for gynaecological problems. There is also considerable interest in the medicinal fungi used in Eastern medicine such as shiitake and maitake, both best known in the West by their Japanese names.

The Oriental fashion is also influencing herbal product suppliers and a number of Chinese-style over-the-counter remedies are now appearing which contain plants that would have been quite unfamiliar a decade ago.

Western interest is also growing in India's Ayurvedic medicine which is a combination of very ancient health and philosophical traditions – dating back to around 5000 BC – overlaid by later Islamic influence and Unani (Greek) medicine. Like Galenic medicine, Ayurveda is based on a model of elements (also five), bodily humours (*tri doshas*) and a need to maintain the inner life force (*prana*) which is believed to give rise to the fire of digestion (*agni*) and mental energy. The three humours of Ayurveda are: *pitta* (bile linked to the fire element), *vata* (wind associated with the air and aether elements) and *kapha* (phlegm or dampness, ruled by the elements of water and earth). *Prana* is linked to breath or oxygen which feeds the fire and, if the fire is weak, then the body is weak.

Around 800 herbs are used in the "great tradition" of Ayurvedic medicine, although there is also a strong regional folk tradition covering around 2,500 medicinal herbs which are used in what is known as the "lesser medicine". Each family will have its own *maharastra* or "grandmother's purse", filled with healing herbs for the household, and the traditions of how to use these have been passed continuously from mother to daughter for generations in the manner of native healers everywhere. Some Ayurvedic remedies, such as turmeric and basil, have long been familiar as culinary seasonings; others, such as gotu kola and *ashwaghanda*, are more recent arrivals.

herbal remedies in the home

While many of these more exotic remedies can be found in health food shops, familiar European garden and culinary herbs should not be forgotten. Medicinal herbs can be, and often are, used as foods or culinary flavourings, and what nicer way to take your daily dose than in a warming cup of tea or added to the evening's meal? Equally, one must remember that many foods also have their own potent therapeutic effects and that some – in high doses – can be extremely toxic. It is unlikely that if the potato were discovered today it would be passed as fit for human consumption because of the toxic alkaloids it contains.

In the past, knowledge of the healing properties and use of plants was something handed down between generations: the family "receipt" book with its mixture of supper dishes, jams and cough mixtures was commonplace and brewing up a healing gruel to combat colds and chills was as much a part of everyday life as baking a cake.

The seasonal use of particular plants was common knowledge, as was the intrinsic character of the food and flavourings – be they hot, damp, dry or cooling – and the likely effect they could have on healthy natural balance. Today, factors such as central heating, air conditioning and air-freighted exotic foods tend to make our living conditions and diet much the same throughout the year and we have forgotten not only the healing skills of our great-grandmothers, but nature's own rhythms as well. Many people would regard gathering wild plants and eating them as a certain way of contracting food poisoning while others regard brewing tea as a major culinary achievement: we have lost both the confidence to use nature's remedies and the intuitive skill to know when we need them.

Rather than expect the health care professional – be that an orthodox GP or a herbal specialist – simply to prescribe a wonder cure, we need to reclaim the responsibility for our own well-being that our ancestors took for granted. Taking the time to brew skullcap and lemon balm tea at the end of a busy day, and then do nothing but sip it for 10 minutes, is just as valuable for the over-stressed, anxiety sufferer as the herbs' sedative properties. Active involvement in our own cure is essential. Taking the herbal medicines prescribed by a specialist is just part of the cure, it might also involve changing diet, taking more exercise, or learning to relax with yoga or t'ai-chi classes.

Taking responsibility for your health means listening to your body: learning to identify the early signs of illness – the sore throat that will turn into laryngitis, the minor twinge that could become a frozen shoulder – and taking action at that stage, rather than waiting until professional help is the only solution. Obviously there are times when urgent medical attention is essential, but for the sort of commonplace, self-limiting ailments that send some to the local chemist for over-the-counter cures and others to their GP's surgery for yet another course of antibiotics or tranquillisers, herbal home remedies can provide an ideal alternative.

This book cannot pretend to be comprehensive – there are many thousands of plants with therapeutic properties and several hundred of these could be used as household remedies. Instead it focuses on some readily available plant products – be they found in the kitchen store cupboard, stacked on the greengrocer's counter, growing as garden plants or wild in hedgerows, or neatly labelled as medicines in the health food shop.

cautions

People are often fond of saying that "herbal medicine is safer" – certainly herbs can have fewer side effects than some orthodox drugs but, as Paracelsus always reminded us, everything is toxic to a greater or lesser degree. Just because herbs are natural plants rather than laboratory concocted chemicals does not mean that they are totally harmless. Healing plants are powerful and need to be treated with respect.

plants from the wild

when gathering, always check identification very carefully and don't assume that a plant has always been correctly labelled by the nursery or seedsman when planning to grow them at home. Use a good wild flower key or illustrated herbal to confirm identity. I once planted a packet clearly labelled as catmint seeds which once fully grown proved to be marsh woundwort.

ready-made products

when using, always follow recommended dosages and never exceed the general guidelines given in Part 3 of this book on "Making and using herbal remedies". Always seek professional help for any persistent symptoms or if there is a sudden change in condition as well as for acute pain or prolonged high temperatures.

orthodox medication

a few herbs can conflict with orthodox medicine such as feverfew with blood-thinning drugs, so seek professional advice if you are on long-term medication and would like to use home-made remedies.

herbs to avoid in pregnancy

the list can appear excessively long but in most cases concern is over high, therapeutic doses. A few of the herbs listed have been reported to cause foetal abnormalities but most act as uterine stimulants so can increase the risk of miscarriage. As a general rule avoid taking any medication (herbal or otherwise) during the first three months of pregnancy unless recommended to do so by a health care professional.

plants to avoid totally in pregnancy

aloe
arbor vitae (*Thuja occidentalis*)
autumn crocus (*Colichicum autumnale*)
barberry (*Berberis vulgaris*)
basil oil
beth root (*Trillium erectum*)
black cohosh
bloodroot (*Sanguinaria canadensis*)
blue cohosh (*Caulophyllum thalictroides*)
broom (*Cytisus scoparius*)
bugleweed (*Lycopus virginicus*)
clove oil
comfrey
cotton root (*Gossypium herbaceum*)
devil's claw
Dang Gui
false unicorn root (*Chamaelirium luteum*)
feverfew
golden seal
greater celandine
gurmari
juniper
kava
lady's mantle (*Alchemilla xanthoclora*)
liferoot (*Senecio aureus*)
mistletoe (*Viscum album*)
mugwort
pennyroyal (*Mentha pulegium*)
Peruvian bark (*Cinchona officinalis*)
Peruvian cat's claw
pokeroot (*Phytolacca decandra*)
pseudoginseng (*Panax notoginseng*)
rue (*Ruta graveolens*)
sassafras (*Sassafras albidum*)
shepherd's purse
southernwood (*Artemisia abrotanum*)
squill (*Urginea maritima*)
tansy (*Tanacetum vulgare*)
wild yam (*Dioscorea villosa*)
wormwood (*Artemisia absinthum*)

plants to avoid in pregnancy in regular large or therapeutic doses

some of theses plants are suitable for use in labour, and culinary herbs on the list are safe in the sorts of quantities used for flavouring.

alder buckthorn (*Rhamnus frangula*)
angelica
anise
bitter orange
caraway (*Carum carvi*)
cascara sagrada (*Rhamnus purshiana*)
celery seed
chamomile oil
chili
cinnamon
cowslip (*Primula veris*)
elder bark
fennel
fenugreek
garlic
gotu kola
jasmine oil (*Jasminium officinale*)
Korean ginseng
lavender
liquorice
lovage (*Levisticum officinale*)
marjoram
motherwort
myrrh (*Commiphora molmol*)
nutmeg
oregano
parsley
passion flower
peppermint oil
rhubarb root (*Rheum palmatum*)
rosemary and rosemary oil
saffron (*Crocus sativa*)
sage
senna (*Senna alexandrina*)
vervain
white horehound (*Marrubium vulgare*)
wood betony
yarrow

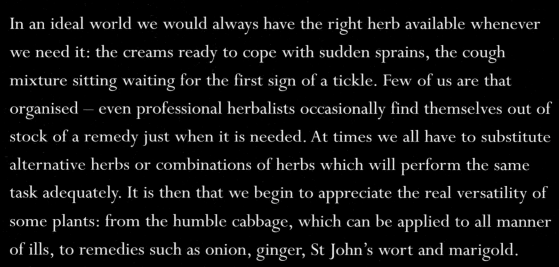

using herbs for common ailments

In an ideal world we would always have the right herb available whenever we need it: the creams ready to cope with sudden sprains, the cough mixture sitting waiting for the first sign of a tickle. Few of us are that organised – even professional herbalists occasionally find themselves out of stock of a remedy just when it is needed. At times we all have to substitute alternative herbs or combinations of herbs which will perform the same task adequately. It is then that we begin to appreciate the real versatility of some plants: from the humble cabbage, which can be applied to all manner of ills, to remedies such as onion, ginger, St John's wort and marigold.

For home use herbal choice is limited as much by such practicalities as the size of the bathroom cabinet as by what is available from local health food shops, the garden or growing in local hedgerows. If you do not have the plants recommended in this section available, check the list of especially relevant herbs included within each ailment group. These are featured in Part 2 of this book and can help you find a suitable substitute from the remedies you have to hand.

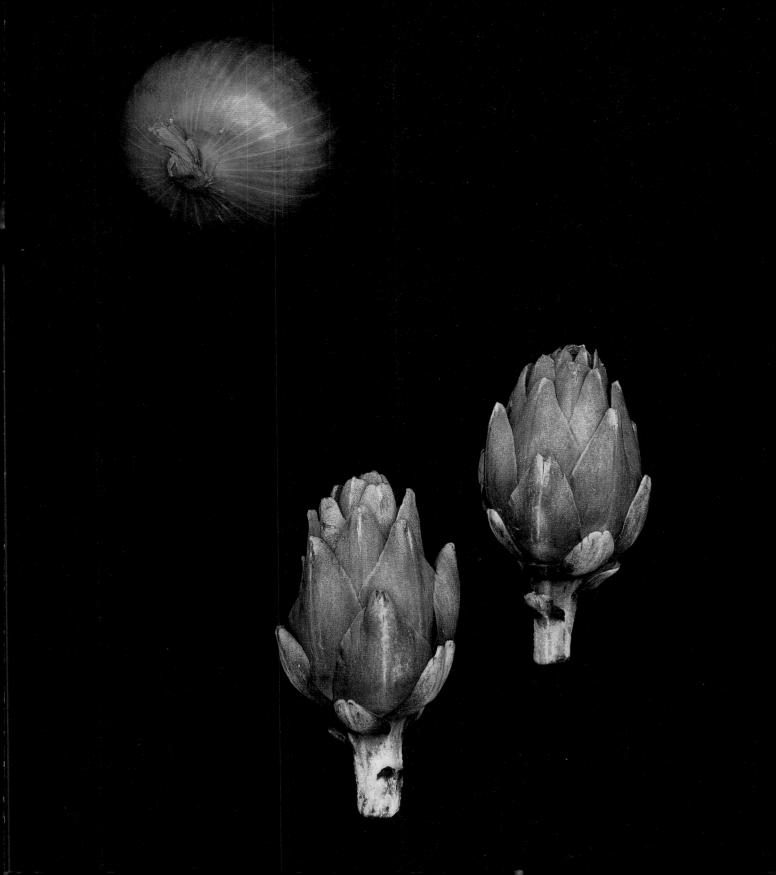

aches and pains

No matter how healthy their lifestyle sooner or later most people have some experience of muscular aches and pains: it could be a pulled muscle or ligament due to accidental injury, the wear and tear of osteoarthritis or even that new ill of our technological age, "repetitive strain injury". Or it could be a less localised problem – a systemic disorder such as rheumatoid arthritis or, more commonly, a nagging backache which seems to have no obvious cause.

Orthodox treatment usually focuses on "painkillers", but pain is only a symptom, there to remind us that the body is out of balance and in need of rest and repair. Sometimes the pain and the cause are closely associated – slipped discs cause back pain, fractured wrists hurt – but it is not always the case. In traditional Chinese medicine five-element theory (see page 10) the liver is associated with the tendons, the kidney with the bones, and the muscles or flesh with the spleen. Unexplained joint or muscle problems can therefore suggest a primary weakness in one or other of these organs. This is often seen with knee pain and liver disharmony: the knees contain rather a lot of tendons, so if there is any liver weakness, they can be the first joints affected. A typical result of liver abuse – in the form of too much alcohol or rich food – can often be aching knees the next morning.

The same applies to those vague backaches: often they can be related to energy imbalances elsewhere in the body and can be significant signs of these disorders. Kidney weakness or problems with the urinary system, for example, can be accompanied by lower-back pain or the ache could be related to a gynaecological problem.

The sorts of aches and pains that respond well to home remedies include sprains, strains, traumatic injuries including bruises, and those occasional twinges caused by old injuries – usually when the weather changes – that can lead to osteoarthritis in later life: all the sorts of ailments, in fact, that the orthodox first-aider would treat with aspirins or painkilling sprays.

First choice in herbal first-aid remedies often lies with the essential oils. These are the "magic bullets" of the herbal repertoire: quick-acting, entering the bloodstream almost immediately when applied to the skin, and – having bypassed the liver – quickly unleashing potent chemicals into the circulation. Essential oils are expensive and can be subject to adulteration by the unscrupulous, with synthetic chemicals added on a massive and hazardous scale. For home use choose branded products offering some sort of quality guarantee and always dilute in a carrying medium, such as sweet almond oil or water, before use (see page 226).

sprains and pulled muscles

Pulled muscles and twisted joints can be acutely painful and if they result from some accidental, traumatic injury, an X-ray is often necessary to identify fractures or cracked bones. Strains involve a slight tearing of a muscle or the tendon attaching it to a bone and are generally caused by over-stretching. Sprains are a tear in the joint capsule or associated ligaments caused by twisting.

Comfrey and arnica are ideal for treating any damaged tissue: apply a little cream, ointment or infused oil and rest the injured area as much as possible. Arnica can be particularly useful for relieving pain, while comfrey increases cell growth and so speeds healing. Avoid using both ointments if the skin is broken: arnica can be irritant, while comfrey is under suspicion for containing toxic alkaloids (see page 204) and it can also speed healing to such an extent that dirt may be trapped in cuts and grazes leading to abscesses. Both herbs also work well used in cold compresses (see page 230).

Twisted or strained muscles often respond well to herbal rubs. Massage oils containing eucalyptus, lavender, marjoram, thyme or rosemary essences can also be effective.

For accidental sprains and pulled muscles a useful massage oil can be made from 0.5ml/10 drops each of essential oils of rosemary and lavender with 5 drops each of essential oil of thyme, marjoram and eucalyptus, mixed with 25ml/1fl oz of good quality carrier oil, such as sweet almond or wheat germ oil, or infused comfrey or St John's wort oil (see page 226). Massage the mixture gently and frequently into the affected area for 24-36 hours to provide pain relief and encourage repair.

A useful alternative is simply to apply a cabbage poultice; crush a leaf with a vegetable mallet and wrap it around the injured limb, securing with a loose bandage. Fresh comfrey leaf, crushed daisies or hot mashed potato can be used in the same way.

backache

Backache is one of our most common ailments: causes can range from pulled muscles and damaged discs (the spongy plugs that separate the vertebrae and act as shock absorbers) to poor posture, kidney disease, gynaecological problems or simply sitting in an awkward position for long periods.

Some sorts of backache are dignified by rather grander names: "lumbago" simply means pain in the lower back (the lumbar region) from whatever cause, whereas "sciatica" is a pain felt along the back and outer side of the thigh, leg and foot, with accompanying back pain and stiffness, often caused by a damaged disc putting pressure on the sciatic nerve. "Fibrositis" is an inflammation of fibrous tissue, especially muscle sheaths, which often affects the back muscles. It leads to pain and stiffness and can be treated with anti-inflammatories and those remedies recommended for rheumatic disorders (see below).

All these various sorts of backache require very different treatment, so accurate diagnosis is important if therapy is to be at all relevant. If the problem originates from mechanical damage in the back itself, treatment from an osteopath or chiropractor can often solve the problem; massage from a remedial masseur or physiotherapist can also give relief, while poor posture can be helped by learning the Alexander Technique through a series of lessons.

For persistent backache with no obvious cause, changing sleeping arrangements can sometimes help: mattresses should give support (they don't have to be hard!) and an extra pillow under the mattress to raise the top of the bed is worth trying. It can also be useful to alternate lying on your back with knees bent and then curling into a small ball with the spine curved, as in the foetal position, as you fall off to sleep.

As well as using massage oils containing juniper, rosemary, lavender, marjoram, thyme or eucalyptus, add 2-3 drops of these same essential oils to a hot bath. For backache related to kidney weakness, drinking buchu and cinnamon tea can be helpful: use one teaspoon of buchu leaves and a generous pinch of dried cinnamon to a cup of boiling water and infuse for 10 minutes. Repeat up to three times a day for up to a week.

rheumatism and arthritis

Rheumatism is a very imprecise term used to describe various chronic muscular aches and pains. It can include fibrositis and lumbago and may be referred to as "myalgia", which just means pain in the muscles. Arthritis simply means an inflammation of a joint, although as there are various types of arthritis requiring rather different treatment it is important to be sure of the exact diagnosis.

Osteoarthritis is generally due to "wear and tear" – youthful injuries to joints that have never fully healed or obesity putting excessive strain on the weight-bearing joints. Typically in osteoarthritis the protective cartilage surrounding the bones of a joint becomes damaged and wears away, causing the bones to rub together and become deformed. Joints often creak, become stiff and painful, while movement is often limited.

Rheumatoid arthritis (RA) is a more serious and potentially crippling disease that always requires professional treatment. It is an inflammatory problem and may be hereditary. The cause is often unknown but it affects joints symmetrically, commonly attacking both hands, both knees or both sides of the jaw. Inflammation leads to destruction of cartilage and eventually bone, with severe bone deformity.

Arthritis can also occur in children and may be of the inflammatory rheumatoid variety or a more complex syndrome. Juvenile arthritis also needs professional medical treatment.

Chronic arthritis may be related to food intolerance and eliminating possible allergens – especially dairy products, wheat, gluten, beef or pork – can prove extremely helpful. Many arthritics also find that refined carbohydrates (such as products made from white sugar and white flour), citrus fruits, tomatoes and excessive amounts of red meat increase symptoms, while studies suggest that generally reducing animal fats in the diet can bring relief.

There is also some evidence that arthritic problems of sudden onset could be triggered by bacterial or viral infections, so it can be worth adding echinacea, garlic or shiitake mushrooms to the diet to boost the immune system.

Localised osteoarthritic problems can respond to topical, long-term treatment. Comfrey, for example, helps to repair the damage from old injuries and rubbing a little comfrey cream into the joint each night can, over a period of many months, bring relief.

As an alternative to the orthodox painkillers and anti-inflammatories, try hot herbal massage oils and poultices. Essential oil of rosemary (0.5ml/10 drops to 10ml/2tsp of carrier oil) makes an ideal lotion for "rheumatic" twinges. If used as soon as symptoms appear, it can generally stop those nagging aches from developing to the stage when painkillers would usually be needed. Equally effective are hot infused oils made from chili, ginger, horseradish and black pepper (or a combination of all of them), which will encourage blood flow to the area and warm cold joints. These oils should be used in moderation as they can cause skin blistering in some people.

Longer-term herbal treatment usually involves the use of cleansing herbs to remove any chemical toxins lingering in the tissues. Herbs which increase urination and perspiration as well as digestive or circulatory stimulants and laxatives can all be helpful in treating chronic conditions. Relevant plants include angelica, birch, borage, burdock, celery, cucumber, grapes, meadowsweet, pears, pineapples, rosemary, watercress and yellow dock, which can be added to the menu or taken in teas. Over-the-counter herbs, like devil's claw or black cohosh, which reduce inflammation can also help, while many people successfully use feverfew for arthritis, although it can have side-effects (see page 158).

There are also suggestions that congenital rheumatic conditions (especially RA) may be due to the body's inability to manufacture the important chemical, *gamma*-linolenic acid (see page 153), so supplements of evening primrose or borage oil can be worth trying. Extra calcium may also be helpful, especially among post-menopausal women.

In Ayurvedic medicine, joint pain is a characteristic of *vata* – air or wind – and arthritis is termed *amavata* or toxic air. It is associated with injury or with weak digestive fire leading to a build-up of toxins which are eventually carried to the joints. Arthritis can be further classified by the three Ayurvedic humours (air, water and fire): the *pitta* or fire type is what we would term rheumatoid arthritis, where the pain is relieved by cold compresses rather than rubefacients; *kapha*-type involves more joint swelling and oedema (an excess accumulation of fluid in the body tissue) and is worse in damp weather; while *vata*-type is more cold and dry in character. The cold-damp variety (the sort most likely to be seen in a cold, damp climate) is treated much as Galen would have recommended with hot, dry herbs like turmeric, mustard and ginger, while patients are recommended to avoid damp and heavy foods – a category which in Ayurveda includes meats, cereals, nuts and milk.

In traditional Chinese medicine, arthritic or rheumatic aches and pains are termed *Bì Zheng*: *Bì* is usually translated in the West as "pain" and *Bì Zheng* as "painful obstructions". Although the term can refer to any disease associated with obstruction, *Bì Zheng* is usually taken to mean diseases which in the West would be classified as arthritis or rheumatic disorders.

Bì Zheng can sometimes be blamed on attack by external "evils". These evils may have been successful because the energy protecting the body – the *Wei Qi* – is weak (hence the usefulness of immune-stimulants and anti-bacterials in therapy). Several variants of *Bì Zheng* can be identified, including "wind" (hence the shifting nature of the arthritic twinges afflicting different joints at different times), "cold and damp", which is comparable to osteoarthritis with joint swellings, and "hot", which is a more apt description of rheumatoid arthritis.

Traditional Eastern therapies thus see an apparently localised condition such as osteo-arthritis not as an isolated joint problem, but as an ailment of the whole person and treat it by correcting the surfeit of cold, damp humours.

gout

Gout is usually included in the "arthritis" group and is an acutely painful disease caused by a build-up of uric acid crystals in the joints (commonly the big toe). It is associated with an inability to break down a group of chemicals called purines that are found in shellfish, red meats and certain other foods – hence gout's association with over-indulgence and rich food.

Eliminating purine-rich foods from the diet will often reduce symptoms, as will cutting down on fruit sugars (including sweet wines and port). Oxalic acid is another food residue that can build up in the joints, so avoid rhubarb, sorrel and spinach in which it is found.

Herbal remedies for gout generally contain celery seed, which can help clear excess uric acid from the system. Other useful diuretics and anti-rheumatic plant medicines worth trying include artichoke, carrot, cabbage, cucumber, leek, turnip, stinging nettles, birch, bear's breech and marsh woundwort.

bruises

A bruise is an area of skin discolouration caused by blood escaping from damaged underlying blood vessels following injury, while a tendency to bruise easily can be related to problems with the blood's ability to clot or may simply suggest that small blood vessels are thin and easily damaged. If your blood does not clot readily – or you are on blood-thinning drugs – avoid taking herbs like feverfew which can slow down clotting still further.

An ice pack in the form of a packet of frozen peas provides an ideal emergency treatment to relieve the pain of a new bruise; better still, keep an ice-cube tray of frozen distilled witch hazel in a plastic bag in the freezer and rub the ice cubes on the affected area instead. Alternating an ice pack with a hot water bottle can help encourage reabsorption of blood and bring more rapid relief. Arnica or comfrey cream applied to unbroken skin will also encourage healing, while if the bruise is the result of a traumatic accident then taking homoeopathic Arnica 6X internally can speed recovery.

Ointments or creams made from daisies or elder leaves were among traditional remedies for bruising and are well worth trying.

cramp

Cramp is a sudden contraction of the muscles; commonly this occurs in calf muscles which become hard and tense. It can be caused by unusual exercise, stress, tiredness or poor posture, or there may be an imbalance in body salts. In hot weather cramp is often due to a shortage of salt related to dehydration and taking salt tablets can be useful for those prone to cramps. Rubbing the muscle vigorously can bring rapid relief.

Herbal massage oils can be helpful to relax muscles – both marsh woundwort and parsley teas were once popular folk cures for the problem.

repetitive strain injury

In recent years RSI has become a *cause célèbre* generally associated with using computer keyboards for lengthy periods, although the disorder was reputedly first noted among copper beaters in ancient Babylon. In the past similar ailments tended to be categorised by occupation – "upholsterer's hands", "fisherwoman's fingers" and so forth – but any repetitive task, be it typing or playing a musical instrument, can lead to physical problems. RSI often manifests as cramp-like pain or a burning sensation in the hands, arms, shoulders or back, leading ultimately to fatigue, an inability to work effectively and depression.

Appropriate herbal medicines will generally include anti-inflammatories and cleansing remedies, as with arthritic problems, but there will also be emphasis on tonic and immune-stimulating herbs, and relaxing nervines, such as vervain and valerian. Muscle relaxing remedies generally used for muscle cramp, such as wild yam (*Dioscorea villosa*) or cramp bark (*Viburnum opulus*) can also be worth trying. Suitable immune tonics include astragalus (*Huang Qi*), maitake or shiitake mushrooms and ginseng.

Baoding balls – Chinese massage balls slightly larger than golf balls – can help. These need to be rotated in the palm for 5-10 minutes each day – a slightly cumbersome skill but one that is not difficult to learn. Start with smaller table tennis balls if you prefer.

Massage oils containing lavender, thyme, rosemary or eucalyptus can also provide some relief, while internal muscle-relaxing remedies such as nutmeg are worth trying.

headaches and migraines

Headaches are generally symptoms of some underlying disorder rather than illnesses in their own right. Causes are numerous and the location and character of the pain is often an indication of what that underlying problem might be. Those centred behind the eyes, for example, can suggest a digestive disturbance, while headaches that seem to start at the back of the neck and creep forward are generally tension related. Pain and sensitivity around the eyes or above the nose can be caused by a sinus problem (see page 26).

For some people, tension headaches are extremely common at stressful times; others may find that stress highlights a different area of weakness with stomach upsets or urinary problems. Relaxing herbs such as vervain, wood betony, skullcap, chamomile, lavender and St John's wort can ease symptoms, while Siberian ginseng can improve one's stress tolerance and thus reduce the risk of headaches in the first place.

Muscle strain in the shoulders and neck can also contribute to head pain. Sitting or working awkwardly, hunched over a desk or computer keyboard, can easily lead to headaches. Massage oils containing herbs such as thyme, nutmeg, lavender, eucalyptus, marjoram or juniper rubbed into the affected areas can help prevent headaches developing.

Migraine is an especially common problem and is typically preceded by visual disturbances: jagged lights at the edge of the visual field or a sense that there is a strange out-of-focus area in what one sees. Identifying the cause is again important: this may be food intolerance or

(continued opposite)

stress-related. Red wine, chocolate, pork, citrus fruits, coffee and cheese are all common culprits.

Many sufferers find that chewing feverfew leaves can help prevent attacks, although this herb can cause ulceration of the mucous membranes (usually in the form of mouth ulcers) in sensitive individuals and it should not be taken if this side-effect develops. Lavender oil massaged into the temples can sometimes help prevent an attack developing, while valerian and wood betony taken internally can also be useful.

Persistent or sudden unusually severe headaches lasting for three days or more should be referred to a medical practitioner.

neuralgia

Neuralgia means nerve pain and usually involves an inflammation of the nerve fibres. It can occur anywhere in the body but is most common as an inflammation of the facial or trigeminal nerves which run along the side of the face and scalp. The pain is often exacerbated by cold and draughts and in very severe cases surgical treatment is recommended to cut the nerve.

A useful and often surprisingly effective treatment is simply to dab the area with a little diluted lemon oil or warmed lemon juice; alternatively, try infused St John's wort oil or hot infused chili oil with a few drops of lavender essence added. Internally, nervines such as vervain, oats, skullcap, or St John's wort can help, as can circulatory stimulants such as ginger and chili. Jack-by-the-hedge is a traditional remedy for neuralgia and was used in hot poultices.

assorted inflammations. . .

bunions

are painful swellings of the joint between the big toe and the adjoining bone which can be caused

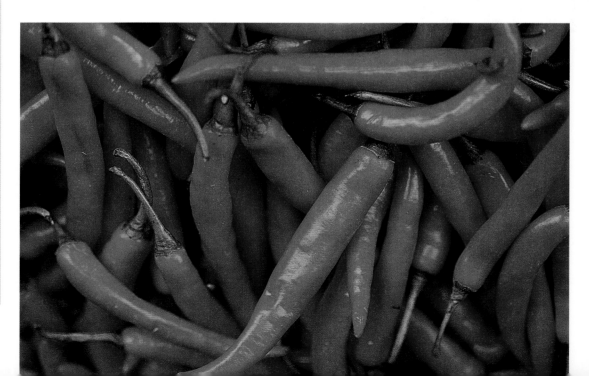

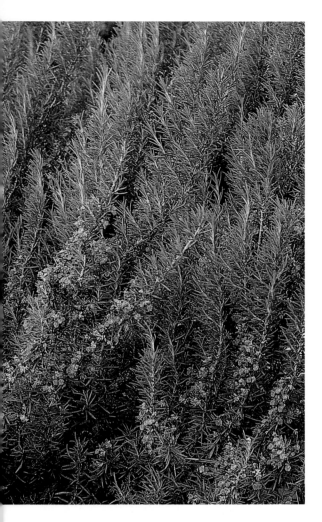

◄ Rosemary *Rosmarinus officinalis*

associated with the backward stretching of tendons. Like "housemaid's knee" (more accurately inflammation of the bursa in the prepatellar region of the knee) it is a painful inflammation usually caused by excessive exercise. As bursitis is an inflammatory problem, herbal anti-inflammatories applied topically can often be helpful.

External massage with a mixture of 5ml/1tsp of St John's wort oil containing 1ml/20 drops of chamomile oil and 0.5ml/10 drops of lemon oil can help to relieve local pain, discomfort and inflammation. Arnica creams and compresses soaked in dilute arnica tincture can also help. Internally a mixture of meadowsweet, black cohosh and St John's wort can be taken along with devil's claw tablets and magnesium supplements. Acupuncture can help to ease pain in chronic or persistent cases and sufferers need to try to reassess their regular movements if possible to avoid repetition.

frozen shoulder

(capsulitis of the shoulder) is a painful stiffness which can follow injury, stroke or heart attack or may simply develop for no apparent cause. Viewed holistically the problem seems often to be associated with over-controlled anger – the sufferer would unconsciously love to throw a right (or left) hook at someone, but social niceties restrain the motion and the subconscious control leads to stiffness. It can often be helped by remedies which improve liver energy flow – the Chinese associate anger with the liver – so try vervain or self-heal teas as well as external massage rubs containing thyme, yarrow or chamomile oils.

by badly fitting shoes. Comfortable shoes are essential, while comfrey, marigold or St John's wort creams can ease inflammation and blistering.

tennis elbow

is a type of "bursitis" which involves inflammation of the radiohumeral bursa (a small sac of fibrous tissue lined with synovial membrane and filled with fluid which helps to reduce the friction in the joint) and is

◄ Chili *Capsicum frutescens*

coughs, colds and catarrh

There are still those who at the first hint of a snuffle or sneeze head for their GP's surgery expecting antibiotics to cure the incipient cold overnight. Certainly antibiotics have a vital role to play in life-threatening diseases, but for common colds and chills herbal remedies can be equally effective. Ancient medical theories often associated illness with climate: dampness was traditionally associated with phlegm-type diseases such as catarrh; many types of cough tend to be more prevalent in cold, wet weather, while fevers were often linked with high summer and a surfeit of heat.

common colds and influenza

Today most people believe that colds, flu and coughs are caused by bacteria and viruses. In other ages mysterious "venoms" were to blame, while the Chinese describe colds in terms of attack by external evils – wind, cold, damp, dryness, heat and fire. Whatever the cause there are always some people who will "catch anything going", while others seem to go for years without the slightest hint of a sneeze. Perhaps John Harrison in his book *Love Your Disease* has a point:

> The common cold is not a disease, so much as an institution. It is employed skilfully and effectively by those who don't want to be particularly ill but want a period of incapacity. Having achieved

that incapacity they can change whatever's troubling them…in this way the common cold or any minor respiratory complaint is used to rebalance the psyche and the internal organs.

In some cases this can well be true and recognising this aspect of a cold is important: curling up in bed with a hot drink or a good book can be a far preferable prescription to antibiotics or patent cold cures.

The typical symptoms of a cold include sore throat, blocked nose, coughs and sneezes. Science blames colds on any one of hundreds of ever-changing viruses: someone who has caught and recovered from a cold can often succumb again, as any immunity to the original virus will be of little use if there is repeated infection.

Because colds are caused by a virus they cannot – despite the optimistic prescriptions – be treated by antibiotics, which are good only for tackling micro-organisms. Orthodox medicine tends to rely on remedies to ease the symptoms, whereas a herbal approach focuses on strengthening the body's immune system and thus helping it to fight the virus. In addition, a number of plants do show anti-viral activity (including lemons, lemon balm and shiitake mushrooms), so can be of real help in countering infection. Frequent colds can be a sign of weakened immunity – they can also indicate a stressful lifestyle or poor diet and no amount of medicines can solve those.

Combating a cold at the first sign of symptoms is also important. Rather than trying to ignore the increasing catarrh and sore throat until the cold is in full flood, start treatment immediately. Echinacea is one of the best herbs for strengthening the immune system (take three 200mg capsules or 10ml/2tsp of tincture three times daily), while garlic – up to 2g daily – is especially helpful if the cold develops into a chest infection. Hemp agrimony has also been shown to have good immune-stimulating properties and is well worth growing in the garden: summer colds respond well to infusions of fresh hemp agrimony leaves, or the stems can be dried for winter use.

High doses of vitamin C (up to 5g/⅙oz a day) are also often recommended, although current research has raised many doubts over the possible damaging side-effects of such large quantities of the vitamin; lower doses (500mg a day) in combination with zinc supplement would seem preferable to strengthen the immune system. To combat symptoms use anti-catarrhals such as elder flower and yarrow and cut down on refined carbohydrates (sugar and white flour products) as these tend to encourage mucus: eat plenty of fruit – and drink lemon juice – instead.

For feverish chills herbs which encourage sweating are useful: make a decoction of fresh ginger root with a little cinnamon, or try elder flower with vervain, meadowsweet and hyssop as an infusion. A popular all-purpose tea for colds is made from equal parts of elder flowers, yarrow and peppermint. This is reasonably palatable and helps to warm the body while having an anti-catarrhal action. In Galenic terms all three herbs are "drying", so would have been used for clearing phlegm in "damp" conditions.

Herbs can also be used in a symptomatic way for other "cold" problems: for sore throats try gargling with strained and cooled infusions of sage or raspberry leaf, or with lemon juice. A little echinacea tincture added to warm water also makes a good gargle; adding a tiny pinch of chili powder to any of these gargles helps to improve efficacy.

Common colds are often labelled as "influenza" but real flu can be severe and in cases life-threatening, with headaches, muscle pain, weakness and high temperature, as well as all the usual symptoms of a bad cold. An attack will typically last for about a week, but will often leave the sufferer feeling depressed and debilitated for some time. Elecampane decoction makes a useful post-influenza tonic – add hyssop if there is a lingering cough or vervain and St John's wort if depression is severe. Flu can be a particular problem for the elderly, very young, diabetics and those suffering from chronic chest, heart or kidney disorders when professional help is generally needed.

catarrhal conditions

Modern medicine tends to consider "catarrh" as a single, consistent problem; however, for the herbalist it can be either "hot" or "cold". Cold catarrh is copious, thin and watery; hot catarrh is thick, scanty and yellow with more inflammation of the mucous membranes. Those with a tendency to "cold" catarrh are often the cold, damp, "phlegmatic" types, with a sluggish digestion. Hot catarrh is a characteristic of more active, tense, "choleric" personalities. While cold catarrh is more characteristic of common colds, some types of sinusitis would come into the "hot" category with thick, yellow mucus that stubbornly refuses to move.

Persistent or chronic catarrh is extremely common; it often seems to be related to geographic areas (such as damp river valleys) and can also be associated with a variety of allergies – many of them difficult to avoid, like house dust or car fumes.

Hay fever is associated with pollen allergies in the summer months but the symptoms can be triggered by a range of all-year problems and then become labelled as "allergic rhinitis". Typical symptoms include sneezing, sore and watering eyes, running noses and drowsiness. The physical symptoms are largely due to the body's production of histamine as it attempts to rid itself of the allergen and orthodox treatments are generally based on anti-histamines.

The herbal approach involves strengthening the mucous membranes to help reduce the likely allergic response: useful herbs include elder flowers, hyssop and golden seal, while anti-allergenic remedies such as chamomile and yarrow oils can help reduce symptoms.

Catarrh can stay in the upper respiratory tract, causing nasal congestion, or the mucus can affect the lower airways and be coughed up as phlegm. Lingering catarrh also makes an ideal breeding ground for bacteria and can lead to inflammation of the sinuses – cavities in the bones of the face. Inflammation here can lead to severe pain, made worse by bending forward or blowing the nose.

Sinusitis, with its associated headaches, tooth problems and general discomfort, causes much misery to many people. It is often helped by massaging stimulating ointments containing chili or ginger into the sinus areas above and around the nose. From a holistic point of view sinusitis is often associated with tense personalities who tend to hold their emotions under tight check. Relaxing herbs – such as skullcap or lemon balm – can help, but perhaps the best choice is chamomile. Not only is this a good relaxing nervine, but the combination of heat and water used to make chamomile tea (as also in extraction of the essential oil), causes anti-inflammatory and anti-spasmodic substances known as azulenes to be produced. Steam inhalations of chamomile flowers are thus good for both the physical effects of sinusitis and its related emotional cause.

While orthodox medicine treats catarrh as a self-contained problem, the condition can also indicate that toxic material elsewhere in the body is not being disposed of adequately. The digestive system could be sluggish or the kidneys not working as efficiently as they should and cleansing herbs for these areas may solve a persistent catarrhal problem as well.

Whatever the cause, diet is extremely important and, as in the common cold, foods that encourage mucus formation should be avoided. These include refined carbohydrates, dairy products and alcohol. A fruit fast for a couple of days helps to clear any lingering toxic wastes while zinc and garlic supplements will help to strengthen the immune system and combat infection.

Steam inhalations can also help to clear catarrh. Add 5 drops of thyme or eucalyptus oil to a basin containing 1 litre/1¾ pt of boiling water, cover your head with a towel and, leaning over the basin, inhale the steam for 10 minutes.

Excess catarrh in children can all too frequently lead to ear problems – such as glue ear (see page 38) – and even orthodox researchers now acknowledge that food allergy can be a cause of both middle ear and catarrhal disorders. In trials with 28 patients suffering from otitis media (inflammation of the middle ear), 17 people developed nasal symptoms after taking a suspect food, while three-quarters of those also suffered hearing loss or earache as well.

coughs

Coughing is the body's natural response to any blockage of the airway which may be due to dust and traffic fumes or mucus resulting from infection. Coughing can also be a symptom of a number of more serious illnesses, so professional medical attention is needed for any cough which persists for more than a few days or for which there is no obvious cause.

Coughs can be dry and irritating or "productive" with phlegm which can vary in shade from white to green – darker colours generally indicating an infection. Dry coughs can often linger for weeks following a cold and in some cases coughing can become a nervous habit.

In traditional Chinese medicine the lung is associated with the emotion "grief" and chesty coughs or asthmatic problems can often follow some sort of shock, such as bereavement or redundancy. Remedies for the nervous system, such as lemon balm or St John's wort, can be helpful in these cases.

In all cases, the choice of herbal remedy will depend on the nature of the cough – dry or productive – and whether the phlegm is thick and infected or thin and watery. Herbal cough remedies include expectorants which will encourage the coughing response and the production and excretion of phlegm, as well as cough suppressants, such as wild lettuce, which can ease a persistent dry, tickling cough.

Taking the wrong sort of remedy can do more harm than good. If there is an infection, for example, suppressing the cough and keeping the infected phlegm in the lungs is not a good idea. Equally, if there is no phlegm, taking an expectorant will just make a dry cough more violent. Many herbal expectorants are believed to work by irritating the mucous membranes of the gut, and then, by reflex action owing to embryonic links between the tissues, also irritating the bronchial membranes so we cough and clear the phlegm. In large doses these herbs often cause vomiting, so taking extra doses in the hope of clearing the cough more rapidly can lead to nausea.

Herbal expectorants are also sometimes classified as either "stimulating", which encourage ever more productive coughing, or "relaxing", which have a more soothing effect and loosen phlegm rather than encouraging its violent removal. Elecampane is a stimulating expectorant, while coltsfoot, liquorice, marshmallow and hyssop are relaxing. Raspberry vinegar also helps clear phlegm and adding crushed raspberries to the remedy will improve the flavour.

As well as expectorants and suppressants, herbal cough remedies include soothing plants known as "demulcents" which can soothe irritated mucous membranes: marshmallow, liquorice and plantain are all demulcent. There are also anti-bacterials such as thyme, which is especially good where the problem is a deep-seated lung infection, and garlic, which can only be excreted through the lungs or skin, so is

(continued opposite)

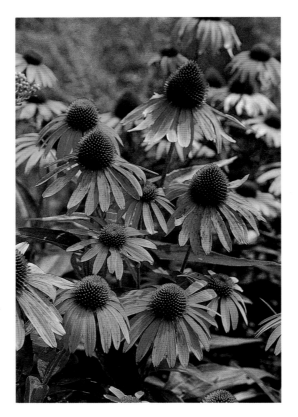

▲ Echincacea *Echinacea* spp.

another good herb for chest infections and one that can be used either as a special "medicine" or simply eaten in lots of very garlicky meals such as *aïoli* or dishes cooked *à la provençale*.

Many cough herbs can be made into syrups – as can onions or leeks – ideally using honey, which is also soothing and healing for the mucous membranes, rather than sugar.

Post-nasal drip – a common cause of coughs – needs an anti-catarrhal approach (see above), but it can also call for expectorants. Hyssop is ideal as it both acts as a gentle, relaxing expectorant and has an anti-catarrhal action. Fennel is also worth considering.

As well as taking cough remedies in teas and syrups, a chest rub can also be useful to help loosen phlegm. The following mixture can be helpful in many cases:

5 drops each of essential oils of fennel and hyssop
10 drops each of essential oils of eucalyptus and thyme

Dilute in 50ml/2fl oz of carrier oil (e.g. sunflower or almond oil) and massage into the chest two or three times a day. Alternatively, put a few drops of the mixture on a handkerchief and use as an inhalant. A few drops in a saucer of water on the bedside table at night can help relieve night-time congestion.

sore throats, tonsillitis and laryngitis

Sore throats can be the first sign of a developing cold, although a tendency to "streptococcal throats" – as they are sometimes labelled – can be associated with underlying food allergy and yeast infections. Sore throats can also herald pharyngitis, tonsillitis or German measles with inflammations caused by viral or bacterial infection. As always, if the problem is recurrent, then the cause may be associated with stress (caused by overwork or food intolerance) or a reduced resistance to infection.

This can be especially true with tonsil problems, since these organs are simply small packs of lymphatic tissue at the back of the throat which help protect the body from infection. Intolerance to dairy products is often to blame in children with a tendency for recurrent tonsillitis; cutting out milk and milk products and using soya or rice substitutes can often solve otherwise intractable problems. In severe cases the tonsil can become filled with pus, causing an abscess or quinsy which can need urgent surgical treatment, so do not delay in seeking professional help if the problem does not show signs of improvement within 24 hours.

Mild sore throats will often clear in two or three days with or without treatment but the discomfort can be eased by gargles using infusions of herbs like sage, agrimony or raspberry leaf. Alternatively, add 5ml/1tsp of tincture to a glass of water – echinacea, thyme or golden seal are effective, although the taste is not pleasant!

Laryngitis is an inflammation of the voice box or larynx and vocal cords usually due to a viral or bacterial infection. It can cause hoarseness or even a complete loss of voice. If symptoms persist for more than a few days then professional investigation is needed in case there is some major problem, such as a growth, causing the hoarseness. Minor cases can be relieved by gargles (agrimony and echinacea work well, either individually or together) and steam inhalations using thyme, peppermint or eucalyptus oil. Soothing foods also help: Juliette de Baïracli Levy – one of herbalism's *grandes dames* – recommends eating plenty of ice cream.

immune weakness

Persistent colds, crops of boils, chronic fatigue or repeated urinary infections, can often indicate reduced resistance. The body's immunity can be stretched by stress, overwork and food allergies, making it harder to combat bacteria, viruses and fungi. Many common organisms are extremely opportunist and while we all harbour numerous potentially lethal bacteria in and on our bodies all the time, if the system is weakened in any way these can very rapidly get out of hand.

Many tonic herbs have a reputation for strengthening the immune system and anyone feeling generally run down or suffering constant minor infections may benefit. Garlic, echinacea and the various types of ginseng have long been used in this way and all are generally best taken for periods of three or four weeks followed by a break. A number of traditional Chinese tonics can also boost the immune system and some are becoming available in the West: the list includes maitake and shiitake mushrooms – now available in numerous supermarkets – which are

▼ Leek *Allium porrum*

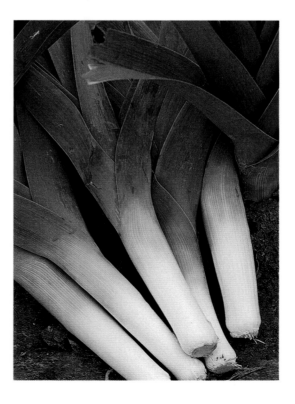

well worth brewing into a soup for those winter days when colds are all too prevalent. Try the following recipe:

Shiitake soup (serves 2-3)
1 medium onion, finely chopped
1 medium potato, coarsely chopped
8 dried shiitake mushrooms
110g/4oz fresh shiitake mushrooms
500ml/18fl oz chicken or good vegetable stock
salt and freshly ground black pepper
15ml/1tbsp olive oil
250ml/9fl oz water heated to almost boiling
1tsp fresh, chopped coriander
whole coriander sprigs to garnish (optional)

Rinse the dried shiitake and soak them in the hot water for one hour. Drain, but keep the strained liquid. Trim the stems of the fresh shiitake and thinly slice the caps. Leave the dried shiitake whole. Heat the olive oil in a saucepan and sauté the chopped onion and potato for 2-3 minutes until the onion is soft and golden. Add the soaked dried shiitake and stock, cover and simmer for 30 minutes. Remove the dried shiitake from the soup and save for use in another dish, as leaving them in this soup gives too strong a flavour.

Allow to cool slightly and process the soup through a blender to create a smooth, slightly thickened soup. Add more stock if the mixture appears too thick for your taste. Return to the heat and add the fresh sliced mushrooms, the reserved liquid from soaking the dried mushrooms and the coriander. Simmer gently for 10 minutes. Season with salt and freshly ground black pepper and serve garnished with whole coriander sprigs.

digestion

There was a saying in mediaeval Europe to the effect that "death dwells in the bowels" – a belief that good health, or the lack of it, was closely linked to good digestion. In Ayurvedic medicine, digestion plays a similar central role with the *agni*, or digestive fire, responsible for preserving health and numerous remedies used to improve and strengthen this vital energy force.

Modern herbalism, too, puts great emphasis on good digestion with a wide range of herbs to stimulate, relax, normalise and generally improve function. As well as those which have a relaxing and antispasmodic action on the gut, herbal digestive remedies are generally classified as:
• bitters – which stimulate the taste receptors leading to increased gastric acid and enzyme production;
• carminatives – which help to relieve flatulence, digestive colic and gastric discomfort by toning the mucous membranes and improving peristalsis (the waves of involuntary contractions in the digestive tract that move

food and waste products through the system);

• astringents – which are usually rich in tannins and help to contract blood vessels and certain tissues, such as the mucous membranes lining the digestive tract, so reducing secretion and excretion. They can be helpful for bleeding, catarrhal discharges and diarrhoea, associated with overactivity of the large bowel; and

• laxatives – to combat constipation by encouraging bowel motion; these range from the most gentle (aperients) to violent purgatives (cathartics) which are rarely used these days. Carminatives are often added to combat the griping pains which strong purgatives can cause.

Where digestive remedies are concerned, too, the boundary between food and herbs as medicine grows notably thin. Many culinary herbs are also carminative (such as dill, parsley and fennel), warming, bitter stimulants (such as fenugreek) or antispasmodics like the mints and rosemary; the French, who seem to have a national preoccupation with the state of their livers, will regularly eat dandelion leaves, which have liver-toning properties, as salad.

According to the Chinese, the liver governs the smooth flow of vital energy or *Qi* through the body, it also stores blood, governs the tendons and is linked with the eyes and poor vision: itching or dry eyes are often associated with liver disharmonies. The Chinese say that the liver "stores the soul" – governing spirit and mental activity: weak liver energy can thus lead to emotional disorders, depression or mental sluggishness. A wide range of apparently disparate symptoms can therefore be linked to basic liver imbalances, so eating herbs (or foods) which help to stimulate the liver – such as artichoke, asparagus and cabbage – can often improve general health as well.

constipation

If concern over their livers is a national preoccupation for the French, then the bowels fulfil the same role for the British: we spend millions of pounds a year on over-the-counter laxatives in an effort to keep "regular". Many of these laxatives work by irritating the bowel to encourage peristalsis: long-term misuse damages the bowel mucosa and weakens the gut, leading to problems like diverticular disease – associated with the development of sacs or pouches (known as diverticula) which develop at weakened points in the colon (lower bowel).

There is no "standard pattern" or "normal" bowel movements. Some people go every day, others every other day or twice a day. Diet is, obviously, significant, with vegetarians and those eating a high-fibre diet likely to have a more frequent pattern of bowel motions than those eating mainly meat and refined carbohydrates. The food we eat also influences how long it can take to be excreted: for people following traditional lifestyles in developing countries it may take about 12 hours or less for food to pass through, whereas for those eating a conventional Western diet it can be as long as 72 hours.

Low-fibre diet combined with a lack of exercise – and often coupled with a sluggish lifestyle or personality – leads to what is sometimes called "flaccid" or "atonic" constipation. Constipation can also be associated with nervous tension and a hectic lifestyle with little time to respond to the normal urge to defecate. The sufferer is often so stressed that the digestive system is unable to relax and allow normal function to progress. In such cases stools are sometimes described as resembling rabbit droppings. This type of constipation can alternate with bouts of diarrhoea and may lead to the catch-all label of "irritable bowel syndrome" (see below).

Atonic constipation can be helped by exercise, a high-fibre diet (or the use of a bulking laxative such as ispaghula) and abdominal massage. Stronger herbal laxatives – such as the well known senna pods (*Senna alexandrina*) – contain chemicals called anthraquinones and work by irritating the bowel. Apricots, bilberries, carrots, figs, grapes, liquorice, olives, pears and walnuts are all rather gentler in action, but can still be helpful in combating constipation.

For constipation associated with nervous tension, bowel relaxants such as chamomile and lemon balm can be worth adding to the mixture. Gentle sources of fibre are preferable in this type of constipation, so conventional "roughage" – such as bran – should often be avoided, as should the anthraquinone herbs, including aloes, rhubarb root and yellow dock, as well as stronger remedies like senna, buckthorn (*Rhamnus frangula*) and cascara sagrada (*Rhamnus purshiana*). Relaxation and a general reduction in stress are also important.

irritable bowel syndrome

Stress and anxiety can also play a part in another common disorder, "irritable bowel syndrome" (IBS) – a name that is often little more than a convenient label for a range of symptoms that can embrace just about any bowel irregularity which does not have a clear pathological cause. Sufferers can complain of numerous problems typical of poor digestive function or food intolerance – including constipation, diarrhoea, bloating, flatulence, stomach cramps, nausea, bowel tenderness, headaches, general tiredness, depression or anxiety. Food intolerance is a common cause: one study suggests that two-thirds of IBS sufferers actually display some sort of food allergy. The main culprits include dairy food, gluten (found in wheat, oats, barley and rye), caffeine-containing drinks, alcohol, cigarettes, eggs and red meat. If food intolerance is the cause, then it is important to identify and avoid the problem categories.

Soothing herbs such as marshmallow and meadowsweet can help to relieve IBS symptoms, as can digestive tonics and stimulants like peppermint and golden seal. Astringents, such as herb Robert, bistort, and agrimony, can be added to these remedies to ease any symptoms of diarrhoea. Relaxing herbs like chamomile, passion flower and lemon balm can be useful, while liver remedies such as milk thistle will help normalise function.

Many women find that irritable bowel symptoms get worse just before a period and a clinical trial at Addenbroke's Hospital in Cambridge used evening primrose oil on sufferers. The researchers based their project on the fact that excess production of prostaglandins-2 (PGE2), a hormone-like chemical, had been linked to some types of IBS. *Gamma*-linolenic acid – found in evening primrose and borage oils – can influence which sorts of prostaglandins are manufactured by the body and the study demonstrated that large doses of the oil (3-4g daily) for at least three months brought significant improvements in IBS when it was related to pre-menstrual problems.

diarrhoea

Nervous tension is a common cause of an over-active digestive tract and a resulting tendency for diarrhoea – although there are plenty of other causes too: infection from bacteria, chills, over-eating, alcohol or other irritant foods can all cause problems. Excessive bowel motions can lead to cramping pains and general soreness in the anal area, while the associated symptoms can include nausea and vomiting.

Sudden diarrhoea is most commonly caused by some sort of gastro-intestinal infection – especially if other people who shared the same meal are similarly affected. This is an all-too-common problem for holidaymakers who may find that local standards of hygiene in exotic locations are not quite the same as back home. When travelling in high-risk areas never eat raw salads, always wash and peel fruit, avoid ice cubes in drinks and regard roadside hawkers selling "bottled water" with some suspicion.

In Chinese medicine, fruits and salads are regarded as "cooling" or *yin* in character and an excess can thus lead to stomach chills and diarrhoea problems – much as John Gerard warned against eating cucumbers in winter back in 1597. Leaving our cold northern isle (*yin* in character) and heading for sunny holiday spots to eat all those exotic fruits can upset the *yin-yang* balance and can contribute just as much to holiday tummy upsets as poor hygiene.

Diarrhoea and vomiting are the body's natural reaction to an infecting organism and are often the best way of getting rid of it quickly: herbal treatment helps with astringent remedies to soothe the digestive tract. Strong, cold, black Indian tea – without milk or sugar – is rich in tannins and can ease an over-worked gut if nothing better is available.

Gastric flu and stomach chills can also lead to diarrhoea. Again symptoms are likely to be short-lived and using astringent herbal mixtures (such as agrimony, bistort, herb Robert or marigold) combined with anti-infection herbs like echinacea or hemp agrimony can help. Diarrhoea is very dehydrating and it is important to increase fluid intake during such bouts – especially with babies and small children.

Regular diarrhoea is more likely to be stress-related. This can range from the irritating, but largely harmless, increased bowel frequency before exams or job interviews, to debilitating disorders such as ulcerative colitis which can lead to long-term, chronic illness and requires professional attention. Sedating herbs can often help: try chamomile, lemon balm, skullcap, valerian or vervain.

piles

Constipation is often associated with piles or haemorrhoids – a type of varicose veins which can easily be felt, like bunches of grapes, around the rectum. Minor cases can often be cured completely, although once formed piles do have a tendency to recur later in life and can often be rekindled by over-exertion as well as by recurrent bouts of constipation. Pilewort is an obvious remedy, although ointments of other astringent herbs, including witch hazel, marigold and agrimony, can also help. Internally, teas of bistort, herb Robert or lady's mantle are useful, as are gentle remedies to combat any tendency to constipation, such as ispaghula.

stomach upsets and gastritis

Minor stomach upsets with abdominal pain, nausea, diarrhoea and vomiting affect most of us at some time. They can often be associated with food poisoning, an excess of rich food or too much alcohol; in such cases soothing herbs like slippery elm and marshmallow can bring relief. Other stomach upsets are linked to chills, when warming herbs such as chili and ginger can be useful.

For some, the problem can be stress related, with any increase in nervous tension or anxiety levels usually accompanied by digestive problems; relaxing carminatives can be useful in these cases. The wide range of herbal relaxants offers plenty of choice depending on individual need and tastes, but a good mixture for nervous tummies is:

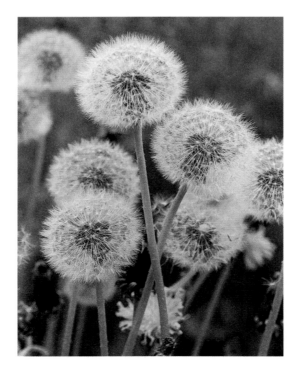

2 parts chamomile flowers
2 parts lemon balm herb
1 part lavender flowers

Use 1-2tsp of dried mixed herbs per cup of boiling water, infuse for 5 minutes, strain and drink.

Nervousness can be one cause of gastric over-activity with excess acid production leading to gastritis or inflammation of the stomach lining. Eventually such damage can lead to ulceration. Other causes of gastritis include over-indulgence in rich foods and alcohol with symptoms similar to those of food poisoning – nausea, vomiting and diarrhoea. Those prone to gastritis should avoid irritant foods – spices, tea, coffee, alcohol, fried foods and pickles – and eat smaller meals more regularly.

An orthodox approach will generally concentrate on antacids to reduce stomach acid, but this can simply encourage even more acid production in an attempt to normalise the digestive process. Herbal remedies will generally include soothing mucilages and anti-inflammatories which can help to protect the stomach lining and encourage healing. Slippery elm is available over the counter in tablets or as powder which simply needs mixing with water. Other suitable remedies include meadowsweet, liquorice, chamomile and marshmallow.

indigestion

There are numerous possible causes of indigestion, including rushed meals, wearing tight belts, eating irregularly or while feeling

◄ Dandelion seedheads *Taraxacum officinale*

tense, and too many rich or potentially irritant foods. The result is a mixture of heartburn, pain in the lower chest, flatulence and nausea that goes under the label of indigestion or dyspepsia.

Herbal solutions include relaxing plants such as chamomile and lemon balm to help to reduce the anxiety and tension which can contribute to indigestion, and aromatic carminatives such as fennel, peppermint, aniseed, dill, or ginger to ease flatulence and nausea. Meadowsweet and slippery elm, can help to protect the stomach from high acid secretions, while bitter remedies such as artichoke, bitter orange, turmeric or cornflower will help to stimulate the digestive process and restore normal function without focusing on stomach acidity.

Heartburn can be a particular problem in chronic obesity and pregnancy where the stomach is forced upwards and the muscle which divides the oesophagus from the stomach is weakened and may eventually lead to a hiatus hernia. Symptoms are often worse at night as there is nothing to stop acid leaking into the oesophagus when sufferers are lying down. Raising the head of the bed by 10-15cm/4-6in by putting normal house bricks under the legs will prevent acid leaking out of the stomach and can prove a very simple way of reducing symptoms. Slippery elm and marshmallow, either combined in capsules or mixed as powders with a little water to form a paste, make a useful combination for regular heartburn and are also safe to take in pregnancy.

The pain of indigestion can be confused with heart pain from disorders like angina pectoris. This sort of pain eases with rest, while heartburn is generally worse when the sufferer lies down. Sudden severe "indigestion" in

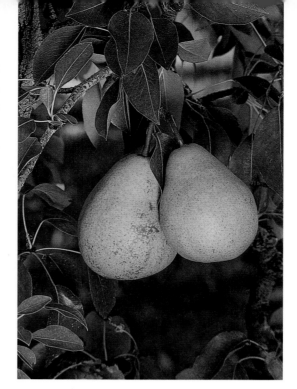

▲ Pear *Pyrus communis*

someone who has previously been symptom free should always be investigated professionally for a possible underlying heart condition. Chronic indigestion can also be a sign of peptic ulcers, gall bladder disorders, liver problems or cancer; expert diagnosis is essential.

An aspect of indigestion is wind — up or down — which is usually more of an embarrassment than an indicator of serious health problems. As the Galenic practitioners knew only too well, certain foods are windy — beans and the Brassica family are common culprits. To combat wind from such cold, damp foods, the mediaeval housewife added warming spices like pepper and ginger. Including fennel, dill, rosemary or sage in our cooking not only improves the flavour but also adds herbs to stimulate and soothe the digestive system and reduce that risk of wind and indigestion.

nausea and vomiting

Nausea and vomiting can be associated with a wide range of illnesses and conditions: from life-threatening fevers and stomach problems to motion sickness, pregnancy, migraines and indigestion. It is important to seek professional help for severe and persistent problems, but minor disorders, with a clear cause, can easily be helped by herbal remedies at home.

For nausea associated with stomach upsets herbs such as lemon balm, chamomile, peppermint, bitter orange, dandelion or marshmallow can be helpful.

Travel sickness – whether it occurs in trains, planes, shops or cars – is especially prevalent among children and soon becomes a problem for the entire family. Symptoms start with pallor, sweating and nausea and lead to vomiting and, sometimes, fainting. The disorder is generally to do with the delicate balance mechanism in the inner ear, and since children's ears tend to be more sensitive the problem is more commonplace among the young.

The best herbal remedy for all types of nausea is ginger – in capsules, tinctures or even in the form of sweets, ginger drinks and ginger biscuits. Ginger beer is ideal for children; alternatively, travel with a small dropper bottle of ginger tincture and simply put a few drops on the tongue before the journey and as needed during the trip.

eyes and ears

Herbs have a long history of use in treating eye and ear problems: before the days of universally available hearing aids and spectacles, itinerant herb doctors would often specialise in eyes or ears and travel the countryside treating patients with brews designed to improve sight or hearing rather than simply alleviate the sort of minor ailments we would treat in this way today.

Old herbals are full of remedies – the vast majority unproven – for restoring sight to the blind and curing tinnitus or deafness. Some, such as the often-repeated tradition that greater celandine seeds will restore sight to blind swallows, go back to ancient times and were once very widely used remedies. Some traditional cures have been shown to have a more solid scientific basis: eating carrots certainly has a role in improving night vision, since vitamin A is needed to maintain the relevant parts of the retina.

In Chinese theory the eyes are associated with the liver and the ears with the kidneys. They are links which one can well understand: excess alcohol, for example, usually leads to an overworked liver and sluggish, bleary eyes. Traditionally, too, the kidney is the home of the body's "reproductive energy" which inevitably runs down as we reach middle age and the menopause. As we get older hearing problems become more commonplace so, again, it is understandable how these connections were first formulated.

This traditional approach can be effective: in China, for example, chrysanthemums (see page 211) are used to treat various liver complaints and are also recommended for eye weaknesses, while herbs which warm the kidneys – such as buchu and cinnamon – can be usefully added to remedies for earache and other weaknesses.

For home use, however, it is best to limit the use of herbal remedies to minor, self-limiting conditions: eyes and ears are sensitive and precious and using impure or crude remedies can do more harm than good.

eye problems

blepharitis
This is an inflammation of the eyelid which can be caused by an allergic reaction to cosmetics and is often accompanied by white scales on the lashes. In chronic cases the eyelid can become ulcerated with a yellow crust, the eyelashes are often matted and may fall out. Marigold is very effective but should be made into a decoction rather than an infusion for use in eye-baths to ensure that it is sterile and clean. Decoct 5-10g/⅙-⅓oz of marigold petals in 500ml/1pt of water (see page 216) and then thoroughly strain the mixture. Allow the decoction to cool and then bathe the eye every few hours.

conjunctivitis,
Also known as pink eye, conjunctivitis is an inflammation of the fine membrane (conjunctiva) covering the eyeball. Sufferers usually complain of severe pain, watering and a "gritty feeling" on blinking. Again, a well-strained decoction of marigold is normally recommended for use as an eye-bath, but decoctions of herb Robert or toadflax can be used in similar ways.

styes
These are an acute inflammation of a gland at the base of an eyelash usually caused by bacterial infection. They can indicate lowered resistance due to stress, overwork or repeated infection. A little marigold cream or tea tree cream can be applied to the site of infection, but take great care not to smudge the creams into the eye itself as they can sting. Aloe sap can also be soothing. Alternatively, use the same sorts of astringent and antiseptic decoctions suggested for conjunctivitis. Taking garlic or echinacea internally can help combat the infection and improve immunity.

tired eyes
We've all suffered from sore, tired eyes after too much reading or too much time spent in a highly polluted atmosphere: close the eyes and cover with slices of cucumber or try used tea-bags of green tea, fennel or chamomile.

ear problems

earache
This is common, extremely painful and distressing (especially in children) and needs great care in treating as infection can lead to perforated eardrums and the risk of permanent hearing damage. The cause is usually an acute local infection, which can be related to sinus or catarrhal problems, and use of anti-catarrhals

plants that can help with
eyes and ears

the following herbs can
be helpful – refer to
Section 2 for details of
use

aloe p.140

beetroot p.111

carrot p.124

cornflower p.176

cucumber p.121

dandelion p.205

fennel p.82

ginkgo p.146

herb Robert p.186

leek p.105

onion p.104

shepherd's purse p.176

toadflax p.190

walnut p.126

witch hazel p.149

wood betony p.202

and suitable steam inhalants (see page 228) can help. If there is any discharge or possibility that the ear drum has burst then seek immediate medical help. For minor cases ear drops using infused oils of mullein or St John's wort flowers are safe for home use. Put a few drops in the ear and then insert a cotton wool swab. Repeat three or four times a day as needed. Massaging the mastoid bone (behind the ear) with antiseptic oils such as lavender and tea tree can also help. A traditional cure was to insert the heart of a freshly boiled onion into the ear – a suitably hot and ideally shaped healing poultice if nothing else is available.

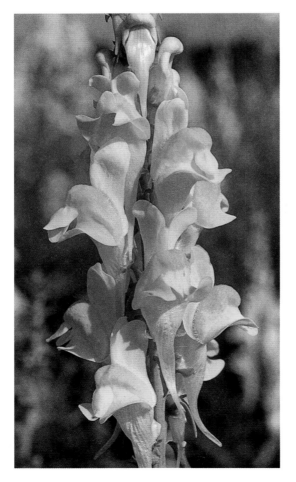

glue ear

A common problem in children, this involves an inflammation of the middle ear (otitis media) with a build-up of fluid leading to deafness. It is often associated with food allergy and can improve significantly if the sufferer tries a milk-free diet. Orthodox treatment usually involves surgery to insert grommets into the eardrum to relieve the fluid pressure; these generally have to be replaced after a few months as they tend to fall out. Anti-catarrhals such as golden seal and ribwort plantain taken internally can often help.

tinnitus

Irritating whistling and rattling sounds affecting one or both ears can be caused by nerve damage (common in those who work in noisy environments) or labyrinth disorders like Ménières disease. Some argue that tinnitus is associated with stress, anger and psychological problems and will disappear once sufferers learn to relax and solve their emotional disturbances. This can sometimes be true, especially where there is no apparent pathological cause, but in cases involving nerve damage is generally not so. Some suggest that the noise is related to the sound of blood flow around the ears and ginkgo has been variously reported to help the problem by improving cerebral circulation. Wood betony has similar properties. These remedies can be worth trying, as can Chinese kidney tonics such as cinnamon or even the traditional cures of drinking plenty of beetroot juice and eating leeks: occasionally the result is significant improvement – but tinnitus is a stubborn condition and there is often no easy solution.

◄ Toadflax *Linaria vulgaris*

heart and circulation

Today, thanks to modern science, we generally regard the heart simply as a powerful muscle to pump blood around the body. Traditional medicine has a rather different view: to the Chinese the heart controls the life process, co-ordinates the activities of all the other organs and manages mental activities and consciousness. It stores *Shen* – a sense of appropriateness and right behaviour – so that what we term mental illness is often seen in Chinese medicine as due to disharmonies in the heart upsetting *Shen*.

Ayurvedic medicine puts the heart in a similar central role: it is the dwelling place of the *atman* – the divine self or spirit of immortal life – controlling consciousness and affected by spiritual weakness. Western Ayurvedic experts like David Frawley argue that the high level of heart disease in Western society is due to our over-preoccupation with personal achievement and material wealth: he suggests that a heart attack is really a problem of "spiritual starvation" and loss causing a broken heart.

Like modern allopathic medicine, much Western herbalism is rather more concerned with symptomatic relief of cardiovascular problems than with the spiritual aspects of the heart and few would consider heart problems as suitable candidates for home remedies. Self-help is, however, possible – either from an orthodox standpoint using herbs to improve circulation, strengthen the heart muscles or reduce cholesterol levels or adopting a more traditional approach and feeding the heart on suitable spiritual remedies.

high blood pressure

Until the invention of the sphygnomanometer we had no accurate way of measuring blood pressure and so pressure problems passed under a variety of other names. Today, DIY blood-pressure machines seem to have taken over from the "speak your weight" scales that used to lurk on every railway station and passers-by can be suitably terrified by instant readings which declare them to be "high". Isolated blood pressure readings really mean very little: several consistently high ones are needed before applying the label "hypertension" and mild cases can often be controlled by simple dietary measures.

Coffee, for example, contains caffeine which stimulates the heart to beat faster, pumping blood through the vessels and kidneys more energetically. The result, even in the healthy, can be an abnormally fast pulse, irregular heart beat, raised blood pressure and increased desire to urinate. Often simply cutting down on coffee – along with tea, cola drinks and chocolate, which contain similar chemicals – is all that is needed.

Herbal infusions make an ideal alternative for those prone to high blood pressure. Suitable remedies include many relaxing herbs as well as those which are "hypotensive" or actively lower blood pressure generally by relaxing blood vessels or slowing heart rates. Typical options include skullcap, passion flower, celery seed, yarrow, vervain, hawthorn, self-heal, valerian or linden flowers. Diuretics can also help if the heart's performance is weak and fluids tend to accumulate in the system. Dandelion leaf is ideal because it contains a good supply of potassium which can be lost when urination is increased by the use of diuretics. A typical infusion for raised blood pressure is:

2 parts hawthorn flowers
2 parts lime flowers
1 part dandelion leaf
1 part yarrow
1 part vervain

One teaspoon of the mixture infused with a cup of boiling water to be taken two or three times a day.

Much modern advice for maintaining a healthy heart usually includes cutting down on fatty foods which could increase the blood's cholesterol levels. Cholesterol is a complex fatty substance which is essential for physical health. The average body contains about 150g/5½oz of the stuff and it plays an important role in maintaining membrane fluidity, as well as providing the raw material for manufacturing many hormones and bile acids. This useful substance can, unfortunately, encourage fatty deposits to develop in blood vessels, which in turn leads to hardening of the arteries and increased blood pressure. Recent studies suggest that cholesterol may not be quite so awful as orthodox health advisors would have us believe and even that artificially reducing it with drugs might just encourage the body to produce yet more. The debate continues, but the anti-animal-fat messages which were so common a few years ago are being modified and there is a growing realisation that a little cholesterol in the diet may be no bad thing.

Numerous herbs can, however, help to control the levels of surplus cholesterol in the blood and encourage its excretion; much research has focused on garlic, which has been proven to help reduce the risk of a further heart attack in those already suffering problems with damaged blood vessels and hardened arteries. Daily doses of 1-4 cloves per person have been suggested as ideal – which is no more than one could easily use in cooking. German trials suggest that 2g a day of powdered garlic is sufficient to achieve notable therapeutic effects.

Other foodstuffs which have been shown to have a similar cholesterol-modifying action include chickpeas, kidney beans, navy beans (the sort that go into cans of baked beans), lentils, soya beans and alfalfa sprouts. Herbs showing the same properties include nutmeg, sage, linden, thyme, liquorice and ginseng. Also important is tea: research suggests that green and oolong teas are the most effective at controlling cholesterol levels. Traditionally a Chinese oolong tea called *Pu Erh* has been regarded as a good digestive remedy after rich meals. In the early 1980s French researchers reported a reduction of 25% in cholesterol blood levels in a group of high risk patients after a month of *Pu Erh* drinking. The tea, available from specialist Chinese herb suppliers, needs to be taken black, as any milk added will precipitate the tannins which are believed to be mainly responsible for this cholesterol-lowering property.

circulatory problems and chilblains

Poor heart function can contribute to numerous circulation problems which may include severe pain in the legs while walking (intermittent

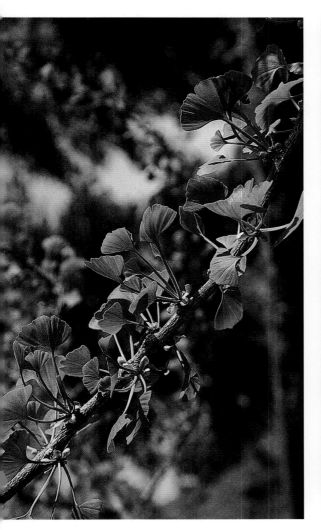

▲ Gingko *Gingko biloba*

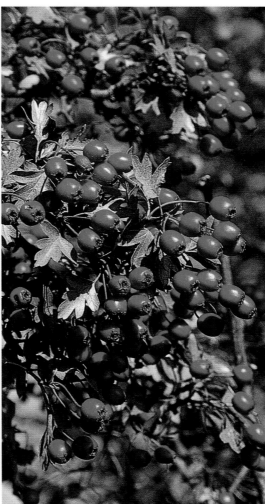

▲ Hawthorn *Crataegus monogyna*

Plants that can help with
the heart and circulation

The following herbs can
be helpful – refer to
Section 2 for details of
use

apple p.130
arnica p.141
basil p.92
borage p.77
celery p.108
dan shen p.98
dang gui p.141
fig p.124
galangal p.106
garlic p.75
ginkgo p.146
ginseng p.153
golden seal p.150
grape p.137
hawthorn p.178
lemon p.119
linden p.99
marigold p.78
motherwort p.189
oats p.110
olive p.131
onion p.104
passion flower p.154
self-heal p.198
shepherd's purse p.176
Siberian ginseng p.145
skullcap p.201
turmeric p.80
valerian p.161
walnut p.126
wood betony p.202
yarrow p.167

claudication) and Buerger's disease (common among heavy smokers); this can eventually lead to gangrene and limb amputation.

Among more minor circulation problems are chilblains, which are generally associated not with failing hearts but with cold, as the body responds to falling temperatures by limiting blood supply to remote toes and fingers in order to keep vital organs and deep tissues warm. Wearing adequate clothing on cold days is the easiest way to avoid occasional chilblains, while habitual sufferers can improve their circulation with stimulating herbs like ginger, cinnamon, horseradish and chili. Recent research also suggests that ginkgo can improve the peripheral blood circulation, although it is more traditionally used for stimulating the blood supply to the brain.

Arnica cream can help relieve the discomfort of chilblains once they've appeared, but should not be used on broken skin. Other helpful herbs to relieve symptoms include aloe vera and pot marigold. Warming herbs such as ginger, cinnamon or chili can be helpful if circulation is generally weak – especially in the elderly.

anaemia

While science has simplified the heart's role to that of pump, we now know that blood chemistry is extremely complex and the cause of numerous disorders. Iron-deficient anaemia is one of the most common and is widespread among women of child-bearing age.

The traditional Western herbal approach includes adding numerous iron-rich foods to the diet – such as apricots, asparagus, beetroot, carrots, stinging nettle and watercress – while the Chinese concentrate on herbs which help "nourish" or manufacture blood. One of the most popular is *Dang Gui* which is now widely available in prepackaged, over-the-counter products from health food shops and chemists. It is useful for anaemia as well as various menstrual disorders, and contains vitamin B_{12} and folic acid, which can counter some types of anaemia.

varicose veins

Varicose veins are usually visible as tortuous, knotted veins on the surface of the legs. They can ache or the surrounding area can be prone to swelling and the flesh can often feel hot.

Veins, unlike arteries, have to help force blood back to the heart rather than depend on the impetus of this powerful pump. The muscles surrounding deep veins can help considerably, but the superficial veins in the legs often have little support for forcing blood back to the central pumping system and over the years they can become distended, lengthened and tortuous.

Deep breathing can help encourage the return of blood from the peripheries while a tendency to varicose veins can often be countered by alternately hosing the legs with a hot and cold shower several times, for 1-2 minutes at a time, each morning. Using bricks to raise the end of the bed to aid venous return at night can also help. Useful external treatments include distilled witch hazel, lemon juice, infusions of vine leaf, agrimony or pilewort, and fig poultices.

Varicose ulcers generally occur in the elderly and are associated with poor circulation, with reduced blood flow to an area often making healing difficult. Professional treatment is usually essential, but using infused oils containing heating herbs like chili, pepper or ginger as a gentle massage around the ulcer (not on it) can help stimulate blood flow to the area to encourage healing.

Internally herbs which contains chemicals called flavonoids and coumarins – which are known to strengthen blood vessels and also reduce the risk of clots – may be helpful. Traditional specific remedies include horsechestnut (*Aesculus hippocastanum*) and melilot (*Melilotus officinalis*, also known as king's clover). Herbs such as rue (*Ruta graveolens*) and buckwheat (*Fagopyrum esculentum*) are high in rutin (a flavonoid) which can help to strengthen blood vessels.

mouth disorders

In Chinese theory the mouth is associated with the spleen – an organ traditionally linked with digestion, so red, lustrous lips suggest that food is being well digested and assimilated, while pale lips indicate poor spleen energy with a weak appetite and abnormal digestion. The condition of the gums, too, is indicative of the state of the digestion: red, swelling and bleeding gums indicate excess stomach heat, as do mouth ulcers around the lips. Mouth problems are thus often related to other bodily ills and should rarely be considered in isolation.

gum disease

Gum disease is, fortunately, not as commonplace as it once was thanks to better oral hygiene and a more positive approach to conservative dentistry.

Brushing regularly and correctly is important, as is eating foods which contain roughage and can help clean the teeth as they are chewed. The traditional "apple a day" is an extremely effective herbal remedy, as is a piece of cheese (without biscuits) after a meal or – even better – a cup of unsweetened green tea at the end of a meal: this is rich in fluoride and has been shown to prevent tooth decay.

Herbal mouthwashes can help with minor problems of localised bleeding or inflamed gums – infusions of sage, bistort, agrimony or marigold can all be effective.

➤ Sage *Salvia officinalis*

bad breath

Just as the state of the gums is associated with digestion, so too the breath: the characteristic pear drop odour that can suggest disordered blood sugar levels or the unpleasant smell of "bad breath" typical of stagnating food in the digestive tract. Bad breath can often accompany constipation or gastritis or may simply be the result of eating highly spiced foods or garlic, smoking or tooth decay.

One of the traditional remedies to sweeten the breath is chewing fennel seeds – they have a

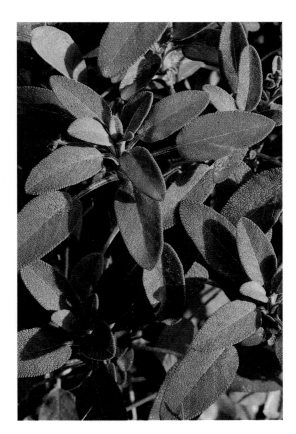

plants that can help with mouth problems

the following herbs can be helpful – refer to Section 2 for details of use

agrimony p.168
aniseed p.94
birch p.175
cloves p.98
daisy p.174
fennel p.82
feverfew p.158
grape p.137
greater celandine p.177
herb Robert p.186
linden p.99
marigold p.78
rosemary p.95
sage p.97
self-heal p.198
thyme p.98
wood avens p.187

pleasant aniseed flavour and the same seeds were once also recommended to stave off hunger pains during lengthy Sunday morning sermons. Sucking peppermints is a common choice for bad breath, but peppermint sweets are generally high in sugar, which is damaging for the teeth, while too much peppermint oil can be irritant on the mucous membranes of mouth, upper respiratory tract and stomach.

Using an unsweetened herbal infusion as a mouthwash is a good way of combating mouth infections and tooth decay: try sage, thyme or rosemary. Chewing parsley leaves can often help to reduce garlic smells.

If the problem is associated with stagnation in the digestive tract, with food taking too long to pass through, then gentle laxative remedies, such as yellow dock, or liver stimulants, such as toadflax or dandelion, can be useful as well.

mouth ulcers

Mouth ulcers — or aphtha — commonly start with a sore red patch of blisters erupting to produce a greyish white ulcer. They will usually clear of their own accord after a week or so, but can be so painful that eating becomes almost impossible.

No one really knows why mouth ulcers occur: the Chinese blame stomach heat but others maintain they are due to low-grade fungal infections, excess sugar or may indicate a weakened immune system. Recurrent bouts of mouth ulcers can suggest some underlying weakness and a course of immune-stimulant herbs and tonics can help: taking garlic or ginseng for a month can boost the system and herbal mouthwashes using sage, birch, cloves, rosemary or echinacea can help relieve symptoms.

nervous disorders, anxiety and stress

While a certain amount of stress is essential to keep us alert and active, an excess is probably one of the most pervasive ills of the late 20th century. We live in an age in which people frequently describe themselves as "time poor, cash rich" — too busy working and earning to spend much time relaxing and enjoying life.

Taking soothing remedies is only a small part of the solution. Many of the ills caused by stress could be solved with a little relaxation — time spent on learning to relax with yoga or t'ai-chi classes or going for unhurried rambles in the

fresh air. Instead of resting on the seventh day we spend it in supermarket queues, making endless home improvements or catching up with the housework. We all — even the busiest parent — need to find space for ourselves each day in order to cope and a few minutes of relaxed deep breathing or listening to a favourite piece of music will work wonders.

An holistic approach always focuses on the needs of body, mind and spirit and this is especially true with any condition labelled as "nerves". Physical manifestations of "nervous disorders" may include insomnia, palpitations or headaches; emotional aspects can include irritability, depression, feelings of anger or guilt, while the lack of determination, emptiness or sense of purpose felt by so many people can typify the spiritual vacuum at the centre of many modern lifestyles.

Herbs can be equally holistic, operating on the same three levels (mind, body and spirit) to improve well-being: vervain is a good example. It can be considered as a liver tonic and relaxing nervine. Taken in Bach Flower Remedy form (see page 48) it is suitable for the perfectionist, slightly obsessional personality who tries to do too many jobs at once and runs each task to death, like a dog worrying a bone. On a spiritual level vervain can increase understanding and psychic awareness: it was once used in crystal-gazing and some maintain that it will repair holes in the human aura (a layer of psychic energy which surrounds all living things and is seen in Kirlian photography).

In Chinese and Ayurvedic medicine emotional imbalance is well accepted as a possible cause of physical disease: the Chinese associate the emotion "fear" with the kidneys, for example, and panic attacks could be a sign of kidney imbalance. "Anger" can have a similar effect on the liver, while what the Chinese describe as "joy" (but may be better translated as "over-enthusiasm") can lead to heart disorders.

Herbal nervines work on several levels, including:
• herbal sedatives and relaxants which can ease tensions, feelings of anxiety or help with insomnia;
• herbal tonics and stimulants which will provide an additional short-term energy boost;
• herbal remedies which can act on the emotions or spirit in some way as part of a total holistic approach.

They can be used much as orthodox sedatives, hypnotics or anti-depressants: skullcap is a sedative, for example, passion flower a hypnotic – to dull the senses or induce sleep – and St John's wort a potent anti-depressant. Such herbal remedies should not, however, be seen as a complete alternative to professional counselling or psychotherapy for those who really cannot cope with their lifestyles.

anxiety and tension

Taking the time to brew a relaxing herbal tea and then do nothing but sit, sip it and unwind is a far more therapeutic way of combating tension than popping a couple of tranquillisers and carrying on with the normal frenetic daily routine. Suitable herbs to add into the relaxing brew include lemon balm, skullcap, chamomile, wood betony, valerian and vervain.

Herbal baths are equally effective: use either 500ml/1pt of an infusion of a highly aromatic relaxing herb – such as chamomile, lavender or lemon balm – or else a few drops of the essential oil.

Tension often leads to headaches as the muscles at the back of the neck stiffen. Massaging that area and the temples can help: use lavender oil diluted in a vegetable-oil base. A 50:50 combination of wood betony and lavender as an infusion is another good remedy for tension headaches, although it is always best to take the tea as soon as symptoms start to appear rather than waiting for a major headache to develop.

Anxiety and worries can lead to depression and unhappiness. Severe depression needs professional help but for minor "downs" lemon balm and borage can be especially uplifting. In recent years St John's wort has gained a reputation as equivalent in effect to many orthodox drugs while kava is especially popular in the USA as a calming remedy. These herbs can also be supportive for those undergoing professional treatment.

Old herbals often describe how even looking on cheerful plants can lift the spirits and "comfort the harte". Perhaps it is worth remembering part of an old Persian poem:

If of thy mortal goods thou art bereft,
And of thy store, three loaves alone are left,
Sell one, and with the dole
Buy hyacinths to feed the soul.

insomnia

The amount of sleep we each need varies considerably and sometimes we require rather more sleep than at others. Sleeplessness only becomes a problem when sufferers feel tired and unable to concentrate during the day or when it becomes a worry in itself. There are many causes for disturbed sleep patterns: heavy meals late at night can lead to disturbed digestion; painful joints and muscles or irritating coughs will keep most people awake, while catnapping during the day simply fills up the sleep quota.

Insomnia is commonly associated with tension, worries and a failure to relax before bedtime. The majority of herbal remedies for sleeplessness are based on sedative and relaxing herbs which will help to reduce anxieties, calm an over-active mind and encourage sleep. Unlike orthodox treatments they are non-addictive, although some people find that the potency of an insomnia remedy is reduced if they take it regularly, so it can be worthwhile changing the mix from time to time if long-term use is likely.

As always with herbal medicine, it is far better to identify and treat the cause of a problem rather than simply tackling the symptoms, so if inability to relax or over-anxiety is the root cause of insomnia, meditation classes or a review of lifestyle concerns might provide the solution. Vervain taken in its Bach Flower Remedy form (see page 48) can be particularly useful for such tense individuals. Other suitable remedies include hops, wild lettuce, passion flower or Californian poppy.

improving energy levels

Herbal stimulants are, of course, familiar to all: coffee, tea and chocolate, which are rich in caffeine, theobromine and related alkaloids, are regularly used as a short-term restorative to keep students and night owls awake. They are, however, superficial remedies offering no real long-term benefits when it comes to improving energy levels and strengthening the nervous system. A better alternative is rosemary, which contains a stimulant called borneal. Take it as an infusion or add a few drops of rosemary oil to stimulating baths. Guarana, a popular over-the-counter restorative, is another where the action is largely dependent on caffeine-like stimulants

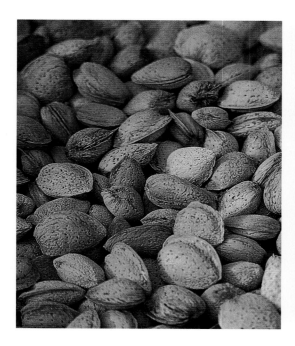

▲ Almond *Prunus dulcis*

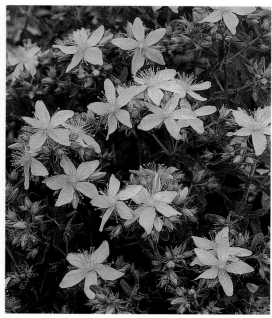

▲ St John's wort *Hypericum officinalis*

although in this case the guaranine alkaloid is much slower to metabolise so has a gentler, more sustained effect.

Longer-term energy tonics are often a better option: Korean ginseng is now well established in the West as a tonic remedy. In traditional Chinese medicine, ginseng tends to be regarded as boosting the masculine (*yang*) energies and, while it can be taken by women, other tonics are often preferable. Siberian ginseng is traditionally feminine (*yin*) in character and so can be more suitable for women, while in China *Huang Qi* is often preferred for younger people. A favourite Chinese tonic for women is *Dang Gui*, now more widely available in the West. Other tonic herbs worth considering include *ashwagandha*, *shatavari*, paratudo, shiitake mushrooms, elecampane, oats, almonds, grapes, thyme, liquorice, *amachazuru* and sage.

If a stressful time is looming – such as exams or a heavy work period – it is worth taking tonic herbs before the event to provide an energy boost, rather than depending on short-term stimulants once the stresses mount. Siberian ginseng is particularly useful for helping the body cope more efficiently with stress and improving performance: it was widely used in the 1960s and '70s by Soviet athletes and long-distance lorry-drivers to increase stamina.

mind and spirit

Western practitioners often avoid discussions of spirituality which, like death, is one of our 21st-century taboo subjects. Using herbs such as kava or *ashwagandha* can help to strengthen the spirit and give a patient the will and self-determination to make the major lifestyle

plants that can help with the nervous system

the following herbs can be helpful – refer to Part 2 for details of use

almond p.134
apricot p.133
ashwagandha p.162
basil p.92
borage p.77
butterbur p.194
californian poppy p.180
cardamom p.81
chamomile p.86
coffee p.120
damiana p.159
gotu kola p.143
guarana p.156
hawthorn p.178
kava p.155
lavender p.86
leek p.105
lemon balm p.87
lettuce p.128
linden p.99
marjoram p.92
nutmeg p.91
oats p.110
paratudo p.155
passion flower p.154
rosemary p.95
shatavari p.142
Siberian ginseng p.145
skullcap p.201
St John's wort p.150
turmeric p.80
valerian p.161
vervain p.100
wood betony p.202

bach flower remedies

remedy	Dr Bach's suggested use	remedy	Dr Bach's suggested use
agrimony	for those who suffer mental torture behind a "brave face"	mustard	for deep gloom and depression
aspen	for vague fears of an unknown origin	oak	for those who struggle on against adversity
beech	for critical intolerance of others	olive	for complete exhaustion
centaury	for the weak-willed	pine	for feelings of guilt and self-blame
cerato	for those who doubt their own judgment and seek advice of others	red chestnut	for excessive fear for others, especially loved ones
cherry plum	for fears of mental collapse	rock rose	for extreme terror
chestnut bud	for a refusal to learn from past mistakes	rock water	for the self-repressed who overwork and deny themselves any relaxation
chicory	for possessiveness and selfishness	scleranthus	for uncertainty and indecision
clematis	for the inattentive and dreamy escapist	star of bethlehem	for shock
crab apple	a cleansing remedy for those who feel unclean or ashamed	sweet chestnut	for extreme anguish; the limit of endurance
elm	for those temporarily overcome by feelings of inadequacy	vervain	for tenseness, over-enthusiasm and over-effort
gentian	for the despondent and easily discouraged	vine	for the dominating and inflexible
gorse	for hopelessness and despair	walnut	for protection at times of change such as the menopause or during other major life stage transitions
heather	for the self-centred obsessed with their own troubles	water violet	for the proud and reserved
holly	for those who are jealous, angry or feel hatred for others	white chestnut	for mental anguish and persistent nagging worries
honeysuckle	for home sickness and nostalgia	wild oat	for uncertainty about which path to take; an aid to decision taking
hornbeam	for "Monday morning feelings" and procrastination	wild rose	for the apathetic who lack ambition
impatiens	for the impatient	willow	for the resentful and bitter who are fond of saying "not fair"
larch	for those who lack confidence		
mimulus	for fear of known things		

Having chosen a suitable selection of remedies put 4 drops of each into a 10ml/2tsp dropper bottle and then fill this with spring water. Take drop doses of the remedy on the tongue as required.

changes essential for long-term recovery. A few drops of rose oil in the bath water can perform small miracles for those who believe themselves unloved or unlovable.

Herbs can also be used to strengthen the *chakras* – the body's spiritual centres defined in Eastern philosophy. The familiar culinary herb basil is believed to reinforce the root, second and third *chakras*, while plants like lavender and elecampane are said to act on the crown *chakra,* which is associated with the pineal and pituitary glands (pea-sized bodies that secrete various important sex hormones and a hormone-like substance called melatonin). Using these types of herbs in conjunction with remedies for physical complaints can be very effective.

Modern science also has to accept that herbs can affect the mind and emotions in ways which we are only beginning to understand. There have been reports of aromatic chemicals from essential oils travelling through the olfactory system to reach parts of the limbic centre in the brain – an area which in humans acts as a focus for emotions. Aromatherapy tends to be regarded in the UK as a massage-based technique, but purists in mainland Europe prefer to think of it – as the name implies – as a therapy associated with smells. Smelling certain oils can be stimulating and uplifting, while others have a more soothing and relaxing effect. Using oils in diffusers to scent rooms or adding a few drops to bath water are easy ways to influence the emotions. Among the many herb oils that can be used in this way are chamomile, lavender, marjoram, melissa (lemon balm) and neroli (bitter orange).

Among the West's favourite remedies for emotional problems are the Bach Flower Remedies – discovered by Dr Edward Bach in the 1930s and used since then for soothing worries, fears and ill temper. The remedies are essentially the dew collected from particular plants preserved with brandy and seem to contain some invisible energy from the plant. They should be further diluted in water before being taken in drop doses. By this stage the remedies are in homoeopathic dilution and many are sceptical of their action. However, Bach Flower Remedies can be extremely helpful for a great many people and are worth trying.

skin problems

Our skin stands between us and the outside world: it must be porous enough to let out unwanted moisture in the form of sweat, but prevent us from being sodden in a rain shower. It has to provide protection from micro-organisms and pollution and it needs to be sufficiently soft and supple to allow a full range of energetic motions.

In Ayurvedic medicine, skin diseases are classified in terms of the three humours: too much *pitta* (fire) causes the blood to over-heat and poison the skin; too much *vata* (wind) causes dryness and itching, while *kapha* (damp) skin problems are related to weeping or oozing sores. Treatment focuses on balancing the offending humour.

The traditional approach of Western herbal medicine is to consider skin problems as related to blood impurities or circulating toxins, using herbs described as "depuratives" and "alteratives" to cleanse the system. Herbs like burdock, stinging nettles or cleavers are common favourites, while folk traditions include the use of carrots, grapes and turnips. These sorts of cleansing herbs are often combined with others to stimulate the liver and digestive function and thus also improve elimination of toxins – laxatives such as yellow dock are often added. Circulatory stimulants can be added to encourage a healthy oxygen supply and improve the quality of the tissues.

Although Western herbalists tend to emphasise internal remedies, external creams and lotions also have their place, especially for dry and scaling skin problems. Marigold, elder flower and chickweed creams are widely used. Aloe vera is another favourite. More recently evening primrose and borage oils with their high *gamma*-linolenic acid content have moved into pole position and are recommended both internally and externally for numerous skin conditions, although they are really best for chronic, scaling, atopic eczema where a metabolic problem may be involved.

acne and blemishes

The characteristic pimples and blackheads of acne are all too familiar to teenagers. Inflamed sebaceous glands – at their most active during puberty – are at the heart of the problem. The concentration of sebaceous glands varies over the body, so acne patches tend to be localised on the face, back and chest, although larger sebaceous cysts are more likely to occur on the scalp and genitals.

The conventional herbal approach is to cut down on the foods which might encourage sebaceous gland activity. This means reducing intake of refined carbohydrates (typically sugar and white flour), fried foods and animal fats. Sweets and chocolates also tend to aggravate the condition – as does excessive intake of alcohol and sweet, sugary drinks.

Herbalists generally recommend the use of immune-strengthening and anti-bacterial herbs – such as echinacea – both internally and externally to combat the infection that results from excess sebum blocking hair follicles and causing pus to accumulate. A traditional stand-by is to rub a garlic clove on to the acne pustule each night – an effective cure, but one that rarely proves popular with spotty teenagers. Washing in – and also drinking – cabbage water is another rather unpleasant folk cure: it does work well, but a slightly more acceptable alternative is cabbage lotion made by pulping cabbage leaves and distilled witch hazel in a food processor. Use this to cleanse and astringe the face twice a day.

Rather less aromatic are remedies such as diluted tea tree oil and marigold. Steaming the skin with a mixture of hot water and a few drops of essential oils such as marigold, chamomile or lavender makes a good deep-cleansing treatment, or use facial washes containing a little finely powdered oatmeal instead of soap.

In Chinese medicine the exact location of the acne pustules is significant as it suggests where in the body there may be excess heat, believed in traditional Chinese medicine to contribute to the problem. Pimples around the mouth, for example, can imply an over-heated stomach, while those around the nose are associated with the lung. Relevant cooling herbs for these organs are then added to the mix.

eczema

Eczema and dermatitis (which simply means inflammation of the skin) are both terms used to describe non-contagious inflammatory skin conditions. The skin is usually red and itching with a rash, or there may be spots which can resemble small blisters that "weep" – oozing clear fluid to form a crust. "Dry eczema" involves a thickening and drying of the skin and is often characterised by dry, flaky patches.

Allergies – to chemicals, metals or certain foods – are a common cause of eczema and in children milk intolerance (especially among those who have not been breast-fed) is often the culprit. Since human milk is an excellent source of *gamma*-linolenic acid (GLA, see page 153), the condition has more recently been regarded as a failure in GLA metabolism. Persuading children to drink soya milk instead is not always easy, although it can often help. Food allergy also has aspects of addiction and dependence and children can literally be hooked on milk so, when the food is withdrawn, they can become irritable and unpleasant – much to their parents' despair.

A recent Government-sponsored study in the UK also found that nine out of 10 children developing nut allergies had previously suffreed fron childhood eczema and suggested a link between the use of eczema lotions and creams containing peanut (*Arachis hypogaea*) oil, also known as groundnut, money nut or arachis oil. Around one in 100 British children now suffers from peanut allergy, which in severe cases can be fatal. Although the research, based at St Mary's Hospital in London, is continuing and remains controversial, as it is easy to avoid eczema remedies which contain peanut oil, it would seem sensible to do so.

Other likely dietary culprits include wheat, eggs and fruits that are rich in salicylates (especially tomatoes, oranges, berry fruits, peppers and aubergines), or shellfish. Tension and anxiety can also be contributory factors, and eczema sufferers often find symptoms increase when they are worried or under additional work or family pressures.

Once the cause has been identified, treatment usually involves use of cleansing herbs to clear the body of any toxins, as well as creams which soften and help repair skin damage. A tea containing burdock, dandelion and yellow dock can be helpful; eat plenty of turnips and carrots and try lotions containing almond oil and evening primrose oil with essential oils of lavender, marigold or chamomile. Chickweed cream can help to relieve itching, and borage juice lotion can also help cool and ease highly irritant flare-ups.

In the elderly, poor circulation related to weakened veins can lead to yet another type of eczema – varicose eczema – which may be associated with a tendency to develop varicose ulcers. Here, circulatory stimulants like ginkgo, ginger, galangal, and cinnamon can help.

If stress is a problem, add soothing teas of chamomile, lemon balm, skullcap, vervain, or wood betony to the regime.

(continued opposite)

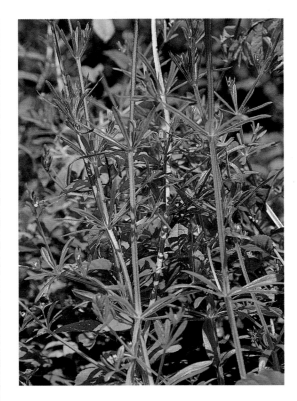

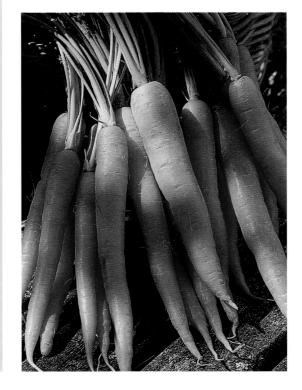

◄ Cleavers *Galium aparine*

psoriasis

Emotional stresses also play a significant role in psoriasis – an extremely common condition associated with the failure of skin cells to develop normally. It is characterised by itchy, dry skin covered in silvery scales that flake off to reveal inflamed, red areas. Knees, legs, elbows, forearms or scalp are most frequently affected.

There is usually a family tendency for the problem and in some cases it can be associated with arthritis. Psoriasis generally first appears in the late teens or 20s and can then become a life-long problem. It tends to come and go for no apparent cause and will often disappear completely in the summer in response to plenty of sunshine and sea-bathing. Psoriasis can often have an emotional dimension sending out messages of "keep away, do not touch me" which can often be helped by Bach Flower Remedies – Larch, Crab Apple or Red Chestnut may be appropriate in some cases.

Herbal treatment usually involves the same sort of cleansing skin herbs used for eczema, as well as relaxing nervines to combat any stress. Alcohol should be strictly avoided as it dilates the peripheral blood vessels and encourages skin cell production still further.

An ideal treatment for minor cases is to apply a cream made from cleavers to small psoriatic patches as soon as they appear. Repeat two or three times a day. For psoriasis affecting the scalp, try hair rinses of a standard rosemary infusion (see page 214) with 5 drops of cade oil added. Cade oil can be added to baths or creams.

◄ Carrots *Daucus carota* ssp. *sativus*

urticaria and hives

Highly irritant weals which can suddenly appear on the skin are variously described as urticaria, hives or nettle rash. They are often associated with an allergic reaction to some substance — either something taken internally or with which there has been skin contact. In severe cases there is also swelling of the hands, face, arms, eyelids or throat and there may be painful joints or breathing problems which can require emergency treatment.

Some people are sensitive to shellfish or molluscs, others blame strawberries. However, a reaction to strawberries can also suggest an intolerance of foods containing salicylates (chemicals occurring widely in fruits, vegetables and many herbs as well as forming the basis of aspirin — another common cause of urticaria). Other drugs, including some antibiotics, can have a similar effect, so always check with your doctor if skin rashes follow a new prescription.

In traditional Chinese theory, nettle rash, which can affect different parts of the body at different times, is often blamed on "wind" – one of numerous evils which can attack us. Herbs to strengthen the immune system (the surface defence energy or *Wei Qi*) are thus recommended. Possibilities for home use include echinacea, *Huang Qi,* maitake or shiitake mushrooms. A favourite in China is schizandra fruit (*Schisandra chinensis*). The Chinese name for another useful herb, *Wu Wei Zi,* means "five taste seed", as it supposedly incorporates all five of the classic Chinese tastes — sweet, sour, salty, pungent and bitter — and it is a good *yin* tonic, promoting body fluids, encouraging secretions and strengthening energy levels. It can be quite effective for many allergic skin conditions.

Contact irritants can also cause urticaria — stinging nettles themselves are an obvious culprit. Their hairs actually contain histamine, a chemical normally present in the body, but one that in excess can trigger the characteristic allergic response. Orthodox remedies are thus generally based on anti-histamines and will work quickly and effectively. Other possibilities include insect stings (including bee stings and bee products), cosmetics, perfumes and a large number of common garden plants such as hops, runner bean tendrils, borage, yarrow, chamomile and rue (*Ruta graveolens*).

Urticaria is usually self-limiting and will clear in a few hours, but herbal remedies can provide soothing relief: useful remedies include chickweed cream, borage juice, fresh plantain leaves, lemon juice, sage ointment and distilled witch hazel.

assorted infections

The skin is always contaminated by a large number of micro-organisms which generally cause us few problems. Stress, exhaustion or a weak immune system usually gives them the opportunity they need.

athlete's foot (*Tinea pedis*)

This is a very common fungal infection affecting the space between the toes and also the toenails. Depending on the infecting fungus there may be inflammation and itching or else scaling skin and general discomfort. Like all their species, the yeasts causing athlete's foot thrive in warm, damp places, so good, sensible foot care — making sure the toes are well dried after bathing and that shoes are comfortable – is important.

Creams based on anti-fungal herbs, such as tea tree, marigold and echinacea, can help.

boils

These are very tender inflamed areas of skin containing pus, generally caused by a bacterial infection of a hair follicle or a break in the skin. A cluster of boils is known as a carbuncle. Boils are usually a sign of reduced resistance to infection – perhaps because of general debility, chronic illness, exhaustion or overwork. There could also be some deep-seated septic focus such as a dental abscess adding to over-all toxicity. Frequent outbreaks of boils can suggest a more serious underlying cause – possibly diabetes or kidney disease. Unskilled lancing of boils can spread infection and is best avoided. Herbal treatments include poultices or drawing ointments accompanied by antiseptic creams or lotions to encourage the boil to discharge. Effective external options include slippery elm, chickweed, tea tree and echinacea, with herbs such as hemp agrimony, garlic, maitake or echinacea taken internally to boost the immune system and combat bacterial infections.

cold sores

These are caused by the *Herpes simplex* Type I virus, which is believed to be carried by around 50% of the adult population. The sores are always quite localised and take the form of tiny blisters which usually start with a tingling sensation and rapidly develop to inflamed, red areas generally occurring around the mouth. Once a person has been infected, the virus can remain dormant in the body for years, usually causing a recurrent outbreak of sores if the sufferer is at all run down or over-tired. Women sometimes find that cold sores will coincide with menstruation and they can often herald a cold or flu simply because both can occur when resistance is weakened by exhaustion. The virus is extremely contagious during the blistering stage and can spread in saliva or by contact, so it is important to avoid touching the cold sore and spreading the infection to other parts of the body. Cold sores are more of a nuisance than a serious health hazard: try applying tea tree, melissa, marigold or lavender oils or creams as soon as the initial tingling sensation starts.

dandruff

This is simply larger-than-usual flakes of dead skin which in the normal course of events would be more discreetly replaced every 28 days or so. It can be associated with seborrhoeic eczema where over-production of sebum (the natural oil secretions which lubricate the skin and hair) leads to oily, yellow flakes and often sore red patches on the scalp. Dandruff is believed to be caused, in part, by a fungal infection (due to *Pityrosporum ovale*), although it is not contagious and seems to depend on an individual over-response to the fungus. Wearing hats can make dandruff worse as the hot, damp environment they cause encourages fungal growth. Use of medicated shampoos can also worsen the condition because of the aggressive effect of detergents on scalp secretions and natural bacteria. Use the same sorts of cleansing remedies as for eczema (see page 51) and add infusions of rosemary leaves, chamomile flowers or stinging nettle roots to hair rinses to improve scalp quality. Gentle, soap-based shampoos should be used rather than detergents: soft soap available from pharmacists is ideal.

head lice

Epidemics of these tiny brown insects are commonplace in schools. Lice lay six to eight eggs a day at the base of the hair shafts (usually at the nape of the neck or behind the ears). These hatch to produce white nymphs and discarded egg husks (nits). These live for about 20 days in an immature form – happily feeding on blood from the scalp – before pupating to the mature insect. Tea tree is an ideal remedy: simply put a few drops of oil on a fine comb and comb the child's hair thoroughly night and morning, or add 0.5-1ml/10-20 drops of tea tree to 500ml/1pt of hot water and use as a final hair rinse.

warts

These are benign lumps in the skin caused by a virus which makes the cells multiply abnormally quickly. Common warts are usually found on the hands, knees and face and are mildly contagious, spreading as the virus comes into contact with damaged skin or when flakes from the wart touch other moist skin areas. Although they can be unsightly and a nuisance, these sorts of warts are usually quite harmless and most will disappear of their own accord. Useful herbal remedies include the sap of both greater celandine and dandelion, which can be squeezed on to warts two or three times each day until they disappear. The common garden weed, wood spurge (*Euphorbia amygdaloides*), is also known in some country districts as wart weed from the tradition of using its juice in a similar way. Professional help is needed for warts which appear to erupt on the site of moles or which start to bleed or change colour.

verrucas

Also known as plantar warts, verrucas occur on the soles of the feet. Because they are always being walked on, the small growths can become painful and are often covered by thickened areas of skin or calluses. Readily available ring plasters and callous pads can provide some relief. The constant pressure also makes these warts grow inwardly rather than erupting outwards as with common warts; persistent cases usually need treatment from a chiropodist, although tea tree creams can help.

urinary problems

Western medicine tends to regard the kidneys as mainly involved in water metabolism, although Ayurvedic medicine sees the kidneys as also influencing the nervous system and reproductive organs. In Chinese medicine, the kidney is believed to control the vital essence or *Jing* which affects both creative and sexual energies. The Chinese believe that if kidney energy is strong, an individual will show "determination" – be enthusiastic, clear thinking, vigorous and make "wise counsellors". Weak kidney energy leads to poor memory, few ambitions, low spirits or depression. In traditional Chinese medicine, the kidneys are associated with hearing and hair – it is a good sign when a baby is born with lots of hair as this indicates strong kidney *Qi* and *Jing*. Traditional Chinese medicine also links the kidneys with the emotion fear and maintains that they can be damaged by over-anxiety.

Persistent urinary problems can be seen as a weakness in kidney energy, so adding warming kidney tonics such as cinnamon to the urinary antiseptics and diuretics is often helpful.

cystitis

Cystitis – literally inflammation of the bladder – is one of the most common "chronic" conditions affecting women. It is generally caused by infections ascending through the urethra – the tube that links the bladder to the outside world – to affect the bladder lining, so tends to be more common in women as their urethras are much shorter than men's: around 3½cm/1¼in compared with about 20cm/8in. The symptoms will be familiar to many: a burning sensation on passing urine, a frequent need to do so and a dull ache in the lower abdomen.

Like all opportunist infections the bacteria which cause cystitis tend to get out of control when the sufferer is run down, so the problem often occurs when we are tired, overworked or under additional emotional stress. For many women cystitis follows sexual intercourse with monotonous regularity, which can put considerable strain on a relationship.

Washing the area between urethra and anus (the perineum) after each bowel motion can help reduce the risk of counter infection, as can emptying the bladder within 10 or 15 minutes of intercourse and again washing the area. Bacteria thrive in warm, damp conditions so wearing loose panties, preferably cotton, and stockings instead of tights can help to keep the area around the urethra cool. Maintaining a more alkaline urine also discourages the bacteria, so opt for a more vegetarian diet, limiting meat intake and avoiding acidic foods like rhubarb, oranges and pickles.

Western herbal medicine has a wide range of herbs which modern science classifies as "urinary antiseptics" – usually herbs which include some chemical or other which is not broken down in the body and is excreted in the urine, thus producing a sort of internal disinfectant. Typical is cowberry or red whortleberry which has been found to contain 7% arbutin – a potent urinary antiseptic – in its leaves. Recent work in the USA has focused on the cranberry, a close relative of the cowberry. One study showed that clinical improvement was reported by 73% of cystitis sufferers given 480ml unsweetened cranberry juice a day for 21 days.

Herbal remedies for cystitis also include diuretics, designed to flush out any toxins or infecting bacteria: buchu is one of the most useful as it is an antiseptic, diuretic and also warms the kidneys. Parsley is another good diuretic and, as with other herbs that "rob the soil", it is rich in minerals and vitamins so is useful in debilitated conditions: very large quantities of parsley, especially the seeds, are contraindicated in pregnancy as the herb may act as a uterine stimulant. Other useful diuretics likely to be found in the household medicine chest include celery seed, leeks, pineapple juice, dandelion leaves and white deadnettle – all can be helpful for cystitis.

Astringents and wound herbs like agrimony, yarrow, purple loosestrife and shepherd's purse can also be useful in severe cases where there is blood in the urine. Echinacea is effective at combating kidney and urinary infections, so taking three 200mg capsules, three times a day, in acute cases can bring rapid improvement.

prostate problems

Many men from their middle 40s onwards suffer from enlargement of the prostate gland. This sex gland sits beneath the bladder, surrounding the urethra, and contributes an alkaline fluid to the semen. As it enlarges it constricts the urethra, leading to hesitation in flow, dribbling and increased frequency of the need to urinate; while retention of urine can result in low grade urinary infection with lethargy and tiredness and, in severe cases, it can become a clinical emergency. Professional diagnosis is always needed because of the possibility of prostate cancer – a common condition in older men but one which has a good five-year survival rate.

Physical inactivity is sometimes a trigger for prostate problems especially in the newly retired who may find it difficult to adjust to a non-work routine: creative energies and vigour seem to deteriorate and decline as a result. The low-grade urinary infections associated with retention can also led to lethargy and tiredness. This in turn contributes to physical inactivity and may be associated with weight gain, sluggishness and stagnation. Keeping active – both physically and mentally – is important to maintain energies and vigour. In Ayurvedic medicine prostate enlargement is also associated with diminished sexual activity – something which older men need not forsake and which can help to maintain kidney energy as well as keep the prostate gland healthy.

Herbal treatment tends to focus on energy-giving herbs, especially Siberian ginseng, and soothing diuretics, such as white deadnettle. One very specific remedy is saw palmetto which has proved very effective in clinical trials. Typical dosage in these tests is generally equivalent to around 10g/⅓oz of the berries twice a day – an extremely high dose – although herbalists often find much lower doses bring about a similar improvement. Recent research also suggests that stinging nettle roots can be effective for treating prostate enlargement.

At any age the prostate gland may also become infected, leading to prostatitis – an inflammation which can have cystitis-like symptoms and is similarly treated with urinary antiseptics, diuretics and soothing anti-inflammatories. Saw palmetto berries and stinging nettles can also be helpful.

▼ White deadnettle *Lamium album*

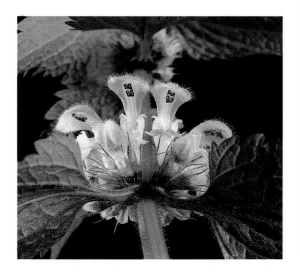

women's ailments

For centuries women had little other than herbs to sustain them through difficult periods, pregnancy and childbirth: the country names of many of our garden and wildflower healers remind us of the fact – lady's mantle, motherwort, mother's hearts, milk thistle, maiden wort, lady's tresses and many more.

Steroidal compounds have been identified in many of these plants, explaining their potent effect on hormones and the menstrual cycle. Chaste-tree berries, for example, stimulate the pituitary gland to produce a variety of sex hormones involved in ovulation, while sage contains oestrogen-like compounds which explain its traditional use in drying up breast milk when weaning a baby and in reducing night sweats and hot flushes at the menopause.

Herbs can, however, do much more than simply provide an alternative to the orthodox emphasis on hormones. Ayurvedic medicine stresses the importance of sexual energy in maintaining health and vitality and offers an impressive variety of herbs designed to help. In Ayurveda sexual energy is often equated with the creative energy used to improve mental or spiritual effort, so using herbs like *shatavari* and basil can be helpful.

Menstrual and reproductive disorders are many and varied and any change in blood flow or sudden irregularity can indicate problems which really need professional help. Self-diagnosis is not to be recommended – but for those commonplace and largely self-limiting monthly problems, herbs can provide a safe and gentle solution.

pre-menstrual syndrome

Bloating, breast tenderness, irritability, anger, clumsiness, inability to concentrate … the symptoms of pre-menstrual syndrome (PMS) are many and varied. The problem can be explained in terms of falling progesterone levels and an orthodox approach thus tends to concentrate on hormone treatments – or use of chaste-tree berries (often given in tincture form, up to 1ml/20 drops each morning) as a herbal alternative. Dietary imbalance and candidiasis can also play a part and there is some evidence that cutting out artificial stimulants (themselves a possible stress on the system) such as caffeine and theobromine in coffee, tea or chocolate can help. PMS has also been linked to various nutritional deficiencies and supplements – notably vitamin B_6 and evening primrose oil – are often successfully used to relieve symptoms.

Herbal medicine can, however, offer a more holistic approach. In traditional Chinese medicine, pre-menstrual syndrome is seen as an energy imbalance often related to liver *Qi* (energy) congestion with symptoms of abdominal bloating, menstrual irregularities and period pain leading to a craving for sweet foods – a common PMS symptom – diarrhoea or constipation and fluid retention. Chinese remedies for PMS therefore focus on energising and tonifying the liver using herbs such as *Dang Gui*. The Chinese consider that pre-menstrual breast distension is associated with rising *Qi*, so they add various bitter orange extracts to the mix to combat this trend. Taking 0.5ml/10 drops of bitter orange tincture in water three to four times a day can certainly help to ease these sorts of symptoms. Parsley tea is another popular remedy for pre-menstrual fluid retention.

Women's monthly cycles have often been associated with the moon, with menstruation traditionally occurring at the time of the new moon and ovulation at the full. Some suggest that this natural rhythm is still followed by women whose main interests lie within the home, while for those more involved with external activities, menstruation coincides with the full moon instead. One way of regulating the menstrual cycle is to sleep with the curtains open, or a dull light glowing, at the time of a full moon and ensure complete darkness at the new moon.

A more recent remedy for menstrual problems has been evening primrose oil – now extensively and expensively marketed in numerous combinations to suit every stage of a woman's reproductive life. The *gamma*-linolenic acid (GLA) it contains is believed to help with production of certain prostaglandins – hormone-like substances that can act as chemical messengers and also cause uterine contractions. GLA is also contained in borage seed oil (often sold as starflower oil) and blackcurrant seed oil (*Ribes nigrum*). Most women, however, are able to produce GLA themselves in a normal metabolic process starting from *cis*-linolenic acid found in leafy plants and seed oils. For those on a tight budget a daily teaspoonful of good-quality walnut or safflower oil can make an adequate alternative to shrink-wrapped supplements.

period pain

Herbalists tend to divide period pain into:
• congestive pain, which builds up shortly before the period starts. It is associated with blood stagnation and blood congestion and can involve bloating and fluid retention. This sort of pain eases once the period has begun; and
• spasmodic pain, due to uterine cramps which start once flow has begun and can be linked to a prostaglandin imbalance and emotional tension.

Relaxing anti-cramping remedies such as chamomile, St John's wort or black haw bark (*Viburnum prunifolium*) are used for the spasmodic sort of pain, whereas more stimulating, hormonal or tonifying herbs like white deadnettle, raspberry leaf, rosemary, *Dang Gui* or chaste-tree can be helpful for the congestive variety.

Period pain can often be eased by exercise: rather than curling up with a hot water bottle and feeling miserable, try a brisk walk in the fresh air. Regular sexual intercourse – especially just before menstruation starts – can also help to reduce period pain, while some argue that intercourse during the period is the best way of easing cramps although there are numerous cultural taboos arguing against intercourse at such times.

Period pain can also – as with PMS – be associated with liver stagnation and so can be exacerbated by alcohol and highly processed foods.

heavy periods

Heavy periods can sometimes indicate some major underlying problems – such as fibroids or

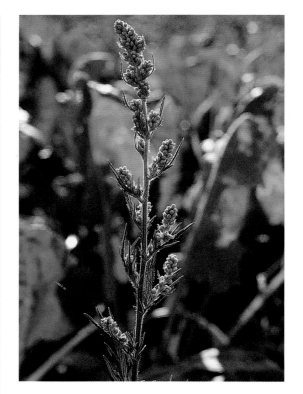

◄ Mugwort *Artemisia vulgaris*

endometriosis – but often they have no apparent cause and are more of an irritant than anything else. Modern medicine tends to respond to complaints of heavy periods with suggestions for hysterectomies which, sadly, many women accept as the only solution. Hysterectomy is something to be avoided if at all possible. In Ayurvedic theory the various energy centres of the body, the *chakras*, start with the root *chakra* which in women is found at the womb. Removing this organ thus tends to leave women feeling "rootless" and can lead to emotional disturbances. Herbs like basil can be helpful to combat this tendency.

Menstrual "heaviness" is also relative: some women always have heavy periods and to them this is normal; others find periods get heavier with age and start to worry. The main thing is to seek professional advice if the pattern of flow changes significantly, but not to be persuaded into unnecessary treatments.

Useful herbs to combat excessive flow include shepherd's purse (also known as mother's hearts), marigold, herb Robert, hawthorn and white deadnettle.

vaginal thrush

Recurrent vaginal thrush often indicates an underlying problem with candidiasis or food intolerance, as the immune system is constantly under stress and unable to combat opportunist bugs such as *Candida albicans*. Taking echinacea or garlic can help counter the infection and

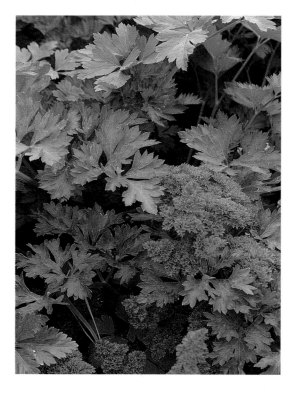

◄ Parsley *Petroselinum crispum*

strengthen the immune system, while anti-fungal creams such as tea tree or marigold can help to give symptomatic relief.

Tea tree has become extremely popular in recent years with commercially made pessaries containing the oil now sold in many health-food shops. Unlike most essential oils, tea tree does not irritate the mucous membranes and most people can tolerate it used neat instead of diluted in a vegetable carrier oil.

A simple application technique is to use a tampon: push it slightly out of the tube and moisten the top with water. Then add 3 drops of tea tree oil to the exposed moist top and insert it in the vagina. Leave for no longer than four hours at a time and repeat twice a day.

pregnancy and childbirth

Herbs have a long tradition of use for easing the pains of childbirth and the ills of pregnancy: for generations of women they were the only available remedies and much folklore – as well as hard scientific evidence – testifies to their efficacy. Today few women in the West have the opportunity to use herbs in this way: childbirth has become a much more orderly and monitored affair.

Using herbs in pregnancy also needs caution: many contain chemicals that will cross the placental barrier, so it is unwise to take any remedies in the first three months unless you really have to. The list of herbs to be avoided in pregnancy is already long and growing as potential new hazards are identified and, frequently, exaggerated (see Cautions, page 13, for details of those to avoid). Many herbs are,

however, perfectly safe to use and even some of those which should be avoided in high, regular doses are fine in moderation or in the sort of quantities used in cooking.

morning sickness,

The nausea which affects many pregnant women in the first three months is generally, fortunately, confined to a few minutes on rising, although with some sufferers it can last all day and extend through much of the nine months. Researchers have found that ginger is extremely effective even in these very severe cases. Up to 1g per dose has been used quite safely in hospital trials. Other herbs that can help include fennel, lemon balm, galangal, bitter orange, chamomile and peppermint. These are best kept as tinctures in dropper bottles on the bedside table and used before rising. Alternatively, leave a Thermos flask of a suitable herbal infusion beside the bed at night so that it is ready to take before rising next morning. Try different remedies as need be – morning sickness may respond well to a particular remedy one day but not the next, so keep plenty of alternatives near by.

digestive upsets

Indigestion and heartburn in pregnancy can be safely treated with slippery elm or marshmallow, while for constipation (often exacerbated by the use of supplementary iron tablets) stay with the gentler remedies – ispaghula, yellow dock or dandelion root.

childbirth

Raspberry leaf has long been used to strengthen the womb ready for childbirth: it helps to tonify the uterus and aid contractions, but should be taken only in the last eight weeks of pregnancy.

During labour many teas have traditionally been used to help relaxation, soothe pain and encourage contractions. In the modern labour ward sipping a home-brewed cup of herbal tea is not always possible, but they can be used in the early stages of labour or where midwives are sympathetic. Traditional choices include wood betony, chamomile, motherwort and basil, with rose petal, raspberry leaf and clove in the later stages. Massaging the abdomen with well-diluted clove or sage oils can also help. To speed recovery from the birth itself, homoeopathic Arnica 30X tablets taken every 15-30 minutes for a few hours will help repair stressed tissues.

breast-feeding problems

Sore nipples in breast-feeding are commonplace: the cause is often poor positioning of the baby, who should suck at the whole areola (the dark area around the nipple) rather than just holding on to the nipple itself. Marigold and chamomile creams can help. Many herbs, including fennel, fenugreek and vervain, also encourage milk flow. To dry up milk at weaning take sage tea.

menopausal problems

For most women the menopause passes by with little more inconvenience than occasional hot flushes and night sweats. For others, it can be a time of major emotional upheaval, depression, weight gain and heavy bleeding.

Today, many of these symptoms may be treated by hormone replacement therapy which boosts oestrogen levels, although critics still have doubts about the long-term effects of such treatment. For some women (including those with a high risk of osteoporosis) HRT can be a preferred solution, but for those who want to complete this transition period in their lives as naturally as possible, then a far better option can be exercise, an increase in calcium intake and herbal remedies – to relieve the more troublesome symptoms and help the body to adjust to new levels of functionality. A normally healthy lifestyle with good diet, a happy and fulfilled outlook and acceptable stress levels is also obviously important. Anyone who starts out being depressed, overworked or malnourished is unlikely to pass through the menopause without trauma.

Traditional Chinese theory associated menopausal problems with a run-down in the kidney's vital energy and using kidney tonics to ease symptoms can be extremely effective. Herbs like cinnamon, fenugreek and buchu which have a tonic effect on the kidneys can be worth trying and there are a number of specialist Chinese tonic herbs (such as *He Shou Wu* and *Dang Gui*) which are now appearing in over-the-counter menopausal products.

Many herbs can be used to ease the more troublesome menopausal symptoms – sage, mugwort and golden seal can help with hot flushes and night sweats; chaste-tree, lady's mantle and black cohosh will help to regulate hormone production, while the emotional ups and downs can be soothed with chamomile, skullcap, borage, St John's wort, vervain, linden or lemon balm. Hawthorn and motherwort are useful for easing menopausal palpitations. Use a combination of herbs to match specific discomforts or take the herbs singly in teas or capsules. Vaginal dryness can often be helped with creams containing vitamin E and marigold.

minor injuries

Herbs have been used for centuries for all sorts of injuries and wounds. Their very names remind us of the fact: yarrow's botanical name (*Achillea*) comes from Achilles, who reputedly used it before the gates of Troy to heal his fellow Greeks while numerous herbs are known as "woundwort" or "self-heal" in country areas. In some cultures a warlike nature tended to dominate views of herbs: the Maori of New Zealand, for example, were always fighting each other and the vast majority of their traditional remedies involve poultices and compresses to heal the injured.

Herbs are still ideal for all sorts of minor cuts, grazes and burns: the choice is wide, so even when you are far from home there is generally a suitably antiseptic healing remedy to staunch blood flow close at hand.

▼ Bear's breech *Acanthus mollis*

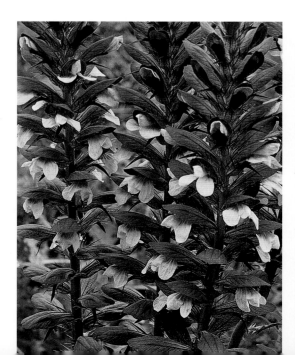

burns and sunburn

Burns are potential medical emergencies and only the most minor should be treated at home. Any burn more than about 5cm/2in across should be seen by a doctor as soon as possible. For less severe injuries running cold water over the affected area or using an ice pack (or packet of frozen peas) will cool it down and ease the immediate pain. Keeping the injury cool for two or three hours can often help significantly.

Useful topical herbs for burns include aloe vera, bilberry, powdered coffee beans, lavender, pot marigold, raw potato, chickweed, white deadnettle, butterbur and St John's wort.

Given the publicity in recent years of the risks of skin cancer from sunbathing in our ozone-depleted environment, one would

▼ Ribwort plantain *Plantago lanceolata*

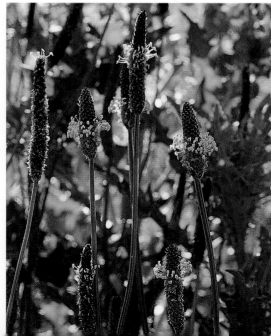

imagine that we would all remain well protected under sun hats and long-sleeved shirts. However, perhaps because the sun's rays are more penetrative in our polluted atmosphere, sunburn seems ever more commonplace. St John's wort oil is a useful standby for emergencies – add 2ml/½tsp of lavender oil to 18ml/½fl oz of St John's wort oil in a 20ml/¾fl oz bottle and include it in the holiday first-aid kit.

cuts and grazes

Herbal alternatives to the usual mixture of orthodox antiseptic creams which fill the average domestic first-aid box are now readily available. Always bathe cuts and grazes by either rinsing the wound under running water or using cotton wool swabs soaked in warm water or an infusion of antiseptic herbs, taking care to wipe from the centre to the edge of the graze to clear any dirt. Pressing a clean tissue or gauze pad over the injury for a few minutes will also stop bleeding. Finally, apply antiseptic creams – marigold (*Calendula*), echinacea, St John's wort (*Hypericum*) or tea tree creams are all suitable and can be used on open wounds.

Aloe vera creams can also be used on grazes and various combinations containing St John's wort are commercially available. In the past, comfrey was generally recommended to encourage healing; however, given recent concerns over the toxic alkaloids it contains (see page 204), many now advise against it being used on open wounds.

The list of wound herbs is long and impressive – if far from home look for agrimony, bear's breech, chickweed, coltsfoot, creeping Jenny, hemp agrimony, herb Robert, Jack-by-the-hedge, marsh woundwort, marshmallow, self-heal, shepherd's purse or yarrow.

insect bites and stings

For most people insect bites and stings in temperate zones lead to little more than local irritation which eases in a few days. However, for an unfortunate minority stings lead to severe allergic reactions which can range from weeping and persistent dermatitis to anaphylactic shock characterised by dizziness, sickness, breathing problems and marked swelling of the affected area. When severe, this can be fatal. Immediate emergency medical treatment is vital in such cases.

Bee stings are acidic and in traditional first aid were treated with blue-bag (an alkaline starch used in laundry) or bicarbonate of soda, while alkaline wasp stings were soothed by vinegar. Both, however, respond well to slices of onion or leek.

To soothe irritant mosquito and gnat bites try rubbing them with fresh common plantain leaves, aloe vera sap, lemon balm leaves, lemon juice, or slices of cucumber or tomato; infusions or ointments containing any of these herbs or sage can also help. If bites become infected, echinacea or tea tree cream can be effective.

Keeping the insects at bay is another way of tackling the problem and several herbal oils will help here: tea tree and lemon balm are ideal sprinkled on clothing; at barbecues or when sitting out of doors, try burning citronella (*Cymbopogon nardus*) candles.

herbs for babies and children

children's dosages

0-1 year
5% of adult dose

1-2 years
10% of adult dose

3-4 years
20% of adult dose

5-6 years
30% of adult dose

7-8 years
40% of adult dose

9-10 years
50% of adult dose

11-12 years
60% of adult dose

13-14 years
80% of adult dose

15-plus
100% of adult dose

Many herbs are quite safe for children – although unfortunately, the taste is often far from pleasant and administering the remedy can prove a problem. Giving babies weak infusions of soothing herbs, such as chamomile or linden, by bottle from a very early age can encourage acceptance of herby flavours, while dosing breast-fed babies can often be best achieved by the mother taking the herbal remedy herself, as many of the active ingredients will then pass into the breast milk. This is an especially neat solution for colic and wind remedies (see below), which can thus be dispensed precisely at feeding time.

Toddlers can be dosed with teaspoons of honey containing herb powders or drops of tinctures, while capsules are ideal and tasteless just as soon as children are old enough to swallow them. Tinctures (neat or dilute, depending on age) given in drop doses on the tongue can also be quite acceptable – the process can even be made into a game that can override the unpleasantness of the taste.

Taste is held to be more significant in some cultures than in others: Ayurvedic medicine, for example, divides tastes into six categories: sweet, sour, salty, pungent, bitter and astringent. A child's healthy growth depends on a good balance of tastes, and special sweets and pills are sold which combine all six tastes with which parents can dose their children.

Herbal dosages need, of course, to be reduced for children. Much depends on the child's size but a general guide is given in the table shown right.

In many childhood illnesses herbs can help to calm over-excitement, ease tension and encourage sleep – which will all significantly aid the healing process. Chamomile, linden and lemon balm are ideal taken in infusions and sweetened with honey. If over-excitement leads to nervous exhaustion then give oatmeal porridge or oatcakes, along with vervain and wood betony infusions. Older children can also be safely given Californian poppy for sleeplessness, while some preparations containing passion flower can be suitable for those aged around eight years old or over.

Children also suffer the same complaints as their elders, so reduced doses of many of the remedies suggested for coughs, minor injuries, constipation, diarrhoea and stomach upsets will generally be suitable. For infections, low doses of echinacea are quite safe. Children can develop dramatically high fevers with the temperature reaching 39°C/102°F or more. Raising the body temperature is part of the normal defence mechanism to combat invading organisms and is not generally a problem. However, if the temperature rises above 39°C/102°F for more than 12 hours, professional help is advisable. For milder cases herbal remedies containing elder flower, yarrow, stinging nettles and linden can be helpful. Peppermint is fine for feverish older children, but should be avoided for toddlers, although especially suitable for children is catmint, which can easily be grown in gardens and makes an ideal tea for feverish conditions and minor stomach upsets.

catarrhal problems

Persistent catarrh in childhood is often associated with milk allergy, so try switching to soya milk instead of cow's. Soya is a good source of calcium and other minerals, so completely eliminating dairy products from a child's diet is unlikely to cause any deficiencies – although if possible you should avoid the genetically modified soya products now coming on to the market. Soya-based yoghurts and desserts which can be suitable for children are also now commercially available. Gentle herbs for catarrhal conditions include elder flower and ribwort plantain. Eliminating milk can also be helpful in many cases of glue ear (secretory otitis media, see page 38).

colic

This is a severe abdominal pain which tends to come in waves a few seconds or minutes apart. In adults it can be due to an obstruction in the intestine or simply to constipation and can need professional treatment. In babies, colic is usually caused by air becoming trapped in the intestines and is generally associated with feeding difficulties – or a failure to "wind" the infant properly after it has finished sucking. Colicky babies often remain so for the first three months of life, which can be extremely wearing on the parents as the child's only reaction to the pain it feels is to cry – loudly. Traditional gripe water is usually based on dill extracts so a suitable alternative is simply to use a weak infusion of dill. Another popular option for colic is homoeopathic chamomile (Chamomilla 3X), available in drops or pillules.

cradle cap

This is a dandruff-like condition that affects young babies and usually starts with scurf on the head followed by the development of yellow, crusted scaly patches. These can spread over the whole head or simply be confined to particular areas. The condition is quite harmless and may be related to over-activity of the sebaceous glands in the scalp, possibly caused by the mother's hormones. A simple remedy is to rub olive or wheat germ oil gently into the baby's scalp, allow it to soak well in and then wash the flakes away; infused marigold or heartsease (*Viola tricolor*) oils and creams can also be safely used.

digestive upsets

Persistent bilious attacks are common with some children and are often identified as a type of migraine. Eliminating the sort of foods that adult migraine sufferers often find trigger attacks (such as cheese and chocolate) can help. The soothing carminatives – lemon balm, chamomile, fennel, dill, coriander – are also worth trying. Childhood constipation needs to be treated with gentle remedies and definitely not the sort of stimulating laxatives that adults may favour (avoid senna and other anthraquinone-containing herbs). Ispaghula seeds are a good bulking laxative. One way to get children to take them is to disguise them with breakfast cereal: put the seeds in the bowl, then add the cereal and milk. The mucilaginous, swollen seeds will generally be swallowed with the soggy cornflakes without too many complaints. Commercial "flavoured" ispaghula remedies are available for children. Yellow dock or liquorice can also be suitable in low doses — or you can opt for the many laxative foods such as apples, figs, pears or dried apricots.

hyperactivity

Food allergies can also account for many cases of hyperactivity — colourants like tartrazine and sunset yellow are particularly suspect. Hyperactivity is explained in Chinese medicine in terms of liver *Qi* disharmonies or flaring of liver fire, so suitable cooling liver herbs like vervain, agrimony or self-heal can be used, often in combination with gentle sedatives like chamomile, lemon balm, Californian poppy or skullcap.

nappy rash

Sore, red bottoms seem to develop in some children no matter how carefully the parent changes and dries the little one. It is important to keep the affected area as dry as possible (even by blowing with a hair dryer set on the cool setting). It is better to use ointments than creams, as they form a protective barrier for the skin whereas creams tend to soak in and soften. Marigold, chamomile or comfrey ointment can be helpful and safe to use, as can aloe vera gel. Bacteria in the faeces can react with urine to produce ammonia and this can encourage fungal infections to develop. If this occurs, use ointments containing marigold or tea tree.

teething

Cutting those first teeth can start from around six months and can be a gruelling time for all the family. Homoeopathic Chamomilla 3X remedies can be very soothing; some babies will take weak chamomile tea from a bottle or it can be added to bath water to encourage more restful nights. Gently rubbing the gums with 1-2 drops of chamomile oil in 25ml/1tbsp of almond oil can also bring relief.

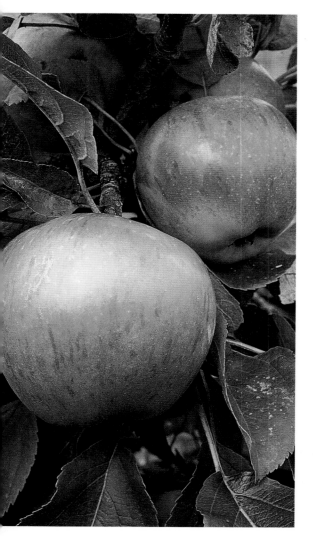

◄ Apple *Malus communis*

the home medicine chest

No one wants to fill the entire bathroom cabinet with herbal remedies, but keeping a limited selection at home to cope with minor ailments and first-aid problems is good sense. The following ingredients are ideal for the home mediicine chest:

arnica is effective in improving circulation and encouraging healing and arnica creams can be used on chilblains, bruises and sprains. The herb should not be applied to broken skin as it is an irritant. Internally, homoeopathic doses (Arnica 6X or 30X) encourage recovery from surgery or traumatic injury.

chickweed cream is made from the common garden weed and is often used to relieve the irritation of eczema, but it is also useful to soothe minor burns, sunburn and insect stings and can be helpful for drawing splinters and boils.

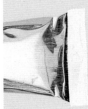

cloves oil is an ideal emergency standby for toothache (apply on a cotton wool swab) or insect bites. The tincture can be used instead of oil and also makes a warming remedy for stomach chills and nausea – use ½ ml/10 drops of tincture in water.

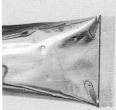

comfrey speeds up tissue growth and repair, so is good for bruises, sprains and even for healing fractures and cracked small bones. It can also be used on clean cuts. Use ointment or infused oil (see page 204-205 for cautions).

echinacea tablets help combat colds, flu and infections. Always keep the first-aid box well stocked with them.

evening primrose or **borage oil** capsules can be helpful as an emergency hangover remedy to help restore normal liver function. Take 2-3g on "the morning after" and try not to do it again! The oil can also be used neat on skin rashes.

garlic tablets are useful for catarrh, coughs, to boost the immune system and to help reduce cholesterol levels. Low doses taken regularly can also help improve digestion function in the elderly.

lavender oil, diluted in a vegetable-oil base, makes a helpful massage for headaches and muscular aches. It can also be used on insect bites and on minor burns and sunburn.

meadowsweet tincture is ideal for stomach upsets associated with eating too much rich or contaminated food. Keep a small bottle in the medicine chest and remember to take it on holiday as well.

passion flower tablets make a helpful sedative for anxiety and insomnia.

slippery elm bark is an extremely mucilaginous herb largely used to soothe and protect against stomach inflammations. The powder can be made into a paste with a little water and taken for heartburn, gastritis, indigestion and for irritant coughs. It can also be used as a poultice or in ointments to draw splinters and corns. Tablets and capsules are a convenient alternative for internal use.

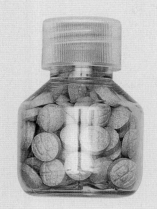

tea tree oil is extracted from an Australian tree and is now known to be one of the most antiseptic and anti-fungal herbs available to us. The oil can be used neat on infected cuts or fungal infections, such as athlete's foot, while three or four drops on a tampon inserted in the vagina will help combat vaginal yeast infections. (Do not leave the tampon inserted for more than four hours at a time.) Creams are commercially available as an alternative.

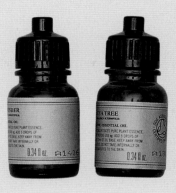

thyme and liquorice syrup is helpful for coughs and chest infections and is available ready-made from health food shops and herbal suppliers.

distilled witch hazel is highly astringent, anti-inflammatory and stops bleeding. It can be used as a cooling lotion for minor burns, sunburn, bruises, insect bites and varicose veins, as well as on cuts, grazes and piles.

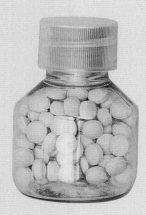

all sorts of remedies

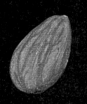

We tend to think of herbs as some sort of "different" category of plants: something to relegate to a dedicated corner of the garden or to buy, dusty and faded, in a specialist shop. Healing plants are not always dreary "green things", they can come in all shapes and sizes from the humble vegetable to an exotic eastern flower. Many have their place in the home medicine chest and give plenty of choice for emergency first aid.

Rather than a simple A to Z of healing plants, the herbs featured in this section are grouped in four broad categories. First are the herbs most common in Western gardens or kitchens: these are mainly plants which could be grown in temperate gardens as culinary herbs. Second are the "household healers" – mainly the fruits and vegetables that would normally be classified as "food". Third are more exotic herbs which would tend to be bought pre-packaged in health food shops and finally there are the hedgerow healers – temperate zone wildflowers and garden flowers common in many parts of the world which have been gathered for centuries to make simple home remedies. For advice on typical dosages and preparing your own remedies, see pages 212-233.

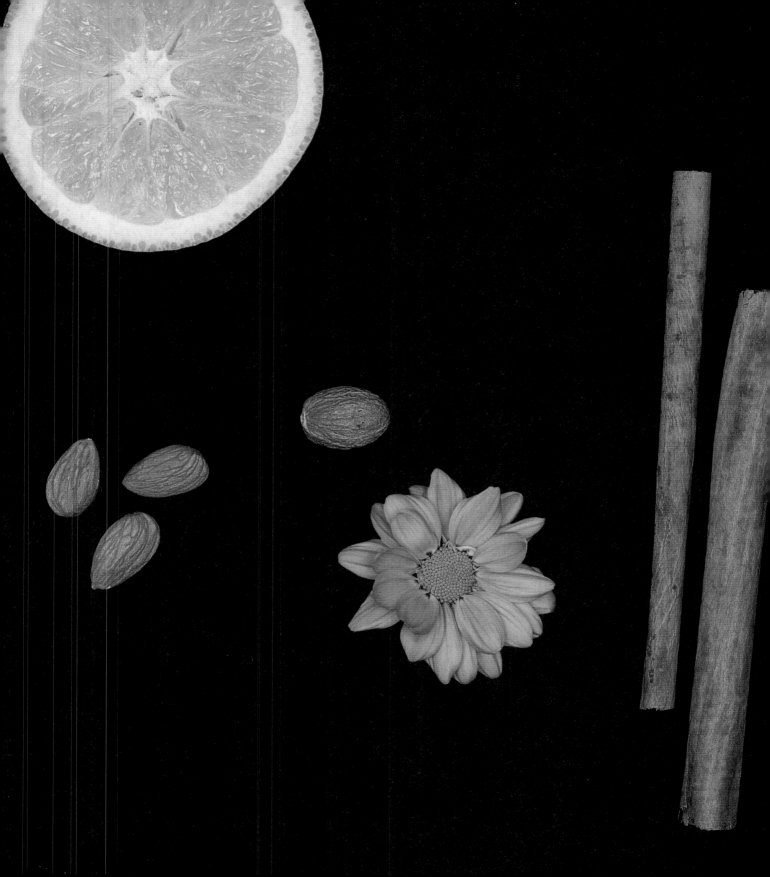

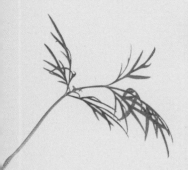

home herbs

Most enthusiastic cooks will have their favourite selection of herbal flavourings, bought freshly cut or dried from the local store, to use every day. The list is likely to include such familiar plants as sage, thyme, parsley, or oregano – all of which not only improve the taste of our meals but also have an impressive array of therapeutic properties to match.

Significantly, many culinary herbs act on the digestive system in some way. Pungent seasonings will help to stimulate the digestive system so that we process the nutrients from our meal more efficiently, others are termed "carminative" which simply means that they help to clear any gas from the digestive tract so helping to prevent flatulence and indigestion.

Until the 17th century when traditional Galenic theories were replaced by modern medicine, culinary herbs were also regarded as performing an important balancing act to prevent particular foods from having an adverse effect on our inner harmony. Cold and damp foods, for example, needed to be tempered by warm and dry foods to avoid creating an excess of phlegm in the body leading to ill health. Certain foods – such as cucumber and strawberries – were known to increase cold and damp humours, so would be avoided in winter when the prevailing climate was already doing just that.

Fragments in old cookbooks and herbals remind us that this balancing act was an everyday activity for household cooks although the precise theories guiding the combinations may have been less familiar. The Italian Giacomo Castelvetro, writing in 1614, urges the use of pepper as a seasoning for numerous cold and damp vegetables – such as beans – which would otherwise cause wind and stomach upsets, and recommends a walnut sauce (reasonably hot and dry) for pork "as an antidote to its harmful qualities". While Nicholas Culpeper in 1653 notes that: "One good old fashion is not yet left off, viz. to boil fennel with fish: for it consumes that phlegmatic humour which fish most plentifully afford and annoy the body with, though few that use it know wherefore they do it." Today, like Culpeper's housewives, we still add fennel to our fish dishes appreciating its flavour and its strong carminative properties rather more than the effect it may have on the long forgotten "phlegmatic humour".

Many of these culinary herbs are easy to grow at home in window boxes, pots or gardens and provide a ready source not just of useful seasonings but of helpful medicinal plants to ease everyday ills: sage is just as effective as a gargle for sore throats as it is in onion stuffings, while rosemary, when not being used to flavour roast lamb, makes a stimulating tonic for the nervous system.

Other garden favourites also have their uses: the bright blue flowers of borage are ideal in summer drinks and salads, while extracts from the plant itself can soothe irritant rashes or strengthen adrenal glands damaged by steroidal therapy. The garden lavender bush will yield a useful tea to ease headaches and migraines.

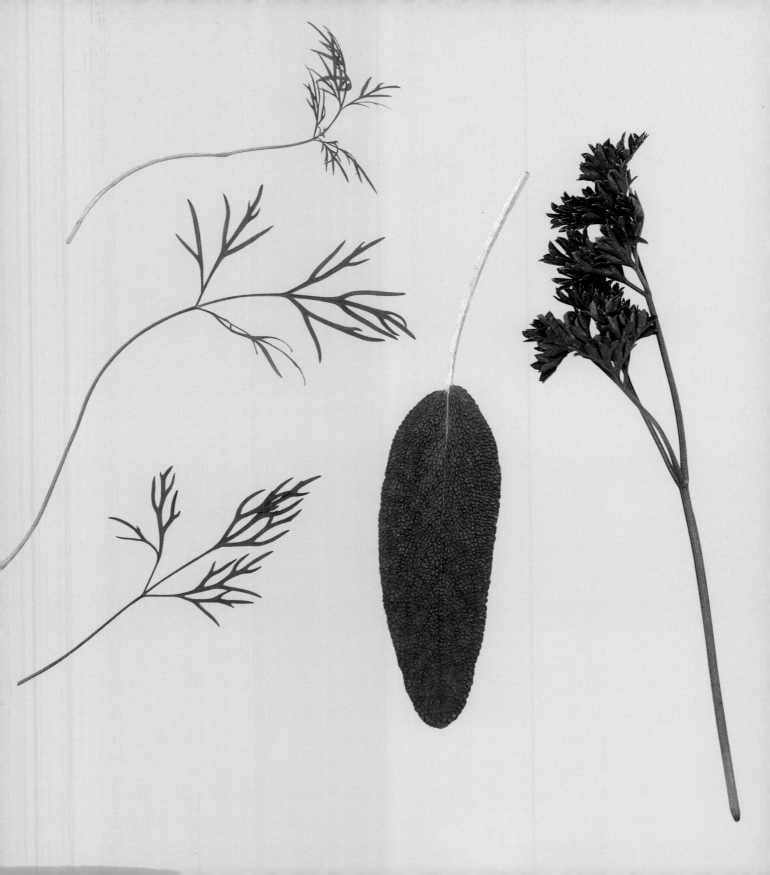

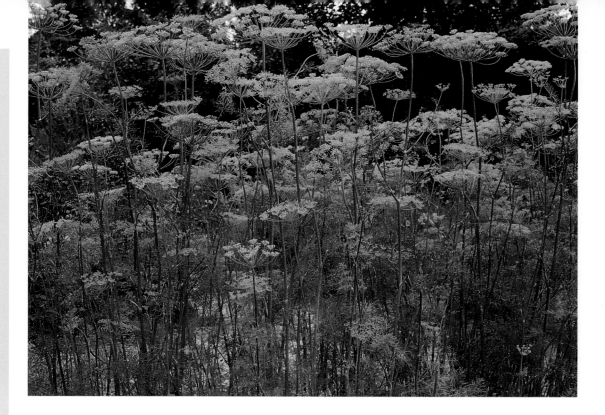

dill

parts used

leaves, seed, essential oil

commercial products

included in some proprietary indigestion remedies but best known as the key herb in baby's gripe water used for flatulence and colic.

how to use

seeds – decoction, 25g/1oz to 750ml/ 1½fl oz of water; *leaves* – freezes well for use in cooking or use dried for infusions (25g/1oz to 500ml/1pt of water).

dill *Anethum graveolens*

Dill has been used since ancient Egyptian times and is believed by some to be the "anise" mentioned in the Bible (Matthew xxiii, 23) which was widely grown in Palestine at that time. Its use as an effective digestive remedy goes back at least 5,000 years.

The Greek herbalist, Dioscorides – who knew the plant as *anethon* – recommended it to stop attacks of hiccoughs and the English name dill is believed to derive from the Anglo-Saxon word *dylle* meaning "to lull" – reinforcing its long-established use as a remedy for noisy and disturbed digestive systems.

Like many traditional medicinal herbs, dill was believed to combat witchcraft and enchantments, or as one mediaeval script puts it: "…to hindereth witches of their will". It was common in magic potions until the 17th century.

using dill

The plant is popular as a seasoning in many parts of Europe and is a traditional accompaniment for cucumbers: in Galenic terms dill is hot and dry so balancing the obvious cold and dampness of the cucumber. It plays a similar role in traditional recipes for cauliflowers and is often combined with mustard in fish sauces.

The leaves of "dill weed" tend to be used in cooking while the seeds are preferred for medicinal remedies: sometimes just smelling these, wrapped in a muslin cloth which was boiled in wine – was believed to be enough to ease indigestion and colicky upsets. Dill is an ingredient in baby's gripe water – although an alternative in breast-feeding is for the mother to drink dill seed infusion so that baby receives its medicinal herbs with the daily milk. The oil is used commercially for scenting soap.

◄ Dill *Anthemum graveolens*

garlic *Allium sativum*

Garlic is one of mankind's oldest medicinal herbs – recipes using the plant have been found in the cuneiform script of ancient Babylon dating back at least 5,000 years.

Garlic was traditionally regarded as a remedy for colds, chest infections and digestive upsets, including amoebic dysentery: today we know it is strongly anti-bacterial and anti-fungal and is active against a wide spectrum of infections. Its characteristic smell is due to a group of sulphur-containing compounds, notably allicin, which account for its medicinal activity. Deodorising garlic by removing the allicin thus makes the remedy markedly less effective. These potent chemicals can only be excreted in sweating or through the lungs so it is a helpful antiseptic for infected lungs and skin problems. Garlic also has some anti-histamine activity helping to reduce the allergic response.

using garlic

Garlic affects the blood and is now known to reduce cholesterol levels, so helping to prevent the development of atherosclerosis which is caused by a build-up of fatty deposits on the inner walls of blood vessels. Studies among heart attack patients have demonstrated that taking garlic can significantly reduce the risk of a second attack. It can also reduce the risk of blood clots, lowers blood pressure and will help to reduce blood sugar levels.

In the East, garlic has long been regarded as an important tonic for the elderly, helping to improve weak digestive function, and researchers have now shown that low doses of garlic (typically a clove each day used in cooking) do indeed have a tonifying effect on the intestine, improving peristalsis and performance.

Recommendations on dosage vary considerably, with some authors suggesting consumption of up to an excessive 1kg/2lb a day although most research involving heart attack patients has involved doses of around 7-15g/¼-½oz daily. Eating parsley can help to reduce garlic odour.

caution high doses of garlic are best avoided in pregnancy and lactation as they may lead to heartburn or flavour breast milk.

▼ Garlic *Allium sativum*

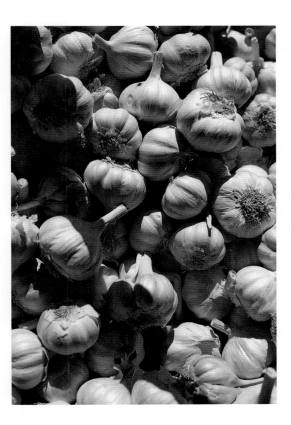

garlic

part used
bulb

commercial products
one of the most widely used herbs in over-the-counter (OTC) products with well over 50 tablet- and capsule-branded simples on the market as well as numerous remedies for colds, heart problems or digestive upsets containing varying amounts of the herb; also available as juice and oil extracts.

how to use
typical recommended doses of garlic in capsules or tablets is generally around 2g per day although clinical trials have involved doses of up to 15g/½oz; *juice* – 10ml/2tsp in water three times a day.

angelica

parts used

root, leaves, essential oil

commercial products

included in a variety of proprietary remedies recommended for coughs, digestive problems or fluid retention; tincture and essential oil available from specialist suppliers; candied stems sold as cake decorations.

how to use

leaves are best used fresh if possible:

infusion – 75g/2½oz of fresh leaves to 500ml/ 1pt of boiling water.

root/rhizome:

decoction – 25g/1oz to 750ml/1½pt of water;

tincture – up to 3ml/60 drops three times daily.

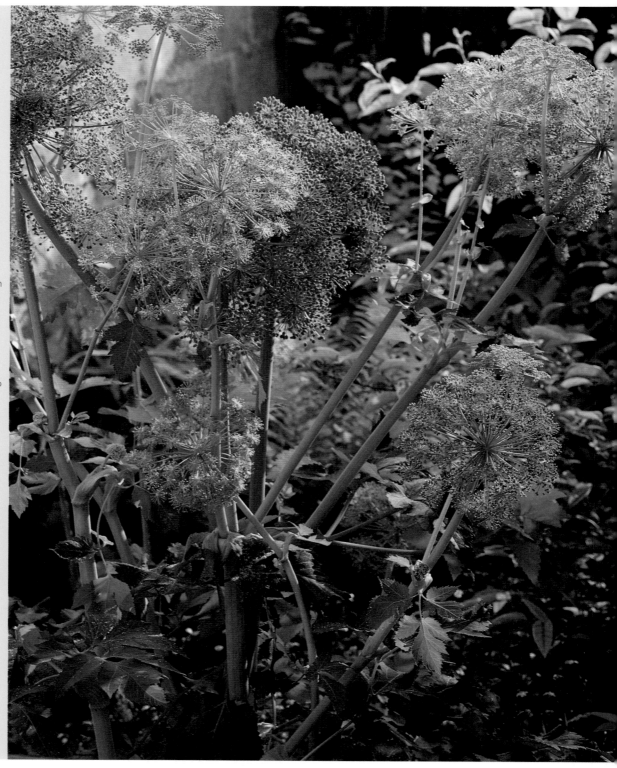

angelica
Angelica archangelica

European angelica is a stately biennial plant that needs plenty of space in the garden and will over-enthusiastically self-seed in fertile soil. The herb is widely used as a flavouring and is responsible for the distinctive taste of the liqueur Benedictine and is also used in making Chartreuse and vermouth. It is a sweet, pungent, warming plant which is familiar in candied form as a green cake decoration.

The plant is believed to take its English name from the fact that it blooms in early May around the feast of St Michael the Archangel (May 8 in the old calender) and was regarded in the middle ages as offering powerful protection against witchcraft and evil spirits. By the 15th century the plant was believed to help combat the plague and it was listed by John Parkinson in 1629 as possibly the most important herb in the repertoire.

using angelica
Angelica will dispel intestinal gas and ease abdominal cramps so makes a helpful digestive remedy for indigestion and stomach upsets; it also helps to stimulate the appetite. Angelica encourages perspiration and urination so tends to be added to cleansing remedies where the aim is to clear toxins from the system; as such, it is useful for both skin and arthritic complaints.

Angelica can be added to mixtures for colds and chills and helps encourage the coughing response so is also used for bronchitis and other respiratory problems. The plant is a uterine stimulant and was used in the past in prolonged labour, it can also be helpful for some menstrual problems.

cautions large doses should be avoided in pregnancy and if taken in excess it may damage the central nervous system. The plant is rich in chemicals called furanocoumarins which can increase the photosensitivity of the skin leading to rashes or inflammation when the skin is exposed to sunlight.

borage *Borago officinalis*

The old country saying "borage for courage" is a rather apt description of the plant since we now know that it will stimulate production of the hormone adrenaline – the "flight or fight" hormone which we produce in moments of stress. Borage has also long been regarded as uplifting for the emotions. It has been identified with the Roman *euphrosynum*, "the plant that cheers", which Pliny tells us was once added to wine to "increase the exhilarating effect", while Elizabethan cooks added blue borage flowers to

◄ Angelica *Angelica archangelica*
➤ Borage *Borago officinalis*

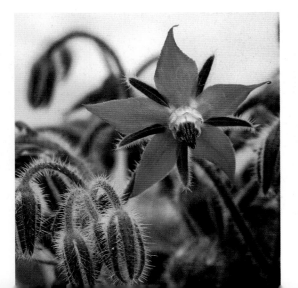

borage
parts used
leaves, seed oil

commercial products
the seed oil is generally marketed as "starflower oil" widely available in capsules, singly or in combination with evening primrose oil; bottled leaf juice is sold by health food shops and the tincture is available from specialist herbal suppliers.

how to use
leaf infusion – 25g/1oz to 500ml/1pt of boiling water taken in three doses daily;
tincture – up to 5ml/1tsp three times daily;
juice – 10ml/2tsp, three times daily;
seed oil capsules – typically 500mg daily.

part used
flowers

commercial products
mainly used in creams, ointments and massage mixtures; both tincture and dried petals are readily available from specialist herbal suppliers.

how to use
infusion – 25g/1oz of dried petals to 500ml/ 1pt of boiling water, taken in three doses daily;
tincture – up to 5ml/1tsp, three times daily (note: commercial marigold tincture is often supplied in 95% alcohol so needs to be well diluted with water);
creams, ointments or infused oil – external use only, apply as required.

salads to "make the mind glad": borage flowers are still traditionally added to summer drinks such as Pimms. The herb is also soothing for irritant tissues, mildly sedative and anti-depressant.

In recent years borage has come to the fore as a rich source of *gamma*-linolenic acid (GLA) an essential fatty acid which is found in the pressed seed oil. Like evening primrose oil (see page 153), borage has thus become a favourite with the health food industry. GLA is needed by the body for a number of metabolic processes and lack of it can be associated with menstrual irregularities, skin problems, irritable bowel syndrome and rheumatoid arthritis.

using borage

Borage oil is often sold as "starflower oil" – this is not a traditional name, but one which probably appeals to the marketeers. It contains substantially more GLA than evening primrose oil, with around 24% (compared with a figure of 9% generally quoted for evening primrose). However, traces of toxic erucic acid (which is known to damage heart tissue) are sometimes found in the oil, leading to claims that evening primrose oil is more efficacious.

Borage is also related to comfrey and traces of chemicals called pyrrolizidine alkaloids – which can cause liver damage in large quantities – have been found in its leaves. It has therefore been banned in some countries, although most herbalists regard it as perfectly safe for regular use. The leaves can be used in teas for stress or to counter the lingering effects of steroid therapy and they can also be added to cough mixtures to help clear phlegm. The juice can be used internally as a natural anti-depressant to improve well-being while externally it makes a

soothing lotion for irritant skin rashes and inflammations.

marigold
Calendula officinalis

Traditional English pot marigolds have been among the herbalist's favourites for centuries. In the 12th century simply looking at the plant's golden colour was supposed to lift the spirits and encourage cheerfulness – or as *Macer's Herbal* has it to "drawyth owt of ye heed wikked

▼ Marigold *Calendula officinalis*

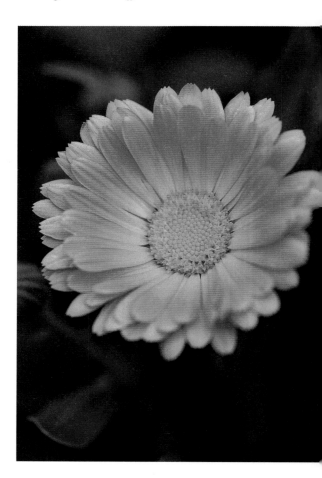

hirores [humours]". By Culpeper's day in the 17th century, marigold was recommended to "strengthen the heart" and was highly regarded as a remedy for smallpox and measles.

using marigold

Marigold is a potent antiseptic which will combat a wide range of bacterial and fungal infections. It will also reduce inflammation and is very widely available – often sold under its botanical name *Calendula* – in creams and ointments for cuts, grazes, fungal infections (including athlete's foot and vaginal thrush) and also for minor burns and skin disorders including dry eczema. Internally it is a useful bitter to stimulate bile production and improve the digestion. It will relieve spasmodic pains and is a good menstrual regulator so is suitable for a number of gynaecological problems, including irregular or painful menstruation. It can also be used for gastric and gall bladder inflammations.

In addition, marigold makes a useful cleansing remedy for swollen or inflamed lymph nodes as in conditions such as glandular fever: lymph nodes are part of the lymphatic system, which transports various fluids around the body, and also form part of the immune system.

Home-made infused marigold oil (see page 224) is a good alternative to proprietary ointments and can also be used as a lotion base – a few drops of tea tree, for example, can be added to make a strongly anti-fungal lotion for athlete's foot. The infused oil can be used to moisturise dry skin, added to bath water to ease eczema, or used as an antiseptic lotion for minor cuts and grazes. Marigold oil or cream is also helpful for soothing sore nipples in breast-feeding – an old-fashioned remedy which some maternity wards have now revived.

cinnamon
Cinnamomum zeylanicum

Cinnamon is widely used as a flavouring in cooking and perfumery, but also has a long tradition as a medicinal plant. A related species, *C. cassia,* has been used in China since at least 2700 BC and it is also listed in Egyptian papyri of 1500 BC as an external remedy for skin disorders and ulcers. The plant is regarded as warming so can be helpful for all sorts of "cold" conditions including chills and rheumatic pains. It also has a stimulating tonic effect and can help to ease spasmodic or cramping pains.

The herb is very warming for the digestive system as well as helping to reduce flatulence. It has been used for centuries to treat nausea and vomiting and is also good for many digestive problems, including diarrhoea and gastroenteritis.

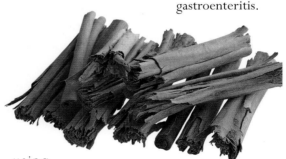

using cinnamon

The Chinese use different parts of the cinnamon plant in two quite different ways: the twigs are seen as warming for the peripheries and used internally to encourage circulation to cold hands and feet. The inner bark is more centrally warming and used to treat cold problems associated with low energy, such as debility, rheumatic problems and kidney weakness.

The plant also shows some anti-fungal activity and is sometimes added to remedies for

cinnamon

parts used
inner bark, twigs, essential oil

commercial products
cinnamon is readily available from supermarkets while Chinese cinnamon (*C. cassia*) is usually sold by specialist herbal suppliers; cinnamon oil is available from aromatherapy suppliers; tincture is sold by specialist suppliers. Cinnamon is included in numerous proprietary remedies for coughs and digestive upsets.

how to use
infusions – add a pinch of powdered cinnamon to other herbal mixtures for colds, aches or stomach upsets; use one small cinnamon stick and a slice of fresh ginger in decoctions for chills; *tincture* – ½-1ml/10-20 drops, up to three times daily.

parts used
leaves, seed, oil

commercial products
included in some proprietary cough mixtures; the essential oil is available from specialist herbal suppliers.

how to use
seeds - decoction, 25g/1oz of dried ripe seeds to 750ml/1½pt of water simmered and taken in three doses; *leaves* - are best eaten fresh or juiced and taken internally (5ml/1tsp, three times a day) or used as a lotion for rashes.

candidiasis; the oil is used to combat infections in aromatherapy. In the home a pinch of cinnamon added to teas for colds, aches or stomach upsets is soothing and warmin. For chills it can be combined in a tea with ginger.

caution high doses of cinnamon should be avoided in pregnancy.

coriander
Coriandrum sativum

Best known from its use in Indian and Middle Eastern cookery, coriander has become a familiar culinary herb over the past few years with a characteristic earthy flavour. Both seeds and leaves can be used in cooking although the seeds are preferred in herbal medicine. Like other traditional aromatic culinary herbs, coriander helps to ease flatulence and indigestion and is sometimes added to laxative mixtures to ease griping pains. The seeds encourage coughing to clear phlegm and make a pleasant tasting addition to cough syrups.

The plant is known as *dhanyaka* in India and is used in Ayurveda for easing heat problems and inflammations especially those associated with the digestive and urinary systems.

using coriander
Recent Japanese research suggests that coriander leaves can accelerate the excretion of toxic metals such as mercury, lead and aluminium from the body. Unless they are trapped and removed by chemicals known as "chelating agents" these heavy metals remain in the body forever with high levels now blamed for certain arthritic condition, depression,

memory loss, muscle pain and weakness. Eating plenty of coriander is thus an inexpensive and easy way to remove (or "chelate") toxic metals from the nervous system and body tissue. Coriander can be especially helpful for anyone suffering from the ill effects of mercury amalgam dental fillings.

The leaves of the coriander plant are fine and feathery and almost disappear once the flowers arrive, but a leafy cultivar (cilantro) is now more readily available and is well worth growing in the herb garden.

The juiced plant is traditionally used in the East as a remedy for allergic problems such as hay fever and skin rashes and it can also be used externally as a lotion for irritant or inflamed skin. Coriander oil, distilled from the seeds, is used in aromatherapy as an analgesic for nerve and muscle pains and to ease digestive upsets.

turmeric *Curcuma longa*

Known as *haridra* in Sanskrit, *haldi* in Hindi and *Jiang Huang* in China, turmeric is one of the more familiar Eastern spices used in flavouring and colouring curries and sauces. Traditionally, it is used in Ayurveda as a digestive, circulatory and respiratory stimulant. It is also used to help cleanse the *chakras,* the seven points regarded in Eastern philosophy as the body's energy centres and running from the crown of the head to the base of the spine.

Turmeric is taken in India as a digestive stimulant and to combat infections as in gastroenteritis and food poisoning. Externally it was used with honey for sprains, bruises and arthritic pains or taken as a milk decoction to cleanse and improve the skin. In Indian folk medicine turmeric is also used to treat parasitic skin problems and poor eyesight, to encourage milk flow in breast-feeding and to ease rheumatic pains. The flowers are used in parts of the country for sore throats and indigestion. In traditional Chinese medicine the herb is mainly used as a blood and energy stimulant and is also regarded as analgesic. It is often used to treat abdominal and chest pain as well as frozen shoulder and a range of menstrual problems.

using turmeric

Modern research has shown turmeric to help combat the natural oxidation of tissues and stimulate bile production; it thins the blood and lowers cholesterol levels in cardiovascular disease and some anti-cancer activity has also been reported.

More importantly, turmeric is now recognised as an effective anti-inflammatory for arthritic conditions. Clinical trials using turmeric extracts for arthritis suggest that the plant is possibly more effective than many orthodox drugs and without the side-effects. Externally, turmeric has shown a "cortisone-like" action so may be worth considering in lotions for conditions such as tennis elbow and other localised joint inflammations. When using turmeric for arthritis it needs to be combined with a painkiller, such as meadow-sweet (page 182) as it has no analgesic properties.

caution turmeric can cause skin rashes in sensitive individuals and may increase sensitivity to sunlight.

cardamom
Elettaria cardamomum

Several very similar botanical plants tend to be labelled as "cardamom": among the most common are what is known as "true" cardamom (*Elettaria cardamomum*) and a bastard cardamom (*Amomum xanthioides*); all tend to be used almost interchangeably in Ayurvedic and Chinese medicine. Several other varieties are grown in different parts of India and commercial suppliers can include a range of these plants.

In Ayurveda, cardamom – known as *ela* – is mainly used for treating digestive upsets helping to stimulate digestive function and clear damp and phlegm (*kapha*) from the system. It is also believed in the East to stimulate the mind and bring clarity and joy. In China bastard cardamom or *Sha Ren* is sometimes used as a substitute for true cardamom in cooking and has been used in Chinese medicine since at least the 14th century. It, too, is mainly used for digestive problems and is also taken in pregnancy for both morning sickness and threatened miscarriage.

Cardamom, a native of Southern India, has been known in the West since ancient times and the *amomi vera* referred to by Pliny were probably round cardamom (*Amomum cardamomum*): he suggested using them – along with "henbane and axle-grease" – as a remedy for joint pains.

cardamom

parts used
seed, essential oil

commercial products
included in several proprietary herbal digestive remedies; essential oil is available from specialist suppliers.

how to use
decoction – 25g/1oz of seeds to 750ml/1½pt of water, simmered and taken in three equal doses.

turmeric

part used
rhizome

commercial products
included in several over-the-counter products for digestive problems and also in external massage rubs for aches and pains; powdered turmeric is available from supermarkets and Oriental grocers.

how to use
the powder can be used to fill capsules, mixed with ghee (clarified butter) or taken in milk decoction with a typical daily dose of 250-1000mg.

fennel

parts used

seeds, stem base as a
vegetable, essential oil

commercial products

included in numerous
over-the-counter herbal
digestion remedies and
laxatives; occasionally
found in external rubs for
aches and pains; bottled
juice from the stems and
essential oil are available
from health food shops.

how to use

infusion – 25g/1oz of
seeds to 500ml/1pt of
boiling water taken in
three equal doses;
juice – 10ml/2tsp, three
times daily.

liquorice

part used

root

commercial products

included in numerous
proprietary mixtures used
for digestive problems or
coughs; capsules and
tincture available from
health food shops.

how to use

tincture – up to 3ml/60
drops three times daily;
capsules – up to 600mg
daily;
decoctions – 25g/1oz to
750ml/ 1½pt water,
taken in three equal
doses.

using cardamom

Today, cardamom seeds are used much like dill and fennel seeds to clear flatulence and ease indigestion; they can be added to laxative mixtures to prevent abdominal griping pains, and will also ease feelings of nausea. The plant encourages both sweating and the coughing response so is also useful for treating colds and catarrh. The essential oil is used in aromatherapy as a nervous stimulant and to ease a range of minor digestive problems.

fennel *Foeniculum officinalis*

Fennel has been cultivated since Roman times – grown for its thick bulbous stems which are used as a vegetable, while the feathery leaves are used in flavouring and the seeds in medicine. The Greeks called the plant *marathron,* which is reputedly derived from a verb meaning "to grow thin" and it seems to have been considered as an early slimming aid. The Roman physician Galen classified it as hot and dry, while later authors recommended it to counterbalance the cool, dampness of fish, as Culpeper recorded in 1653.

Fennel was also associated with fortune telling and was used to decorate houses at midsummer to keep evil spirits at bay. The seeds were traditionally chewed as an appetite suppressant and were a mediaeval favourite on fast days.

using fennel

Today fennel is often used for indigestion, wind or colic and is added to laxative mixtures to ease the griping pains that strong purgatives can cause. Fennel tea bags are readily available and make a good after-dinner drink to ease the digestion. Fennel is also a good mouthwash for gum disease and sore throats and is sometimes included in herbal toothpastes; it will also increase milk flow in nursing mothers. The juice is recommended for nervous stomach upsets, abdominal cramps and chesty colds and has a pleasant aniseed-like taste that is popular with children.

The essential oil is sold commercially and can be added to external rubs for bronchial congestion and digestive disorders; beauticians add it to massage treatment for cellulite – the "orange peel skin" associated with excess fatty tissue.

cautions fennel should be avoided by epileptics and should not be given to very young children. High doses should be avoided in pregnancy.

liquorice *Glycyrrhiza glabra*

Liquorice is one of our most widely researched and respected medicinal herbs: it has been used since at least 500 BC and drugs based on liquorice extracts are still listed in official pharmacopoeia as remedies for gastric ulcers and inflammation.

The Greeks called liquorice "Sythian root" and used it for asthma and coughs, while in traditional Chinese herbalism it is called the "great detoxifier" or "great harmoniser" and is believed to drive toxins from the system and to eliminate harmful side-effects of other herbs.

The variety of liquorice used in Western herbal traditions is *G. glabra:* it originates in the Mediterranean region and Middle East and has

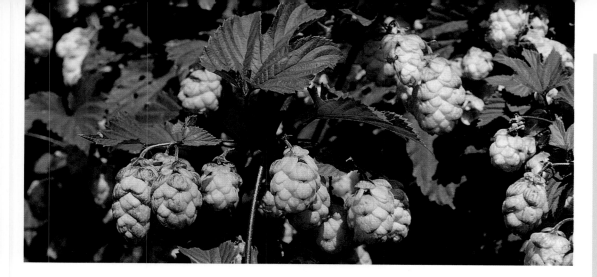

▲ Hops *Humulus lupulus*

been cultivated in Europe since at least the 16th century. The Chinese use an Asian species, *G. uralensis (Gan Cao),* which has similar actions. It is regarded as one of the most important of Chinese tonics – often called "the grandfather of herbs" – and pieces of Chinese liquorice root are often given to children to chew in order to promote muscle growth.

using liquorice

Liquorice has a hormonal effect, stimulating the adrenal cortex due to the presence of glycyrrhizin, which is some 50 times sweeter than sucrose, and encourages production of such hormones as hydro-cortisone.

The plant is very soothing and demulcent, making it ideal for gastric ulceration. It is also a digestive stimulant and laxative and is often used for constipation.

cautions excessive liquorice can cause fluid retention and increase blood pressure and it should be avoided in cases of high blood pressure. It should not be taken by those on digoxin-based drugs. Avoid high doses in pregnancy.

hops *Humulus lupulus*

Although we associate hops with traditional English beer, the plant is a comparative newcomer, introduced from Germany in the 16th century. Enthusing about the hop's many virtues, John Gerard, writing in 1597, urges that "beer" be considered a "phisicall drink to keep the body in health [rather] than an ordinary drinke for the quenching of our thirst", while a few years earlier in 1562 William Turner in his *New Herball* was amazed that, given the herb's numerous properties, physicians did not "use it more in medicine".

using hops

Just as in brewing, the female flowers or strobiles are used medicinally. The plant is strongly sedating, so should be avoided by those liable to nervous depression, although it does have a restoring effect on the nervous system and can be helpful for stress, irritability and anxiety as well as insomnia. It is often used in hop pillows but the strobiles oxidise rapidly, so properties can vary markedly on drying and after storing for any time. The fresher the herb the better it is for insomnia — the hops in

hops

part used
strobiles (flowers from female plants)

commercial products
hops are often sold in pillows to encourage restful sleep; included in many proprietary remedies mainly for nervous tension, anxiety or insomnia; capsules (150mg) and tinctures are available from specialist suppliers.

how to use
tincture - up to 2ml/40 drops, three times a day; *infusion* - 15g/½oz to 500ml/1pt of boiling water taken in three equal doses.

pillows need to be changed every few months to ensure continuing activity – while dried hops tend to be more restorative and stimulating for the nervous system.

Although the research is inconclusive, hops are believed to contain chemicals which are very similar to the female sex hormone oestrogen. In the past, women hop pickers often experienced menstrual irregularities and early periods while working in the hop fields and breathing in the herb's potent aromatic oils. The same constituents may also contribute to the reduced male libido experienced by heavy beer drinkers, with an eventual increase in external female sexual characteristic.

Hops – like the beer they make – are bitter, so make an effective digestive stimulant; like beer, too, they also encourage urination.

caution hops should not be taken by those suffering from depression.

hyssop *Hyssopus officinalis*

The name "hyssop" is believed to derive from a Greek word, *azob,* meaning holy herb, but the famous purging hyssop of the Bible (Psalm 51, v. 7 – "purge me with hyssop and I shall be clean…") is thought unlikely to be the plant we know by that name and was more probably a Middle Eastern variety of marjoram.

using hyssop

Hyssop belongs to the mint family and like many in that group is a bitter digestive herb useful as a robust flavouring in meat stews and casseroles. It will clear flatulence and ease indigestion and is a mild painkiller. It is one of the more important of the 130 herbs used to flavour the liqueur Chartreuse. Today, hyssop is mainly used to encourage coughing and relieve spasmodic pains in a wide range of respiratory tract problems, including influenza, asthma and bronchitis; it is also helpful for clearing nasal catarrh and has some anti-viral properties, notably against *Herpes simplex* which is responsible for cold sores. It is also useful for encouraging perspiration in fevers. Hyssop tea, made from the aerial parts of the plant gathered just before flowering, can be helpful for colds and feverish chills, while a syrup is ideal for coughs.

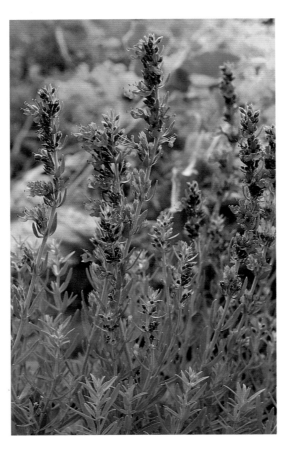

◄ Hyssop *Hyssopus officinalis*

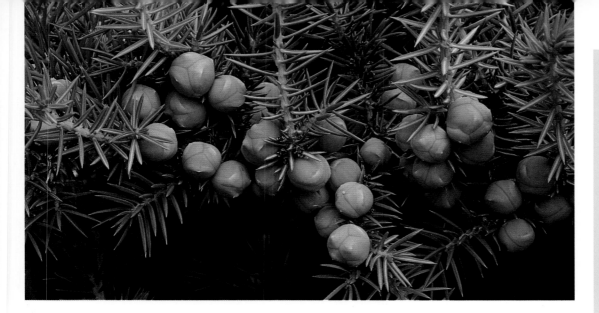

▲ Juniper *Juniperus communis*

The essential oil is available commercially – it is one of the scents used in eau de Cologne – and a few drops can be added to chest rubs for bronchitis and asthma or used as a mild sedative in relaxing baths.

juniper *Juniperus communis*

Juniper berries are a favourite for flavouring game dishes and are often included in marinades for venison or hare. Traditionally the herb has been associated with sacred cleansing rituals and its sprigs are still regularly burned each day in Tibetan temples as part of the morning purification rite.

The Egyptians used the berries in mummification and well into the fifth century AD bodies were covered in juniper berries and salt before burial. Several medicinal recipes also survive in Egyptian papyri dating to 1550 BC. A type of juniper (*J. phoenica*) was grown in Egypt and tomb paintings showing the berries being picked and processed survive in the Saqqara tombs built around 2300 BC.

using juniper

Juniper berries are widely used for urinary tract problems, such as cystitis, and as a cleansing remedy for rheumatism. The essential oil, collected by steam-distilling the berries, is used in aromatherapy both for urinary problems and as a stimulating tonic massage. The same oil is added as a flavouring to London gin – hence the diuretic action of that particular beverage. Another type of essential oil made from juniper is cade oil, produced by dry-distilling the heartwood of various juniper species and used for psoriasis and other skin problems. It contains phenol and is mildly disinfectant.

cautions prolonged use of juniper can irritate the kidneys and any preparation containing the herb should not be taken for longer than six weeks without professional advice. It should not be taken internally by those suffering from kidney disease and must be avoided in pregnancy.

juniper

part used
berries

commercial products
included in numerous over-the-counter herbal remedies mainly for fluid retention and urinary problems and in external ointments and rubs for rheumatic aches and pains; the essential oil tinctures are available from specialist suppliers and the berries are sold as a culinary herb.

how to use
tincture – up to 2ml/40 drops three times daily; *decoction* – 20g/¾oz of dried berries to 750ml/1½pt of water, simmered and taken in three equal doses daily.

lavender
Lavandula angustifolia

The name lavender comes from the Latin *lavare*, to wash, and the herb has been used to scent baths and toiletries since Roman times. Lavender is useful for digestive upsets, nervous tension, insomnia, migraines and headaches. It is a mild painkiller, anti-depressant and will also relieve muscular spasms and cramps; the flowers can be made into a pleasant tasting tea taken at night for sleeplessness or during the day for headaches and nervous tension.

Dioscorides, writing in the second century AD, recommended lavender for "griefs in the thorax", although the plant used by the Greeks was probably *L. stoechas,* generally known today as French lavender and rather less hardy than the familiar English variety. In Arabic medicine this tradition of using lavender for chest problems has continued and it is still used in the Middle East as a cough remedy. Herbalists usually describe lavender as "cooling", suggesting that it is best suited to ease those sorts of headaches that are soothed by cold packs rather than the sort of pain that is comforted by a warm compress.

using lavender
The essential oil is steam-distilled from the flowers and is used in aromatherapy for muscular aches, pains and headaches. A few drops of lavender oil can also be added to creams for eczema or diluted in water to make a soothing lotion for sunburn and minor scalds. Added to bath water, lavender oil is relaxing and soothing for nervous tensions and insomnia; in massage oils it can be helpful for muscular aches and pains, strains and some rheumatic problems.

Lavender is also surprisingly good in cooking – try French lavender sprigs instead of rosemary for roast lamb.

caution avoid high doses in pregnancy.

chamomile *Matricaria recutita / Chamaemelum nobile*

Both German chamomile *(M. recutita)* and its relative Roman chamomile *(C. nobile)* are among the most widely used of medicinal herbs. Their actions are very similar, with Roman chamomile having a slightly more bitter taste and German chamomile being slightly more anti-inflammatory and analgesic. While herbalists may have their individual favourites, the plants are extremely close in action and can be regarded as interchangeable in lay use.

The Greeks knew the herb as "ground apple" (*kamai melon*) – so called because of its characteristic smell – and it is still used for ornamental lawns, giving a hint of apples when walked on. Special non-flowering cultivars have been developed for lawns, but these are useless if you want to use the herb medicinally since it is only the flowers that are of value. To the Anglo-Saxons chamomile was *maythen*, one of the nine sacred herbs given to mankind by Woden and listed in the ninth-century poem the *Lacnunga.*

using chamomile
Both chamomiles are used for nervous stomach upsets, nausea, insomnia, and externally in creams for eczema, wounds, nappy rash, sore

➤ German chamomile *Matricaria recutita*

nipples and piles. The flowers are readily available in tea bags or sold loose for infusions and, although the flavour can be something of an acquired taste, chamomile tea is probably one of the most popular herbal drinks on the market.

Chamomile is also used in homoeopathy and Chamomilla 3X is a valuable standby for babies, used to treat both colic and teething. It is one of the safest herbs for children and babies and some mothers use weak infusions as a night-time drink to encourage restful sleep. The infusion can also be added to bath water to soothe over-excited infants.

Chamomile yields a deep blue essential oil on steam distillation which is very relaxing and useful in skin care. This is used for a range of digestive disorders, inflammations, emotional problems and muscle pains. It is extremely expensive but usually 2-3 drops are sufficient.

The botanists have renamed chamomile repeatedly over the years – Roman chamomile may still be found labelled as *Anthemis nobile*, while German chamomile is often called either *Chamomilla recutita* or *Matricaria chamomilla*.

caution avoid excessive use of chamomile oil in pregnancy.

lemon balm
Melissa officinalis

Lemon balm's botanical name, *Melissa,* comes from the Greek word *mel,* meaning honey, and the herb has a long association with bees and the healing power of their products. It is said to be such a favourite with bees that if hives are rubbed with its leaves the insects will never swarm and always return. Lemon balm was regarded by the Greeks as a cure-all and the herb has been considered over the centuries as being as valuable as honey for treating wounds and equal in tonic effect to royal jelly.

John Gerard declared that it "comforteth the hart and driveth away all melancholie and sadnesse", while it was praised by the German herbalist Paracelsus as an "elixir of youth" which he made into a preparation called *primum ens melissae.* As late as the 18th century lemon balm was still being recommended in "canary wine" to "renew youth".

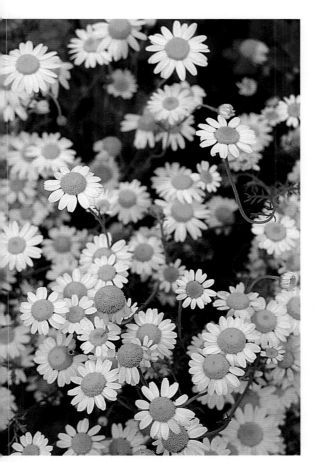

➤➤ Overleaf: Lavender *Lavandula angustifolia*

parts used
flowers, essential oil

commercial products
included in many proprietary mixtures sold as calming remedies for anxiety or insomnia and also digestive remedies; used in several external creams for skin problems; capsules (520mg), juice, tinctures and the essential oil are available from health food shops. Also used in homoeopathic preparations (Chamomilla) for children.

how to use
infusion – 25g/1oz of dried flowers to 500ml/1pt of boiling water taken in three equal daily doses; *tincture* – up to 5ml/1tsp, three times daily; *essential oil* – 2-3 drops to 10ml/2tsp of almond oil used in massage rubs.

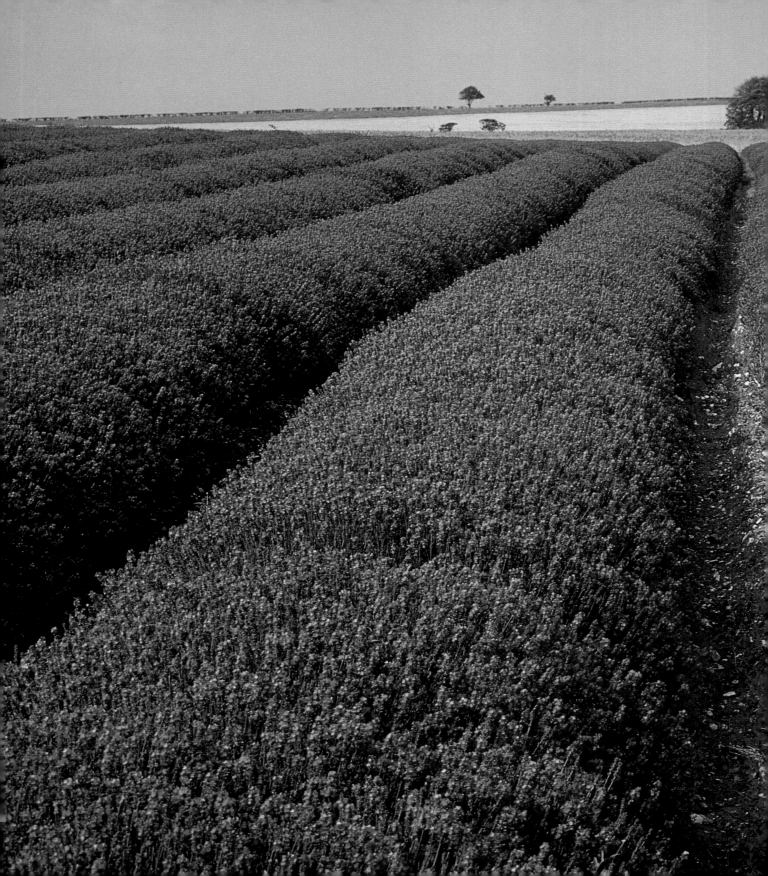

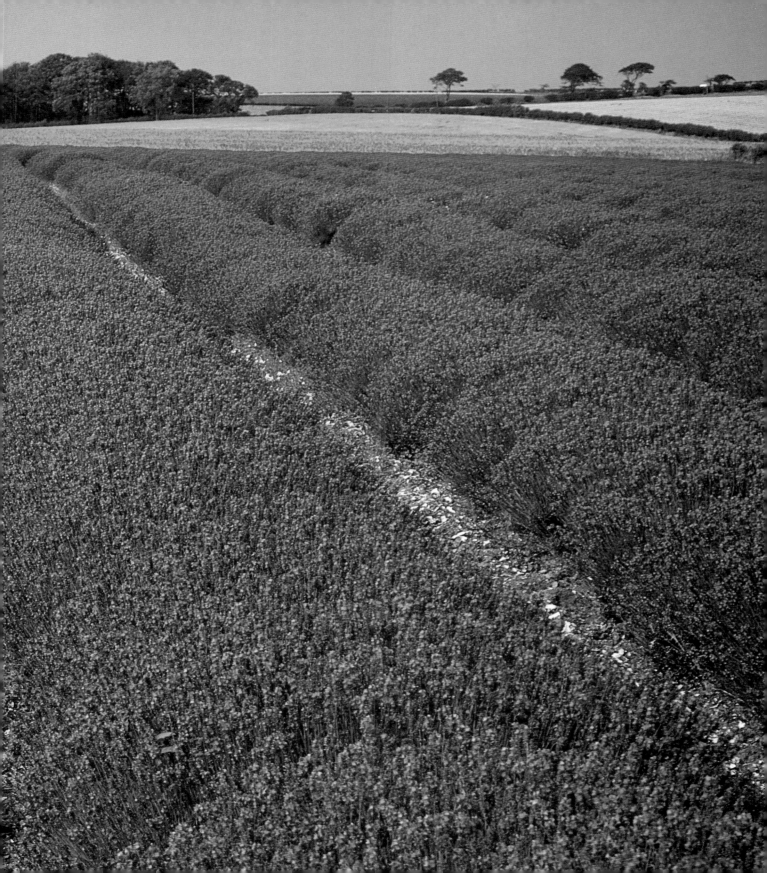

part used

leaves

commercial products

extensively used in over-the-counter herbal remedies often in very small quantities as a flavouring; included in a number of proprietary remedies for digestive problems, coughs and sore throats; capsules of both peppermint oil and powdered herb are made; tinctures and essential oil are available from specialist suppliers while "peppermint emulsion", a mixture of the oil and water, is sold by chemists.

how to use

tincture – up to 3ml/60 drops, three times a day; *infusion* – up to 20g/¾oz of dried herb to 500ml/1pt of boiling water taken in three equal doses; *capsules* – one oil (50mg) or dried leaf (250mg) taken three times a day.

using lemon balm

Today we regard the plant more prosaically as a digestive remedy and sedative; it is a gentle herb for treating nervous tummy upsets in children but is also potent enough to help with depression and anxiety and to relieve tension headaches. It has been used successfully for severe conditions like post-natal depression. Lemon balm is also cooling and will encourage sweating so is useful to reduce body temperature in fevers. Modern research has shown it to be extremely effective against several bacteria and also the *Herpes simplex* virus which is responsible for cold sores. It can also be helpful for other viral infections including mumps and shingles.

Tea made from a handful of fresh leaves makes a refreshing and restorative drink at the end of the day, although it needs to be dried with care to avoid losing too much of the characteristic lemon flavour. Externally, lemon balm creams can be used on insect bites, sores and slow-healing wounds. The essential oil is used in aromatherapy for nervous problems but is also valuable, well-diluted in sprays, for keeping insects away.

peppermint
Mentha × piperita

There are thought to be around 30 different species of mint – but as the plants readily cross-pollinate and hybridise no one is really certain. As the monk Wilafrid Strabo put it in about 875 AD "…if a man can name the full list of all the kinds and all the properties of mint, he must know how many fish swim in the Indian Ocean".

Peppermint is the variety most widely used in herbal medicine, and is believed to be a cross between spearmint (*M. spicata*) and water mint (*M. aquatica*): it has a high menthol content – hence the characteristic smell. Until the 17th century there was little differentiation between the species – peppermint would just as often have been used in "mint sauce" as the apple mint (*M. suaveolens*) we favour today. Spearmint, also

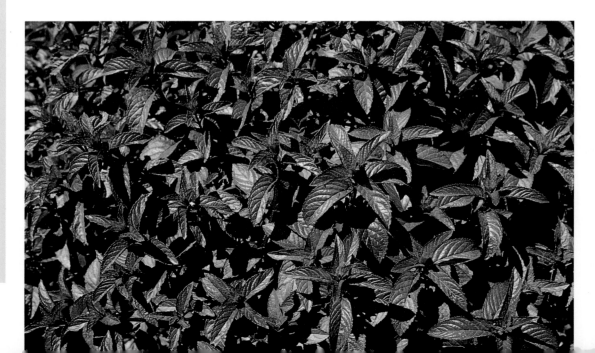

known as common mint or garden mint, is the variety most often grown in gardens and makes an adequate substitute for peppermint used medicinally. It does not have the high menthol content of peppermint, so is far less irritant and is more suitable for children.

using peppermint

In general all the mints will ease flatulence and indigestion, relieve spasmodic pains, encourage sweating and clear nasal catarrh. Peppermint oil is also antiseptic and mildly anaesthetic. Mints stimulate the digestion and are warming and decongestant in colds and catarrh. Peppermint, taken in tea, tincture or tablet form, can help to relieve nausea (including morning sickness), while the oil is used in stimulating rubs to soothe rheumatism and bronchial congestion. A cup of peppermint or spearmint tea after meals is an ideal way to avoid indigestion and abdominal discomfort after eating.

cautions peppermint should not be given to babies or toddlers in any form: excess of the oil can irritate the stomach lining and misuse may lead to ulceration. The herb may cause an allergic reaction. Avoid peppermint oil in pregnancy.

nutmeg *Myristica fragrans*

Nutmegs were first brought to Europe from the East Indies by Arab traders in the 11th century, although the tree was not successfully grown in the West until the 1770s. The nutmeg is the seed of the tree, while mace — also a culinary herb — is the aril.

◄ Peppermint *Mentha* x *piperita*

The herb has a long history as a seasoning, but is quite a potent plant, causing sleepiness and hallucinations in excess. Cases of delirium as a result of over-consumption were reported as early as 1576. The over-indulgence no doubt owed something to nutmeg's erroneous reputation as an inducer of abortion, although 18th-century herbals report cases of drowsiness and delirium after dosages of only around 2 drachms (7g/¼oz).

using nutmeg

The herb is included in digestive remedies for nausea, abdominal bloating, indigestion and colic. Nutmeg kernels have also been used to counter diarrhoea and dysentery and were once regularly chewed by sailors heading north as a stimulant to combat colds and seasickness. The essential oil is used externally to relieve muscular aches and pains and is also traditionally used in many parts of the East as an abdominal massage to relieve pain, including period pain.

A little fresh nutmeg grated over banana, milk puddings or cereal can counter nausea and vomiting and also act as a sedative. Nutmeg can also relieve headaches and relax neck muscles stiffened by tension — a home-made tincture can be especially effective taken in drop doses.

cautions excessive use will cause headaches, dizziness and delirium. Avoid in pregnancy.

nutmeg

parts used
seed kernel, aril (outer seed casing)

commercial products
included in a few over-the-counter remedies for rheumatic pains and coughs and also added to external rubs for muscular aches and pains; the essential oil is available from specialist suppliers.

how to use
buy whole nutmeg and grate a pinch as required to add to infusions for colds, digestive upsets, nausea and poor appetite. Daily dose should not exceed 1g; *tincture* – take in drop doses for nausea and muscular tension.

basil *Ocimum basilicum*

Familiar in Europe as a culinary herb *(O. basilicum)* its close relative holy basil *(O. sanctum)* is regarded in India as a potent tonic – sacred to the deities Vishnu and Krishna, capable of "opening the heart and mind", and second only to the lotus in a hierarchy of sacred plants. In Ayurveda it is believed to bestow love and devotion and is also used in chills to clear excess phlegm and catarrh (associated with the *kapha* humour) from the nasal passages and lungs.

Although basil originates in India, the plant has been known in Europe since ancient times, even so views and traditions associated with it have been mixed: the Greek physician Dioscorides said that it should never be taken internally, while the Roman Pliny recommended it for fainting, headaches, indigestion and other digestive upsets and catarrh, adding that as an aphrodisiac it was especially good for horses "at the time of service". He also reported that many still believed that basil pounded in a mortar and left would "breed a scorpion" if left covered by a stone or "breed worms" if left in the sun. The Greeks and Romans also believed that the more you abused or scorned it the better it grew so planting the seeds was always accompanied with plenty of invective, while in parts of the Middle East it is still planted on graves in loving remembrance.

using basil

Today, basil is generally recommended in the West for digestive upsets and to clear intestinal parasites although it is also important to remember its Eastern attributes and keep a basil plant in the house for its purifying and protective influence. In India basil is made into a tea with honey to promote clarity of mind while the stems are made into rosaries and worn to encourage clarity and compassion. The essential oil is popular in aromatherapy and can be used as a nerve tonic, anti-depressant and digestive remedy or be added to chest rubs for coughs and congestion. The fresh leaves can be useful topically for clear fungal infections on the skin.

caution avoid basil oil in pregnancy.

marjoram
Origanum majorana

Both popular culinary flavourings, marjoram *(O. majorana)* and oregano *(O. vulgare)* are very

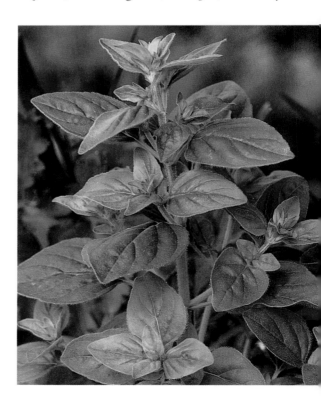

closely related with numerous cultivars largely grown for subtle variations in their flavour. The plants originated in the Mediterranean and the botanical name is derived from two Greek words, *oras* meaning mountain and *ganos* meaning joy; so "oregano" means "joy of the mountain" – reflecting the herb's lush growth in rural Greece and the flavour it gives to sheep and goats grazing on the hills.

using marjoram

Medicinally marjoram and oregano are also used in very similar ways: taken internally for colds and minor digestive upsets as well as to ease respiratory spasms in asthma and persistent coughs. In folk tradition marjoram leaves (preferably secured in a muslin bag) were added to baths to ease aching limbs and the oil can be used in various combinations for muscular aches and pains. Marjoram oil is also used in aromatherapy to ease digestive spasms and period pains.

Like other members of the mint family (notably thyme, sage and rosemary) with a reputation for encouraging longevity, marjoram has been investigated over the past few years for its anti-oxidant properties. Researchers suggest that it can prevent premature ageing of cells so could have a role in geriatric medicine and could be used to combat "free radicals" – chemical groups produced as byproducts of various metabolic processes which can oxidise and damage healthy cells.

caution avoid high doses of both marjoram and oregano in pregnancy.

parsley *Petroselinum crispum*

Parsley seeds reputedly had to visit the devil 13 times before germination, but if they were planted on Good Friday they were excused this chore and so would germinate much more quickly. The plant's development can certainly prove erratic when grown from seed and it is best to plant the seeds where they will grow permanently (they do not transplant well) and water them initially with boiling water.

Like nettles, parsley tends to "rob the soil", concentrating many minerals and vitamins in its leaves – it is rich in iron, calcium, potassium and magnesium, among others – so makes an excellent food for those suffering from anaemia and debility: one should always eat the parsley

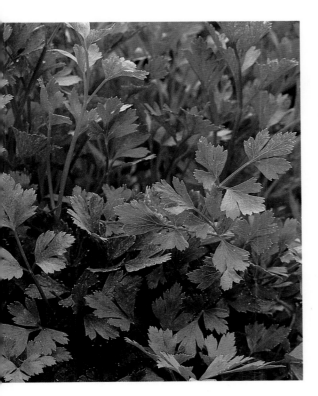

◄◄ Basil *Ocimum basilicum*
◄ Parsley *Petroselinum crispum*

parsley

parts used

leaves, roots, seed, oil

commercial products
often added to garlic remedies to reduce breath odour; included in over-the-counter remedies for fluid retention and urinary disorders; bottled juice is available from health food shops.

how to use

leaves are best eaten fresh but can be made into:
infusions – 25g/1oz of dried leaf to 500ml/1pt of boiling water taken in three equal doses;
juice – 1ml/20 drops, three times a day;
root tincture – up to 5ml/1tsp, three times a day.

seeds, essential oil

commercial products
added to numerous proprietary remedies for coughs, throat problems and digestive upsets; essential oil and tincture available from specialist suppliers.

how to use
decoction - 15g/½oz of seeds to 750ml/1½pt of water, simmered and taken in three equal doses during the day;
tincture - 2ml/40 drops up to three times a day.

pepper

parts used
fruits, essential oil

commercial products
the oil is included in a number of over-the-counter massage rubs and ointments mainly recommended for aches and pains; it is included in cosmetic preparations for cellulite (the orange-peel skin associated with underlying fatty tissues).

how to use
decoction - use 10 black peppercorns per cup of water, simmer and take three times a day;
oil - add 5 drops to 20ml/¾fl oz of infused chili oil as a warming rub for arthritic joints.

garnish rather than leaving such a nutritious plant on the plate! It makes a good nutritious tonic food in convalescence.

using parsley

Parsley leaf encourages urination and is often recommended for fluid retention associated with menstrual irregularities and also in cystitis. It is a useful digestive remedy for colic, flatulence and indigestion and mildly laxative. The plant is a uterine tonic, stimulates menstrual flow and can relieve cramping pains so can be helpful for premenstrual tension, period pains and during the menopause: the leaves were also traditionally made into a poultice and applied directly to the breasts to help dry up milk flow when breast-feeding.

Chewing parsley leaves can help clear the smell of onions and garlic from the breath and parsley is sometimes included in over-the-counter garlic capsules as a deodoriser.

The leaves are generally eaten fresh or can be used in teas, while the root (which can be eaten as a vegetable) and seeds are made commercially into tinctures. The seed oil is used in aromatherapy to encourage urination and to help eliminate fluid from the tissues.

caution avoid large quantities of leaves and both seed and oil in pregnancy or if suffering from kidney inflammation.

anise *Pimpinella anisum*

Anise seeds – or aniseed – has been used as a spice since Egyptian times and is still a popular flavouring for sweets and liqueurs such as the Turkish *raki*. The plant is very similar in many ways to its relatives dill and fennel, and like them is used mainly as a digestive remedy to clear flatulence and to encourage coughing and clear phlegm. The three plants can be fitted on to a simple scale – dill-fennel-anise – with dill the most effective for digestive problems and anise preferred for coughs while fennel is equally useful for both attributes.

using anise

Both aniseed and anise oil in massage rubs can be helpful for various chronic chest problems including bronchitis, whooping cough and asthma. The oil is also strongly antiseptic and has been used topically for lice and scabies (a parasitic skin infection). It is however, toxic in high doses, potentially addictive and one of the more damaging ingredients in traditional French *pastis* drinks.

Aniseed is traditionally used in many parts of Europe by nursing mothers to encourage milk flow and was taken during childbirth to speed delivery. It was also an ingredient in traditional female aphrodisiac brews and modern research indicates that it is mildly oestrogenic.

caution avoid high doses in pregnancy.

pepper *Piper nigrum*

Known as *Hu Jiao* in China and *marich* in Ayurvedic medicine, black peppercorns have been used in cooking and medicine since ancient times. Pliny (AD 79) makes numerous references to pepper which was added to a wide variety of remedies, although he is far from enthusiastic about the plant itself: "It is remarkable," he writes, "that the use of pepper has come so much in favour ...to think that its only pleasing quality is pungency and that we go all the way to India to get this!" The spice was, however, expensive and highly prized and even became a currency during the siege of Rome in AD 408: the traditional "peppercorn rent" did not mean, as we now understand it, a nominal trifle but was once a common way of paying quite sizable sums.

using pepper

Black, white and green peppercorns are all used in cooking and come from the same plant: black are the dried unripe berries, white the dried ripe berries and green the fresh unripe peppercorns. Pink peppercorns often sold among the culinary seasons are quite a different species (*Schinus terebinthifolius*); they have an entirely different flavour and no significant medicinal properties.

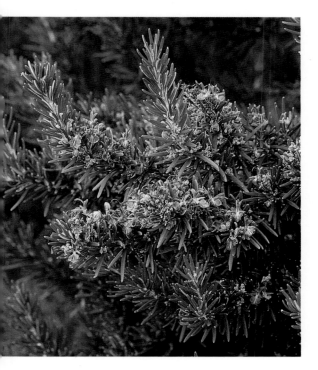

Pepper makes an effective warming stimulant remedy for the digestive tract. It is a warm, dry plant so, following Galenic theory, it was traditionally used in cooking to balance cold, damp vegetables such as beans, with their tendency to cause flatulence and stomach chills.

In Ayurvedic medicine pepper is used to energise digestive energy (*agni*) and clear toxins from the digestive tract. It is also mixed with *ghee* (clarified butter) for use topically on irritant skin rashes.

In China it is mainly used to warm the digestive system and combat nausea, vomiting and diarrhoea associated with cold and chills in the stomach. Pepper oil is used in aromatherapy massage for coughs, chills, digestive upsets, aches and pains.

caution pepper oil can be irritant in large quantities so needs to be used in moderation.

rosemary
Rosmarinus officinalis

Rosemary is traditionally associated with remembrance – sprigs were exchanged by lovers or scattered on coffins. It is an apt association as rosemary has a stimulating effect on the nervous system and a reputation for improving the memory. The plant originates from the Mediterranean area and was first grown in Britain in the 14th century. It was regarded as uplifting and energising – or as Gerard said, "It comforteth the harte and maketh it merie".

◄ Rosemary *Rosmarinus officinalis*

rosemary

parts used
leaves, essential oil

commercial products
included in several proprietary herbal anti-oxidant and tonic mixtures and massage rubs for muscular aches and pains; juice, tincture and essential oil are sold by health food shops.

how to use
infusion - 25g/1oz of fresh rosemary leaves to 500ml/1pt of boiling water, taken in three equal doses;
tincture - up to 4ml/80 drops, three times a day;
essential oil - ½ml/10 drops to 5ml/1tsp of almond oil as a massage for aches and pains.

parts used
leaves, fruits

commercial products
included in several
proprietary mixtures for
menstrual problems but
more commonly sold in
tablets or capsules as a
simple; tincture available
from specialist suppliers.

how to use
infusion - 25g/1oz of
dried herb to 500ml/1pt
of water taken in three
equal doses a day;
tincture - up to 5ml/1tsp,
three times a day.

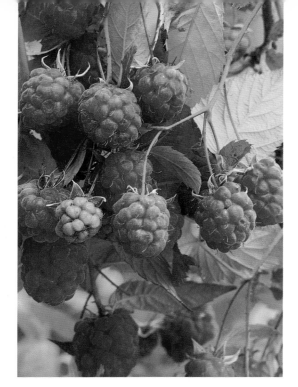

▲ Raspberry *Rubus idaeus*

using rosemary

As a nerve tonic it can be helpful for temporary fatigue and over-work: take rosemary tea to relieve headaches, migraines, mild depression and coldness associated with poor circulation. It is a pleasant-tasting drink and, since rosemary is an evergreen, one that can be made using fresh herb throughout the year. It also makes a good digestive remedy, helping to stimulate bile flow and improve function as well as clearing gas from the digestive tract. It will increase urination and has some antiseptic properties so makes a pleasant tasting addition to teas for ailments such as cystitis.

The essential oil made by steam-distilling the leaves is a valuable remedy for arthritis, rheumatism and muscular aches and pains. Rosemary is also traditionally used to darken hair colour and restore colour to grey hair as well as combating dandruff: add a few drops of oil or a cup of rosemary infusion to rinsing water after shampooing to help clear dandruff and improve the hair quality.

caution avoid high doses of rosemary and use of rosemary oil in pregnancy.

raspberry *Rubus idaeus*

Raspberry leaf is probably best known as a supportive treatment for childbirth, helping to tonify and strengthen the womb in the weeks before the birth is due. The tea is generally taken for eight weeks before the confinement and can also be sipped during labour.

using raspberry

The leaves are astringent, cleansing, encourage urination and will stimulate the digestion so are often included in morning tisanes as a refreshing way to start the day. As a uterine relaxant and tonic, raspberry leaf is also recommended for period pain, while its astringency makes it an ideal gargle for sore throats or a useful addition to remedies for diarrhoea and piles.

The fruits also have a place in the medicine chest: they are laxative and encourage urination and are a sweating diaphoretic so can be an effective cleansing remedy to help clear toxins from the system. They are also a traditional cooling remedy for fevers and cystitis. In addition, raspberries have been recommended for indigestion and rheumatic pains while a vinegar made from them was once a popular folk remedy for coughs – used to "cut the phlegm".

Raspberry vinegar can be made by soaking 500g/1lb of raspberries in 1 litre/2pts of wine vinegar for two weeks. The thick red liquid produced on straining can then be added to cough syrups or diluted with water as a gargle for sore throats. It also makes a pleasant salad dressing mixed with olive or walnut oil.

sage *Salvia officinalis*

Sage is traditionally associated with longevity and there are numerous legends telling of long-lived princes who regularly downed cups of sage tea, while an old country rhyme tells us that "…he who drinks sage in May, shall live for aye".

Like many folkloric traditions this is yet another that modern research is verifying: sage extracts have been used successfully in a number of trials to combat old-age problems including senile dementia, and commercial products for Alzheimer's disease based on sage extracts are now becoming available. The plant is known to contain powerful anti-oxidants which can combat the ageing of cells. It is also rich in oestrogen so could almost be regarded as an early, and very gentle, form of hormone replacement therapy.

using sage

Sage dries up body fluids which, combined with its hormonal action, makes it ideal for relieving night sweats at the menopause and for drying up milk in lactating mothers on weaning. The plant has an affinity with the throat and makes an excellent gargle and mouth wash for minor infections and inflammations.

▼ Sage *Salvia officinalis*

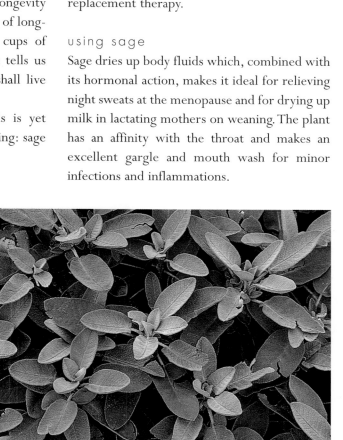

sage

parts used
leaves, essential oil

commercial products
included in an assortment of over-the-counter herbal remedies such as anti-oxidant mixtures, throat lozenges, and anti-catarrh mixtures; capsules, juice, tincture and essential oil are all available from health food shops. *Dan Shen* is available from Chinese herbal shops.

how to use
juice – 10ml/2tsp, three times a day;
tincture – up to 4ml/80 drops, three times a day;
infusion – 20g/³⁄₄oz of dried herb to 500ml/1pt of boiling water taken in three equal doses a day.

clove

part used

flower buds

commercial products

included in many proprietary mixtures for coughs, catarrh, and digestive problems; the essential oil is available from chemists and health food shops.

how to use

add 1-2 cloves to infusions of other herbs for digestive problems or chills;

oil – use neat on a cotton swab placed on the gum to relieve toothache.

The purple variety (*S. officinalis* Purpurascens Group) is often preferred by herbalists, although other cultivars display similar properties. Use in a tea for indigestion or drink a cup regularly as a tonic to combat the effects of old age. In many parts of Europe, sage ointment is a favourite standby for minor cuts and insect bites.

In China the roots of a related plant, *Salvia miltiorhiza*, known as *Dan Shen*, are used as a cooling sedative and energy tonic which will also stimulate blood flow. Studies suggest that *Dan Shen* can be effective in chronic heart conditions such as angina pectoris.

caution avoid high doses of sage in pregnancy.

clove *Syzygium aromaticum*

Cloves have been used for flavouring for around 2,000 years and were known in Roman times as an exotic spice. In China the clove is known as *Ding Xiang* and has been used in medicine since around 600 AD; it is regarded as a kidney tonic, increasing *yang* energy, strengthening for the reproductive organs and ideal for treating impotence. It is also used for hiccoughs, nausea and vomiting associated with cold in the stomach. In Ayurvedic medicine cloves are known as *lavanga* and are regarded as a lung remedy and included in candies for coughs and colds.

using cloves

Clove oil is available from pharmacies and is useful as an emergency first-aid remedy for toothache (put a few drops on a cotton-wool swab and place on the gum nearest to the aching tooth). Cloves are often included in "herbal" toothpastes and dental preparations.

Cloves are helpful for disguising the taste of more unpleasant herbs, so a couple added to a herbal mixture for stomach upsets or chills can often make the brew rather more palatable.

In many parts of the East, clove oil is also used as an abdominal massage during labour to encourage contractions and ease pain. While this is certainly not something the novice should attempt, drinking teas flavoured with plenty of cloves during the second stage of labour can help to ease childbirth pains.

caution cloves should be reserved for labour and childbirth and not taken earlier in pregnancy.

thyme *Thymus vulgaris*

Like many culinary herbs thyme is a soothing digestive remedy which can stimulate the digestion, as it copes with rich foods, and ease flatulence. The plant (particularly the oil) is also extremely antiseptic, will ease muscle spasms and cramps and encourages coughing helping both to clear phlegm and, thanks to its anti-bacterial action, combat chest infections.

It is one of the most popular of herb garden plants with around 40 cultivars available from specialist nurseries. Many of these have distinctive flavours and are valued by chefs. Common or garden thyme (*T. vulgaris*) is the cultivated form of wild thyme (*T. serpyllum*), which is known as

▲ Thyme *Thymus vulgaris*

thyme

parts used
aerial parts, essential oil

commercial products
included in many proprietary cough mixtures and anti-oxidant preparations; capsules, juice, tincture and essential oil are all sold in health food shops.

how to use
tincture – up to 5ml/1tsp, three times a day; *infusion* – 25g/1oz of dried herb to 500ml/1pt of boiling water taken in three equal doses a day; *syrup* – 5-10ml/1-2tsp every 3-4 hours; *essential oil* – ½ml/10 drops in 5ml/1tsp of almond oil as a massage rub.

linden

part used
flowers

commercial products
included in over-the-counter herbal remedies for nervous tension, anxiety, and blood pressure problems; tincture is available from specialist suppliers.

how to use
infusion – 25g/1oz of dried herb to 500ml/1pt of boiling water taken in three equal doses daily; *tincture* – up to 4ml/80 drops, three times a day.

"mother of thyme" – possibly because of its traditional use for menstrual disorders. Wild thyme's botanical name is based on its creeping or serpent-like growth pattern and Pliny – in true Doctrine of Signatures fashion – recommends it as an antidote for serpent bites and "the poison of marine creatures". The Romans also burned the plant in the belief that the fumes would repel scorpions and "all such creatures".

using thyme

As an antiseptic cough remedy, common thyme is useful in syrups and combines well with marshmallow or liquorice for conditions such as bronchitis. Drink thyme tea as a tonic for exhaustion or to regulate the digestion and use fresh, crushed leaves to heal minor wounds and warts. The oil is used in aromatherapy for muscular aches, pains and stiffness and can be added to baths to combat exhaustion.

linden *Tilia cordata*

Flowers from the European lime or linden tree can be collected in late summer to provide a convenient, soothing remedy that can also help combat high blood pressure. The herb is believed to counter the build-up of fatty deposits in blood vessels that can lead to arteriosclerosis or "hardening of the arteries". In France, linden is known as *tilleul* and is one of the most popular of after-dinner tisanes.

using linden

Mediaeval herbalists regarded linden as hot and drying, so it was recommended for headaches caused by cold and was also used for dizziness and epilepsy. It is mildly sedative, encourages perspiration and will also ease muscle spasms and cramps. Although we now use only the flowers medicinally, the leaves were once made into ointments for swellings or sores and used in mouthwashes for minor gum infections.

The flowers combine well with lemon balm for nervous tension and anxiety or can be mixed with hawthorn flowers for high blood pressure. Because it is both calming and reduces blood pressure, lime flowers are ideal for those suffering from high blood pressure which is related to stress. It can also be suitable for digestive upsets, associated with nervous tension, and in feverish colds or influenza.

fenugreek
Trigonella foenum-graecum

The potent aroma and taste of fenugreek are familiar from Indian and Middle Eastern cookery and it gives a spicy flavour to curries, pickles and garnishes. The dried aerial parts (rather than the seeds), known as *hilba*, are used in tea in modern Egypt as a remedy for spasmodic abdominal pain – due to both digestive upsets and menstruation. In Ayurveda fenugreek (known as *methi*) is regarded as a good remedy in convalescence and debility helping to stimulate liver function and ease indigestion. The Chinese also regard fenugreek *(Hu Lu Ba)* as a kidney remedy – to warm the kidneys, dispel cold and relieve pain. It is used for pains in the abdomen and groin associated with kidney weakness.

using fenugreek
The seeds are used in Western herbal medicine and the plant is regarded as a warming remedy, ideal for all sorts of colds and chills affecting the abdomen. It is a soothing and healing remedy for both stomach and intestines: it can be helpful for such conditions as colitis, diverticulitis, irritable bowel, weak digestion and poor appetite. It is also warming for the kidneys and can be supportive in urinary tract infections and lower back pains. It helps encourage coughing to clear phlegm, will encourage milk flow in nursing mothers and also has some anti-inflammatory action.

Modern research has shown that fenugreek will reduce blood sugar and cholesterol levels and it is increasingly used to support dietary control of late-onset diabetes.

caution avoid high doses in pregnancy.

vervain *Verbena officinalis*

John Gerard – who clearly had little time for folk traditions – warns his readers not to listen to "odde olde wives tales" of vervain that told of "witchcraft and sorceries". As late as the 17th century the plant was still being used in fortune-telling rites – a practice that can be traced back at least to Druidic times.

The Romans called it *hiera botane* (sacred plant) and used it to purify homes and spread on Jupiter's altars. Well into the Christian era it was castigated as a witch plant – or as the 11th-century Physicians of Myddfai warn "...give no heed to those who say that it should be gathered in the name of the devil." The Druids, according to Pliny, collected it when the "dog star could be seen in the heavens" and even today many regard it as a strong spiritual herb capable of healing holes in the human aura.

using vervain

Medicinally it is largely used as a relaxing remedy for nervous problems and as a liver tonic – bitter and stimulating for the digestion; it is an ideal tonic in convalescence and debility. Vervain can also be helpful for nerve pains and migraine – taken internally or applied topically in a compress. It combines well with oats in depression and is a useful herb for nursing mothers – relaxing the nervous system to take the tension out of feeding time and stimulating milk flow.

caution vervain should be avoided in pregnancy, but can be taken in labour to stimulate contractions.

ginger *Zingiber officinale*

Ginger originates from tropical Asia, but spread to Europe in ancient times: it is mentioned by the Romans, listed in some of the earliest Chinese herbals, regarded in Ayurvedic medicine as a universal medicine, and was introduced by the Spaniards to America where it is now cultivated extensively in the West Indies.

The plant is useful for controlling both nausea and coughing, it stimulates the circulation, encourages perspiration, relaxes blood vessels and is extremely warming for all sorts of "cold" conditions. Ginger has a distinctive pungent, aromatic flavour and is familiar and widely used as a commercial flavouring.

Gerard described the fresh root as "hot and moist and provoking venerie" and laments his inability to grow the plant in his London garden. As a hot, dry herb he used ginger to warm the stomach and dispel chills. In the 18th century ginger was added to many remedies to modify their action and reduce the irritant effects on the stomach or, as Henry Barham put it in 1794, to "taketh away their malice" – a technique still practised in China, where ginger is cooked with such potentially poisonous plants as monkshood to reduce toxicity.

using ginger

Fresh ginger from the greengrocer can be made into a warming tea for colds and chills or a pinch of powdered ginger can be added to other herb teas to give added stimulation. Ginger oil is used in external remedies to encourage blood flow to ease muscular stiffness, aches and pains. A hot infused oil (see page 224) made with ginger is a home-made alternative to the distilled essential oil.

In Chinese medicine fresh and dried root ginger are regarded rather differently, with the dried believed to be helpful for abdominal pain and diarrhoea and the fresh considered more suitable for treating feverish chills, coughs and vomiting.

As a remedy for nausea, ginger is ideal for travel sickness and has been successfully tested in clinical trials for very severe morning sickness in pregnancy (typical clinical dose is 1g, three times a day). Ginger in capsules is ideal but ginger biscuits, crystallised ginger sweets or ginger beer can also prove effective – especially with children.

---

ginger

parts used
root, essential oil

commercial products
included in a great many proprietary remedies mainly used for digestive problems, colds and infections; easily obtainable as a simple in tablets, capsules and tinctures or as the essential oil.

how to use
capsules (250-300mg) – take one tablet before travelling to combat motion sickness or after meals for indigestion;
tincture – up to 2ml/40 drops per dose, three times daily;
decoction – 25mg of dried or 75mg of fresh root to 750ml/1½pt of water, simmered for 15-20 minutes and taken in wine glass doses for digestive problems and chills;
oil – make a hot infused oil by simmering 25g/1oz of fresh ginger in 250ml/½pt of sunflower oil over a water bath for 2-3 hours and use for cold aching joints.

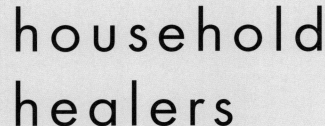

household healers

A very fine grey line divides the concept of "food" from that of "herbal medicine": many plants sit comfortably in both categories and, like garlic, are equally at home on a greengrocer's counter as in a pharmacy.

As well as the many culinary herbs listed in the previous section, plants that we categorise as "foods" also have their share of medicinal properties. Onions, apples, cabbages, even cold tea all have a therapeutic use and make ideal household standbys as emergency remedies.

Equally, we need to remember the actions of these foods, as a surfeit can produce as many side-effects as an overdose of a more orthodox "drug". How many of us have eaten rather too many peaches, nectarines or plums when the fruits arrive in the shops only to wonder at the sudden bout of diarrhoea that follows? All these fruits would be described by orthodox practitioners as "laxative" or encouraging bowel motions – which explains the effect they have on us. To the 17th-century doctor, however, they would have been classified as "cold" and generally rather "moist" as well; the intrinsic coldness of the fruit would be blamed for any troublesome digestive problems that followed.

In Galenic medicine, foods were not only necessary nutrients (see page 9), they each had characteristics that could affect the healthy balance of the system and so they had to be used in moderation or carefully combined to avoid side-effects. Writing in 1597, John Gerard suggests that cucumbers (cold and moist in the second degree) should be added to meat dishes "for the stomacke and other parts troubled with heate". These traditions survived well into the 17th century, although by then, as Culpeper noted (see page 72), the practice was falling from use.

While modern medicine dismisses humoral theories as mediaeval hocus pocus, scientists do at least acknowledge that sometimes foods are not always as safe as we would believe. Man-made hazards (such as BSE) apart, foods often contain toxic chemicals which can do harm as well as good and in excess they can sometimes seem to present as many troublesome side-effects as more orthodox medicines. We also know little of how genetically modified organisms may affect us: some will contain familiar combinations of chemicals, which the body understands, but how the digestive system will cope with the more unusual additions still needs to be investigated.

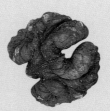

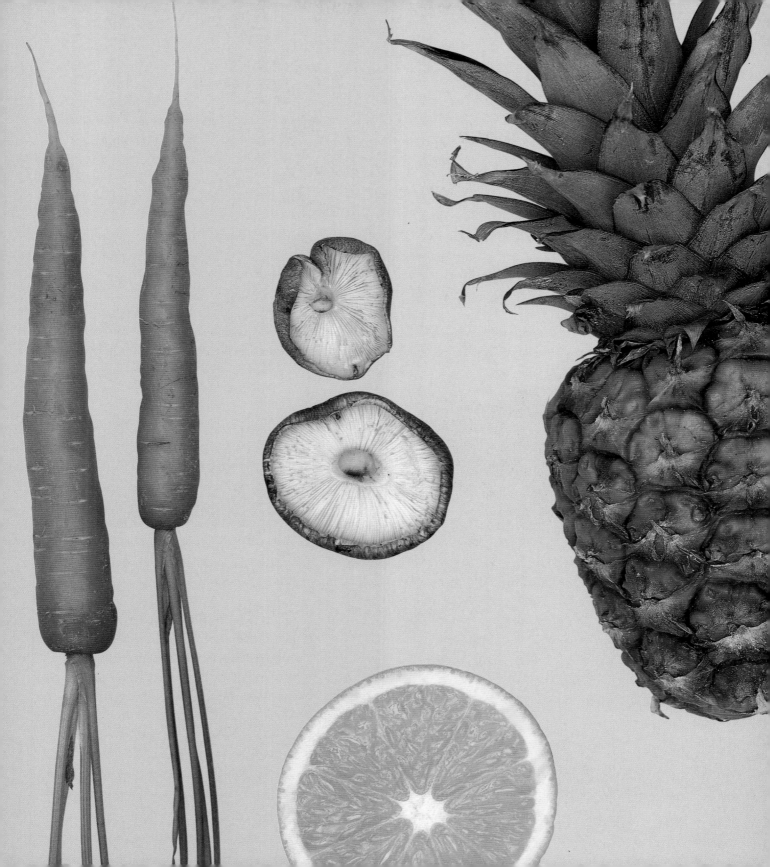

parts used
whole plants

commercial products
dried seaweeds are
available loose from
Oriental grocers; some –
such as *nori* – are now
sold in capsules and
tablets in health food
shops.

how to use
capsules – up to 2g per
dose; eat with food.

onion

part used
bulb

commercial products
bottled onion juice is
available from health
food shops or
pharmacies; it is
sometimes included with
garlic or horseradish in
stimulating cold remedies.

how to use
typical dose of fresh juice
is 10ml/2tsp three times
daily;
onion cough syrup (see
below) – 5ml/1tsp up to
every 3-4 hours;
use fresh onion boiled for
hot poultices or in
cleansing soups.

seaweeds *Algae*

Seaweeds belong to the simplest plant grouping – the Algae – and various types are used both in medicine and Oriental cookery. They tend to be grouped by colour into green/blue weeds such as sea lettuce (*Ulva lactuca*), the brown seaweeds including Japanese varieties such as kombu and wakame, and the red seaweeds such as laver and carrageen (*Chondrus crispus*) which is used in herbal medicine mainly for coughs and irritable digestive problems.

Kelp (*Fucus* spp.) is probably the most familiar in the West as an over-the-counter herbal remedy (see page 146), but other home-grown edible varieties like laver (*Porphyra umbilicalis*) are familiar in some traditional dishes. In Wales laver is boiled and then fried with oatmeal to become laverbread. Increasingly fashionable are the Japanese varieties used in *sushi* – such as *wakame* (*Undaria pinnatifida*), *kombu* (*Laminaria* spp) and *nori* (*Porphyra tenera*) – although the "crispy seaweed" served in Chinese restaurants is actually just fried cabbage.

using seaweeds

Like kelp, all these seaweeds tend to be rich in iodine as well as other minerals such as zinc, iron, magnesium and calcium. They are also a good source of vitamin B_{12}, which tends to be lacking in vegetarian diets, so make a valuable food supplement for non-meat-eaters. Most can be helpful in anaemia or after the menopause as a natural calcium source.

Kombu is a good source of vitamins A and C, but is high in sodium so needs to be avoided by those on low-salt diets or with high blood pressure. It is strongly flavoured and generally used in soups or stock. The flavour is helped by large amounts of monosodium glutamate found in the plant so may be best avoided by those with MSG sensitivity. *Nori* is used in Japanese cooking to wrap sushi and other savouries and can also help to reduce cholesterol levels and strengthen the immune system.

Wakame is probably more palatable for Westerners than some other seaweeds and is used as flavouring in miso soup made from fermented bean curd.

onion *Allium cepa*

Like garlic and leeks, onion has long been used to combat infections, improve the digestion and ease coughs. It is an effective anti-bacterial and can reduce inflammation. Like many foods onion will also help with digestion, stimulating the production of bile by the liver and helping to clear waste products by encouraging urination.

Onions will also stimulate coughing to clear phlegm and one of the most popular traditional recipes for home-made cough syrup was simply to layer slices of onion with honey or sugar and leave overnight. In the morning a clear syrup can be collected which makes an effective – if not particularly pleasant-tasting – remedy for stubborn coughs.

Raw onion was extensively used in folk tradition to ease bee and wasp stings and can be used in poultices for chilblains. The heart of a cooled, boiled onion used to be inserted into the ear to relieve ear ache, while a bowl of hot boiled onions with plenty of pepper was standard fare for any threatening chill.

using onion

Today, we know that the plant will also reduce both blood pressure and cholesterol levels, so can help to combat a tendency to heart disease. Onion juice is ideal for clearing warts and also makes a cleansing internal supplement to help maintain a healthy gut flora (important for those prone to candidiasis) and prevent fermentation.

Like garlic, onion owes much of its smell to a number of sulphur compounds which stimulate the digestive system and have an antibiotic action, preventing decay. Onion soups are ideal for colds and catarrh and the herb's cleansing action makes it a valuable addition to the diet for arthritics, gout sufferers or where fluid retention is a problem.

leek *Allium porrum*

Like other members of the onion family, leeks have a long history of medicinal use – although they had to be taken with caution: Gerard described them as "hot and dry", warning that eaten raw the leek "ingendreth naughtie blood, causeth troublesome and terrible creams, dulleth the sight … and is noisesome to the stomacke".

Once cooked, however, the vegetable became rather more respectable, the juice, mixed with a little rose oil, could be used as drops for ear ache and tinnitus, while made into a gruel with barley it was recommended for bronchial congestion to clear phlegm. In contrast, Coptic medicine (which flourished *c.* 100–400 AD) suggested leek mixed with fresh urine to improve the eyesight – a remnant of ancient Egyptian medicine where leeks had been regarded as a cure for blindness from at least 1000 BC (traditional recipes demanded that the urine had to come from a woman who had never deceived her husband!).

using leek

The contemporary French herbalist Jean Valnet suggests that a leek remedy is as good as taking "the cure at Vichy", a noted French spa. Leeks can be used with honey, like onions (see above), to produce a cough syrup and they make a useful addition to the diet of those prone to catarrh and congestion. They are also laxative (stimulate bowel motions) and help to rid the body of uric acid wastes, so can be supportive for arthritic disorders and gout. Like other members of the *Allium* family, leeks are also anti-bacterial and leek poultices can be used externally as an antiseptic for wounds or to draw pus from boils. A slice of leek can be rubbed into the skin to relieve the discomfort of insect stings.

leek

part used
aerial parts

commercial products
not generally used in commercial medicinal products although fresh leeks can be found in greengrocers in winter and spring.

how to use
use fresh or in soups; home-made juice (10ml/2tsp, 3 times a day) can also be mixed with bread for poultices or with milk as a lotion for skin rashes.

galangal

part used

root

commercial availability

tincture is available from specialist suppliers; included in several products from German or Austrian specialists in Hildegard of Bingen remedies; the root is sold fresh in many supermarkets as a flavouring for Thai dishes.

how to use

decoction – 1-2 slices fresh root per cup; *tincture* – up to 0.5ml/10 drops per dose in water as a circulatory and heart tonic or for nausea, stomach chills and indigestion; 2-3 drops undiluted on the tongue as required for angina pectoris attacks, dizziness and palpitations.

galangal *Alpinia galanga*

Galangal originates in South-east Asia and is important in both Chinese and Ayurvedic medicine. It is known as *kulanjian* in Hindi and is a popular stomach remedy. The dried rhizomes were brought to Europe by Arab traders from the ninth century and were a favourite with Hildegard of Bingen (1098–1179), a German nun, mystic, musician and healer, who used galangal for a wide range of heart disorders. According to Hildegard: "Whoever has heart pain and is weak in the heart, should instantly eat enough galangal, and he or she will be well again." German studies, based on Hildegard's work have confirmed that the herb is effective at easing heart pains, dizziness and fatigue and can combat chronic heart disorders such as angina pectoris.

using galangal

The plant has become familiar in recent years as a flavouring for many Eastern dishes and the fresh root is often found on supermarket shelves. The root can be used much like fresh ginger in warming decoctions for colds or chills or to combat feelings of nausea and travel sickness.

Galangal is still used in India for digestive and respiratory problems and is classified as a *vajikarana* or aphrodisiac tonic. *Vajikarana* take their name from *vaji*, meaning a stallion, and are believed to bring the energy and vitality of a horse – also renowned in Indian tradition for its sexual activity – and focus on reproductive energy to help energise all of the body's tissues. By increasing sexual energy the *vajikarana* not only help to create new life in conception but also help to renew our own lives.

Lesser galangal (*A. officinarum*) is used in similar ways as a digestive remedy in India and is known as *Gao Liang Jiang* in China. It is used as a warming remedy for the digestive system, to relieve cold and pain, and to stimulate *Qi* (energy). Like galangal, this variety is also used in China for indigestion, gastroenteritis, stomach pains, colds and chills.

caution heart problems such as angina pectoris need professional treatment; do not use galangal to replace prescribed medication without consulting your health care professional.

pineapple *Ananas sativa*

Pineapple is rich in an enzyme called bromelain which acts as a digestive stimulant so is ideal for easing indigestion and gastritis. The fruit is also diuretic and cleansing and can be helpful for arthritis, gout and urinary stones. It is nutritious, rich in minerals and a useful food for those prone to iron-deficient anaemia or in debility and convalescence.

using pineapple

Drinking a glass of pineapple juice before meals can help stimulate a sluggish digestion. For the same reason it is sometimes recommended as a slimming aid: the French herbalist Jean Valnet recommends eating "two grilled lamb chops and large slices of fresh pineapple" for lunch and dinner and drinking 2 litres/3½pt of still mineral water each day for three days as the ideal short-term weight-reducing diet.

➤ Pineapple *Ananas sativa*

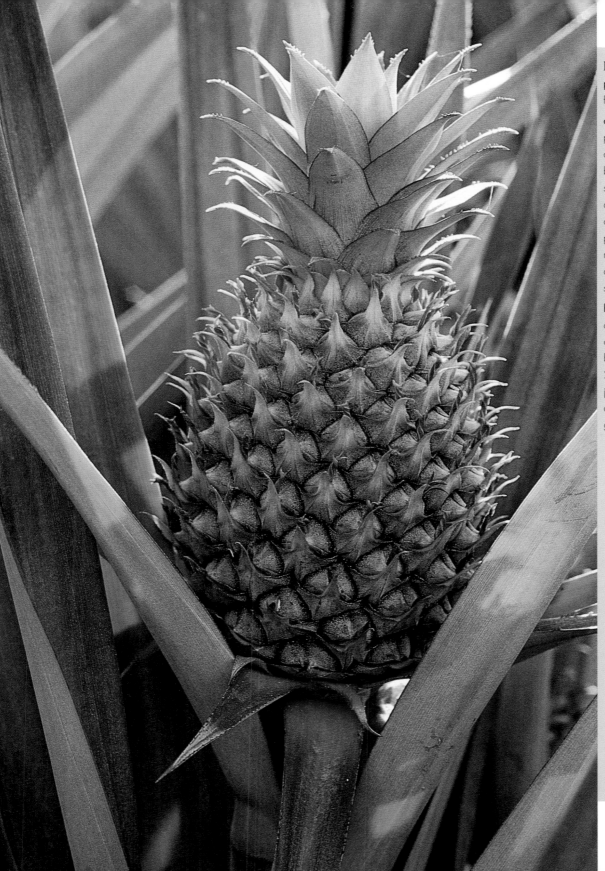

pineapple

part used
fruit

commercial products
pineapple juice is readily available in supermarkets; bromelain extracts are sold in health food shops as a digestive stimulant and capsules of pineapple stems are also made by some suppliers and marketed as a slimming aid.

how to use
capsules generally contain 500mg bromelain (1-2 per day); 2-3 glasses of pineapple juice daily as a general digestive tonic or drink a glass before each meal.

celery

parts used
seeds, stems, oil

commercial products
an ingredient in numerous tablets and capsules recommended for arthritic problems, fluid retention or rheumatism; capsules containing only crushed celery seed are also available from health food shops as is pressed celery stalk juice, celery seed tincture and the essential oil distilled from the seeds. Celery salt is also sold for food flavouring.

how to use
the seed in infusions (1tsp per cup);

tincture - 2½ml/50 drops in water three times daily;

tablets - 600mg daily;

juice - 10ml/2tsp three times daily;

essential oil should be used externally only - 1ml/20 drops per 100ml/3½fl oz of hot water for compresses in urinary disorders, for example.

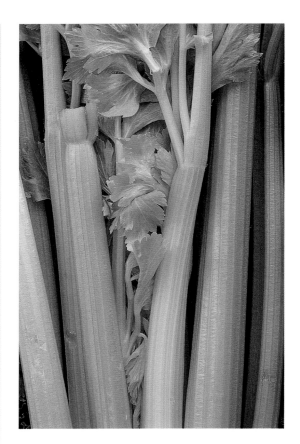

Bromelain acts only on the digestive tract — it is not significantly absorbed into the system, so does not affect the liver. Externally, crushed pineapple is anti-inflammatory and can help to heal ulcers and slow-healing wounds, while the juice can also be used to tonify the skin. Gargling with the juice is a useful alternative for sore throats.

celery *Apium graveolens*

Although it is the seeds of the celery plant that are mainly used as a medicinal herb, both stalk and root of this familiar vegetable have therapeutic properties: the root was once used to treat urinary stones, while the stalks are

◄ Celery *Apium graveolens*

characterised in Eastern medicine as having a bitter-sweet taste, making it a moist, cooling food ideal to balance hot, drying, spicy chili dishes.

using celery
The seeds will encourage excretion of uric acid, which is helpful for a number of arthritic conditions, especially gout. They also help lower blood pressure and are a reputed aphrodisiac. The juice, extracted from the whole plant and roots, can be used as a tonic for debilitated conditions and may also help with joint or urinary tract inflammations. Celery is also helpful to relieve wind and excess gas in the digestive tract and a cup of weak celery tea can make a useful after-dinner drink for those prone to indigestion.

An essential oil, extracted from the seeds is used in aromatherapy for kidney infections and cystitis, often well diluted in hot compresses rather than as a massage treatment. The oil contains apiol, a uterine stimulant also found in parsley seeds, and for this reason large quantities are contraindicated in pregnancy; however, the stalks are perfectly safe for expectant mothers and can also help stimulate milk flow after the birth.

caution avoid seeds and oil in pregnancy.

horseradish
Armoracia rusticana

Horseradish is probably most familiar to us today in jars — creamed to eat with roast beef or smoked fish. Until the 17th century the plant was popular as a garnish in Scandinavia and Germany, but little used in other parts of Europe. The French called it *moutarde des allemands,* while Gerard notes that it will "kill vines if grown anywhere near them", adding that "when made into a sauce for fish and meates", it "doth heat the stomache better and causeth better digestion than mustard".

The root is extremely hot and mustard-like – traditionally classified as "hot and dry in the third degree" – and will blister sensitive skins if a poultice of the root is applied for too long. It is ideal to improve the circulation or to warm "cold" conditions like arthritis, rheumatism, the common cold and some types of catarrh. Gerard recommends it for sciatica and also for colicky pains.

using horseradish

Horseradish encourages sweating and urination and will also stimulate the liver and digestion, so it can be helpful internally for some skin and rheumatic conditions where a build-up of toxins in the system is contributing to the problem. It is also now known to be anti-bacterial.

It needs to be used sparingly, but a little of the decoction is worth adding to cough syrups for bronchitis and stubborn catarrh; it will also stimulate the digestion, making it a very practical and pleasant condiment.

cautions excessive internal use of horseradish can cause vomiting and allergic reactions. It should be avoided by those with stomach ulcers. Externally it can cause blistering in those with sensitive skin.

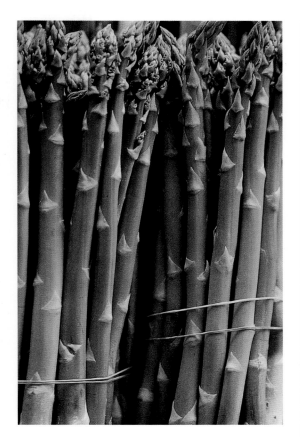

asparagus
Asparagus officinalis

Asparagus is familiar as a seasonal vegetable – a summertime delicacy that is well worth attempting to grow in the vegetable garden, especially by those with plenty of time for weeding. Its action as a medicinal plant will be familiar to most asparagus eaters, who will no doubt have noted the effect its main component, asparagine, has in increasing urination. The characteristic smell it adds to the urine is caused by breakdown of asparagine to a substance called methylmercaptan; this is produced in the urine often within a very few minutes of enjoying a bowl of asparagus spears. Several species of the plant have more

horseradish

part used
root

commercial products
widely used in culinary sauces, the fresh root is sold in good quality greengrocers usually in the autumn or winter; the bottled juice is available from health food shops; horseradish tincture is produced by specialist suppliers; the herb is sometimes included in proprietary mixtures for rheumatic aches and pains.

how to use
juice – 5-10ml/1-2tsp, 2-3 times a day in water;
tincture – up to 2½ml/50 drops, in water 2-3 times a day;
½tsp grated fresh root per cup of decoction;
a hot infused oil containing 15g/½oz of horseradish in 500ml/1pt of oil can be used as a rub to help stimulate the circulation and ease rheumatic pains.

asparagus

part used

stem

commercial products

the bottled juice is sold in health food shops; *shatavari* is sometimes found in capsules in health food shops or is available from specialist Ayurvedic medicine suppliers.

how to use

juice – 10ml/2tsp, three times a day;

shatavari – up to 1g of powdered root per dose, traditionally taken mixed in *ghee* (clarified butter) or in milk decoctions.

beetroot

part used

root

commercial products

not generally used in commercial medicinal products, organic juice is generally stocked in health food shops or make your own using organically grown beets from a greengrocer (see page 221).

how to use

juice – a small wine glass (100ml/3½fl oz) twice a day;

decoction – 75g/2½oz of chopped fresh beet to 750ml/1½pt water (see page 216).

---

significant medicinal properties, including *A. racemosus*, which is an important tonic herb (known as *shatavari*) in Ayurvedic medicine. The name *shatavari* means "who possesses a hundred husbands" and the herb is believed in India to have an extremely beneficial effect on the female reproductive organs. *Shatavari* is commonly recommended for menopausal problems and also for digestive and lung disorders. It is often eaten in a mixture with honey, milk and clarified butter.

using asparagus

Our more familiar Western vegetable – *A. officinalis* – has long been used as a cleansing herb for rheumatism and to support liver function. Asparagus has been promoted as a slimming aid by some producers of over-the-counter products, largely because of its diuretic and laxative action. It can help to disperse urinary stones and, as a good source of vitamins and minerals (including iron), it is ideal for debility and anaemia. Methylmercaptan can be irritant in cystitis, so it is best to avoid eating asparagus when suffering an attack; it also has a high purine content, so needs to be eaten in moderation by gout sufferers. Asparagus soup should certainly be included regularly in the menu of convalescents and anyone prone to iron-deficiency anaemia.

oats *Avena sativa*

Oats – despite Dr Johnson's dismissal as "a grain which in England is generally given to horses, but in Scotland supports the people" – are one of

▶ Beetroot *Beta vulgaris*

---

the world's most important cereal crops, used as a staple food in northern Europe for centuries. Oats are sweet, nutritious and warming – ideal to combat a cold, damp, northern climate. They are rich in iron, zinc and manganese, so are also a good source of many vital minerals.

using oats

Oatstraw, grains, bran and fresh whole plant are all used medicinally in various ways. The

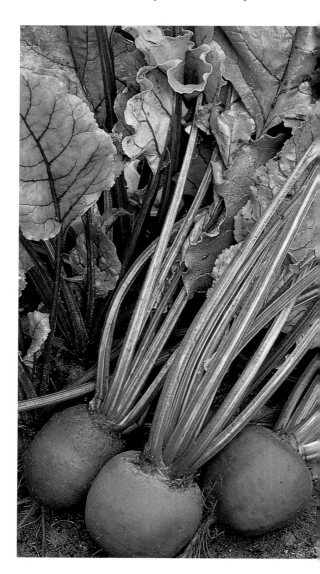

oatstraw and grains are especially anti-depressant and therefore make a good restorative nerve tonic which is regarded as emotionally uplifting, so a bowl of porridge made from good-quality oatmeal is the ideal way to start the day. Oatstraw tincture is generally used in herbal medicine and is often combined with vervain for nervous problems, exhaustion and depression, emotional upsets associated with the menopause, or debility following illness. The juice of fresh oats, pressed when still green, is similarly used as a nerve tonic.

Oatstraw baths are used in folk medicine to counter rheumatic pains and the fresh plant is also used in homoeopathy for rheumatism.

As a home remedy oatmeal is excellent in skin washes for eczema and dry skin – add a tablespoon to a bowl of warm water and use for washing. Gerard certainly considered it as a beauty aid at a time when white skin was highly regarded: "Oatmeale is good for to make a faire and well coloured maide," he wrote, "to looke like a cake of tallow."

Recent research suggests that oatbran (and to a lesser extent oatmeal) can also help to reduce blood cholesterol levels, so should certainly be regularly included in the diet of those at risk from heart disease or atherosclerosis.

beetroot *Beta vulgaris*

While we may consider beetroots – cooked and pickled in vinegar – as a useful addition to cold meat dishes and salads, the ancient Greeks regarded them as an important fever remedy, and in mediaeval times, beetroot was categorised as an easily digested, nutritious food ideal in convalescence and debility.

The Roman writer Pliny (*c.* AD 75) recommended a beetroot decoction as a hair rinse to cure dandruff and as a lotion for chilblains, while ear drops of beetroot juice were used to combat vertigo and tinnitus. Beetroot juice was also used by the Romans as a wound dressing, to relieve toothache, and as an antidote for "serpent bites".

using beetroot

While we no longer regard beetroots as quite such a versatile cure-all, they have been recommended in recent years as an effective digestive remedy and are often included in cleansing naturopathic treatments for chronic illnesses and cancer. It can also be a useful standby for minor wounds as the root really does help to stop bleeding.

Beetroots are rich in vitamins A, B-complex and C, contain several important minerals (including silicon, iron and zinc) and a number of amino acids. Research suggests that beetroot juice can stimulate and cleanse the lymphatic system, increase resistance to infection, and stimulate both kidneys and digestive function. The lymphatic system helps to maintain the body's fluid balance, acting as a drainage network, as well as being home to many of the cells which give us specific immunity against infection. As an easily digested food beetroots are ideal for those with sensitive stomachs, while their generally cooling and immune-stimulant actions also make them a useful addition to the menu for those suffering from colds, coughs and catarrh.

➤➤ Overleaf: oats *Avena sativa*

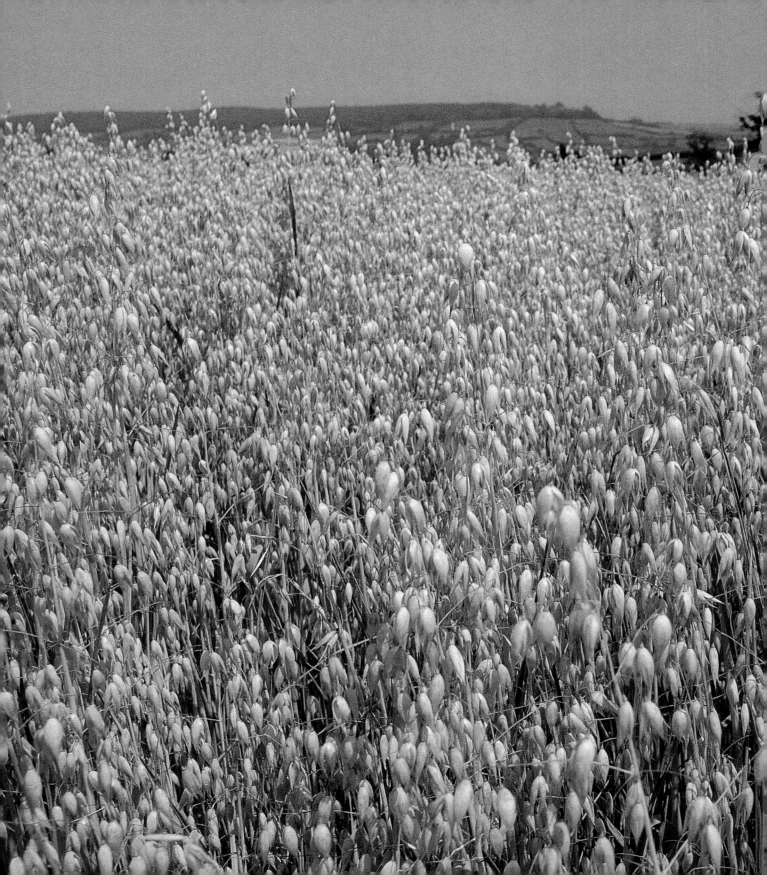

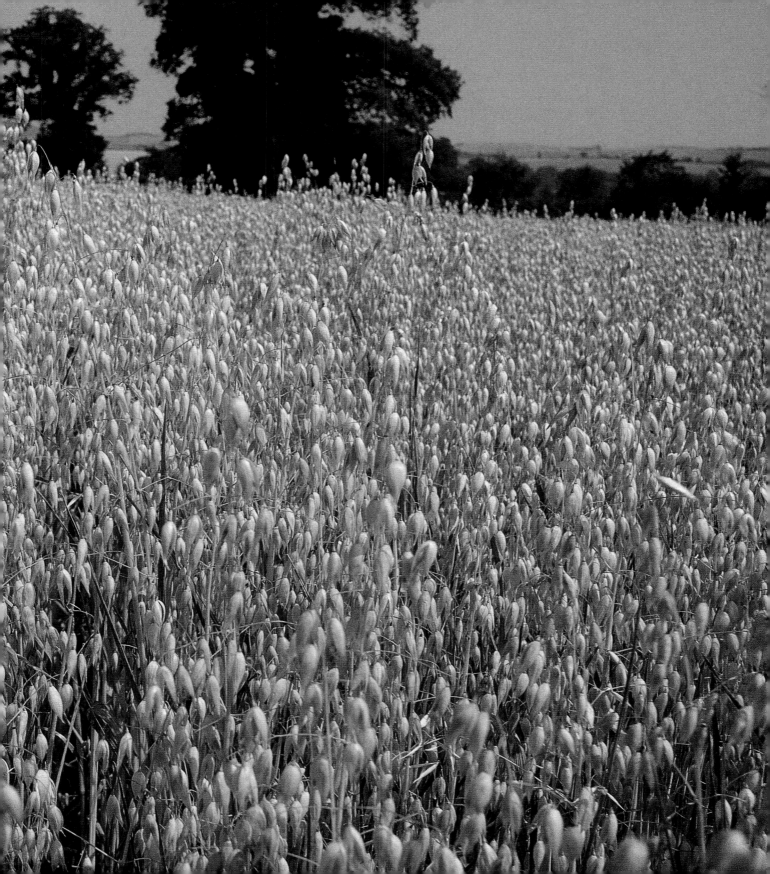

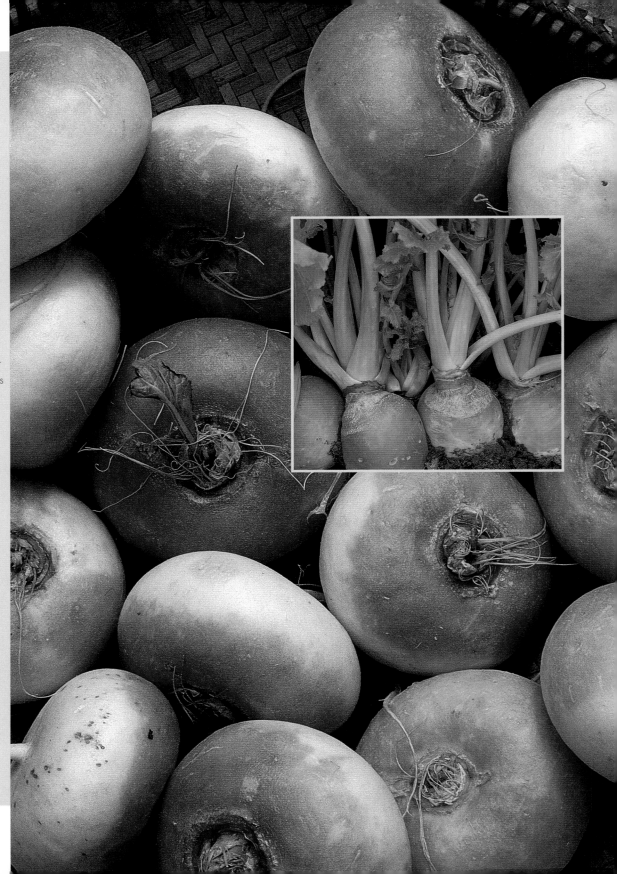

turnip

parts used

root, leaves

commercial products

not generally used in commercial medicinal products although fresh turnips can be bought in greengrocers in winter and spring.

how to use

home-made fresh vegetable juice (see page 221);

fresh root decoction can be made from 75g/2½oz of turnips to 750ml/1¼pt of water or milk and drink 2-3 glasses of the liquid daily for colds, chills and chest problems (see page 216); if you grow your own turnips use the fresh leaves (75g/2½oz to 500ml/1pt of water) in infusions and drink a large wine glass (150ml/5fl oz) three times daily;

turnip syrup – 10ml/2tsp three times a day for colds and coughs.

turnip *Brassica napus*

Turnips were traditionally associated with beauty and generations of women dutifully ate their turnips or drank turnip water (basically the water in which turnips had been previously cooked) each morning in an attempt to grow more lovely. Both root and leaves act as blood cleansers so can help to clear spots and improve the complexion.

The roots are rich in calcium, phosphorus, magnesium and vitamins A, B-complex and C, with iron and copper in the leaves, so turnips are an extremely nutritious and tonic food.

using turnip

Turnips also have a diuretic action, helping to cleanse toxins from the system by increasing urination, and were traditionally used for gout and kidney stones – often associated with excess uric acid. This sort of cleansing action means that turnips are a good food for arthritics and can be helpful for eczema and acne.

Research suggests that eating turnips can also improve the immune system. They have an antiseptic effect on the respiratory system, and are used in folk medicine for bronchitis and other chronic lung disorders. Turnip decoction is used in France as a gargle for sore throats. Turnip syrup is another traditional standby for coughs and can be made by layering slices of turnip and sugar and leaving for four to six hours, as with onion syrup (see page 105).

Externally, turnip can soften the skin and reduce infections; slices can be rubbed on dry skin while poultices can be helpful for boils and chilblains or used on painful arthritic joints.

◄ Turnip *Brassica napus*

mustard

Brassica nigra / Sinapis alba

While today we might be tempted to dismiss mustard foot baths and plasters as a music-hall joke, this homespun folk remedy is well worth remembering as an effective means of stimulating the circulation to help clear colds and headaches. Mustard also stimulates the digestive system and has long been used as a culinary seasoning; it was probably introduced into Britain by the Romans who were enthusiastic mustard eaters. By Elizabethan times, mustard seeds crushed with vinegar made a popular sauce for both meat and fish, "because", as John Gerard put it, "it doth help digestion, warmeth the stomache and provoketh appetite".

using mustard

The seeds of white mustard (*Sinapis alba*) are rather larger in size than those of black mustard (*Brassica nigra*) and tend to have a milder flavour. Both varieties are, however, used in very similar ways: externally they are warming and draw blood to the surface, so are useful for easing cold joints (as in osteoarthritis). As a digestive stimulant, mustard is the ideal condiment for meat that can be difficult to digest; it can also be useful for encouraging the blood flow to peripheral areas of the body, such as fingers and toes, in cases of poor circulation or chilblains.

Mustard foot baths are a traditional remedy for colds and chills: as a means of encouraging blood flow to the feet they can help to reduce over-all body temperature by dissipating heat. Mustard poultices are another traditional favourite, used for rheumatic aches and pains, although the herb can irritate sensitive skins.

mustard

parts used
seeds, oil

commercial products
mustard oil is included in patent remedies for muscular aches and pains; mustard seeds are available in culinary herb selections or from health food shops.

how to use
for mustard baths use 1tbsp of mustard powder or seeds, preferably in a muslin bag, to a bowl of hot water and soak the feet for 10-15 minutes; use 25g/1oz to 500ml/1pt of sunflower oil to make hot infused oils (see page 224) on their own or combined with chili for home use to make a warming rub for muscular stiffness, aches and pains.

cabbage

parts used
aerial parts

commercial products
fermented cabbage
(*sauerkraut*) is available
from most grocers and
delicatessens; bottled
freshly pressed cabbage
juice is sold by health
food shops.

how to use
juice – 10ml/2tsp up to
three times a day;
sauerkraut – one serving
(1-2tbsp) a day;
poultice – use fresh
leaves softened with a
vegetable mallet and
secure with a loose
bandage or sticking
plaster.
lotion – use for skin
problems such as acne.
Process cabbage leaves
in a food processor or
juicer, then cover with
distilled witch hazel and
blend the mixture to
produce a smooth lotion.

Both black and white mustard seeds are ground for use in pickles and sauces.

caution mustards can irritate the skin and prolonged use of poultices can lead to blistering.

cabbage *Brassica oleracea*

Jean Valnet, a notable contemporary French herbalist, has described cabbage as "the medicine of the poor" and it is probably one of the most widely used household remedies in folk tradition.

The cabbage has been cultivated in the West since at least 400 BC, while in the second century AD the Greek herbalist Dioscorides

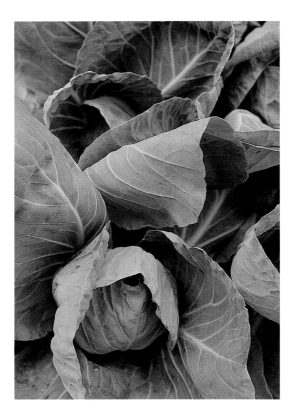

considered it as a digestive remedy, joint tonic and cooling preparation for skin problems and fevers. Raw cabbage eaten before meat was reckoned to prevent drunkenness by over-indulgent Romans. In Germany *sauerkraut*, a fermented cabbage mixture, is regarded as a preventative for cancer, rheumatism, gout and premature ageing.

using cabbage
The vegetable is highly anti-bacterial, encourages healing and tissue growth and will also reduce inflammation and rheumatic pains. The leaves have been used as anti-inflammatory poultices to relieve complaints ranging from arthritis to mastitis, while cabbage lotions were once a regular household standby for skin problems. The plant also helps cleanse the liver and improve digestion. Both juices and infusions can be used to treat a range of digestive problems including stomach ulcers.

The fresh leaves can be used directly on inflammations, aching limbs or arthritic joints while cabbage lotion is ideal for acne.

tea *Camellia sinensis*

When tea was first introduced into Europe in the 17th century it was regarded not as an everyday drink but as a medicinal herb; numerous tea-house advertisements from the time extol the plant's virtues as a digestive remedy and cure for over-indulgence. Tea has been drunk in China since around 3000 BC when a mythical figure, Shen Nong – the "divine husbandman" – supposedly discovered its

◄ Cabbage *Brassica oleracea*

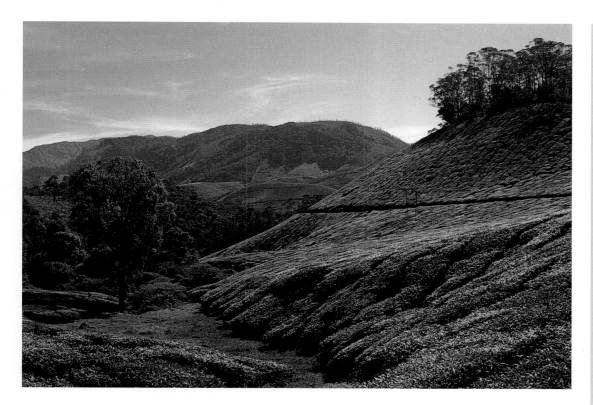

tea

part used
leaves

commercial products
black, oolong and green teas are readily available loose or in tea bags; green tea is increasingly available as a food supplement in capsules or tablets and is also used in a number of cosmetic products.

how to use
infusion – use 1tsp per cup and drink up to four cups a day;
capsules – 600mg up to 3 times a day;
use damp green tea leaves or an infused green tea bag to ease insect bites and stings.

properties when a few leaves fell from an overhanging branch into a kettle of water he was boiling, conveniently, underneath.

using tea

The plant has a stimulating effect on the nervous system thanks to its caffeine-like alkaloids. The caffeine-like effect also encourages kidney function accounting for the common diuretic effect of too much tea drinking. Most of the tea drunk in the West is black tea made by fermenting the leaves, while green tea is made from leaves that have been pan-fried and then dried. Oolong tea comes in between as a partly fermented variation.

Tea is also anti-bacterial and can slow damaging oxidisation in tissue. Green tea is believed to improve resistance to stomach and skin cancers, although there is currently some

▲ Tea *Camellia sinensis*

controversy over research results, and it can also stimulate the immune system. It is rich in fluoride so can help fight any tendency for tooth decay and is also useful for soothing insect bites. Oolong tea is generally regarded as a digestive remedy and is now known to reduce cholesterol levels and so may be useful to combat atherosclerosis. In China, green tea is considered as cooling and is preferred in hot weather, while oolong and black teas are more warming for cold days.

Black tea — most common in the West — is very rich in tannins so is especially astringent and is ideal — unsweetened and without milk — to ease the lower bowel discomfort associated with diarrhoea. It is also a traditional Cantonese remedy for hangovers.

part used
fruit

commercial products
fresh and dried chilis are sold in most greengrocers and supermarkets; capsules and tinctures are readily available in health food shops while small amounts of chili are included in dozens of proprietary herbal remedies mainly for coughs, colds and circulatory problems.

how to use
chili can be irritant so use in small doses;
tincture – 0.5-1ml/10-20 drops three times daily;
capsules (500mg) – one per dose;
infused oil can be made using the hot method (see page 224) with around 50g/2oz of dried chili to 1 litre/1¾pt of sunflower oil.

chili *Capsicum frutescens*

Chili, or cayenne, has become familiar in sauces and flavourings in recent years thanks to growing interest in oriental, Mexican and West Indian cookery. The herb first arrived in Britain from India in the 1540s and was known as "ginnie pepper". Gerard was less than enthusiastic about its properties, declaring that it was an "enemie of the liver" and would also "killeth dogs". He did, however, recommend it for scrofula – a then-prevalent lymphatic throat and skin infection known as the King's Evil and reputedly healed by the touch of a reigning monarch.

Various chili species are available: *C. frutescens* is generally used in medicine while the hotter variety, *C. annuum,* is often used in cooking. Chili became extremely popular in the 19th century with the Physiomedicalists (see page 10), a group of traditional healers originating in 18th-century New England where the icy winters certainly brought plenty of colds and chills to be warmed by spicy herbs. Chili increases perspiration so was a popular component in the "sweating" treatments favoured by the Physiomedicalists and based on the Native American tradition of sweat lodges used to counter various illnesses. Many Western herbalists still add chili to mixtures for treating such "cold" complaints as arthritis, digestive weakness and general debility, and it is regarded as a useful stimulant for both the digestion and the circulation.

using chili

Like many traditional culinary herbs, it also helps expel excess gas from the digestive system, so will reduce the risk of indigestion

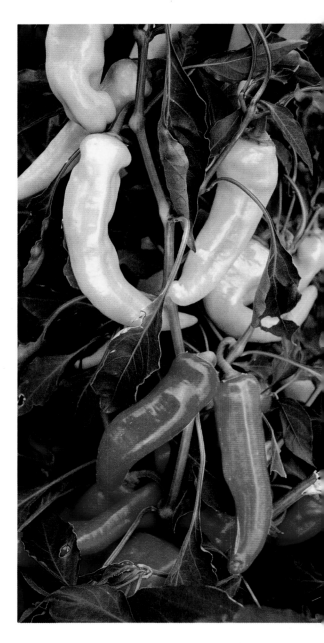

▲ Chili *Capsicum frutescens*

and of abdominal bloating after a heavy meal; chili is also antiseptic and anti-bacterial which may also explain its popularity as a seasoning in combating stomach upsets from food poisoning.

Externally, chili ointments are used to ease

irritation and stimulate blood flow to the skin so may be used for treating chilblains, lumbago, muscle pain, the pain of shingles and nerve pain (neuralgia).

caution avoid high doses in pregnancy.

bitter orange
Citrus aurantium

The bitter, or Seville, orange is familiar from that favourite breakfast delicacy, marmalade. The name reputedly originates from the French *marmelade*, a traditional mixture of stewed apples and quince, although a more picturesque legend has it derived from *mer malade* or sea sickness. This fits in neatly with bitter orange's digestive properties to ease flatulence and nausea making it a potent remedy for both travel and morning sickness as well as digestive upsets.

The plant originated in China – where it is still extensively used to relieve both nausea and coughs – and by the Middle Ages it was a favourite with Arabian physicians. In the 16th century, an Italian princess called Anna-Marie de Nerola is reputed to have discovered an oil – neroli – that could be extracted from the flowers. The princess used her discovery to scent her gloves – today, with neroli oil costing around £1,000 a litre (1¾pt) or more most people would consider it far too precious to lavish on any sort of clothing. Neroli is used in aromatherapy as a calming sedative and tonic and will also ease cramping pains.

using bitter orange
Bitter orange is also a stimulating tonic remedy and will increase the coughing response so is a useful palatable addition for cough remedies; more recent research suggests that it can reduce high blood pressure and it also stimulates urination.

Bergamot oil is distilled from the fruit and is used in aromatherapy for urinary tract problems. It has strong anti-bacterial properties to combat infections and is also the familiar flavouring used to scent Earl Grey tea. Bergamot can increase the photosensitivity of the skin and was once added to sunbathing lotions to speed up the tanning process – although given current concerns over the links between suntan and cancer this practice is now less common. Petitgrain oil is used as a gentle astringent and skin tonic in many beauty preparations.

The sweet orange (*C. sinensis*) is a good source of vitamin C but lacks bitter orange's medicinal properties. Use Seville oranges in cooking for indigestion, nausea or add extracts to cough mixtures.

caution avoid excessively high doses of bitter orange in pregnancy.

lemon *Citrus limonum*

Lemon was considered by the Romans as an antidote for many poisons and in modern Italy eating fresh lemons is still believed, by many, to combat major epidemic infections. They are certainly very rich in minerals and vitamins – including vitamins B_1, B_2, B_3, carotene (pro-vitamin A) and vitamin C (up to 50mg per 100g/3½oz of fruit) – as well as being both anti-bacterial and anti-viral.

bitter orange

parts used
fruit, peel, essential oils

commercial products
sold under the names *Zhi Ke* (ripe orange) and *Zhi Shi* (unripe orange) by Chinese herbalists and sometimes found as tinctures; essential oils are neroli (orange blossom), petitgrain (leaves) and bergamot (fruit peel); fresh bitter (Seville) oranges are sold for marmalade making in January/February.

how to use
tincture – 1-2 drops on the tongue to combat nausea as required or up to 2ml/40 drops, three times daily;
up to 9g/¼oz per dose in Chinese decoctions.

parts used

fruit, essential oil

commercial products

lemon extracts are added to many proprietary cough syrups or sore throat lozenges (often in combination with honey) and the oil is used in insect repellent sprays; commercial lemon juices sometimes contain sulphur extracts as a preservative.

how to use

fresh lemon – use warmed slices or fresh juice to ease neuralgia pains and skin irritations or add to warm water as a gargle;

juice – add 1-2tbsp to herbal infusions for coughs, colds, minor infections or digestive upsets;

oil – dilute 4-5 drops in 1tsp of sunflower oil to relieve insect stings and the pain of neuralgia or use in gargles (see right).

using lemons

Lemons can improve the peripheral circulation and are tonifying for heart and blood vessels; as a venous tonic they may be helpful for piles and varicose veins. In folk medicine, lemons have always been a popular remedy for feverish chills and coughs and 5-10 drops of lemon oil diluted in water (or warm lemon juice) makes a good household standby as a gargle for sore throats.

Lemon has anti-inflammatory and anti-histamine properties and the juice can be used to ease sunburn and irritant skin rashes. It will also help to stop bleeding so can be used on cotton-wool swabs to speed clotting in nosebleeds, or as an emergency antiseptic wash for minor cuts and grazes.

Lemon is also popular in traditional beauty treatments to whiten the skin and teeth, and to encourage freckles to fade. Mixed with equal amounts of glycerine and eau de Cologne lemon juice makes a soothing and softening hand lotion. Rotten lemons can also be used to repel ants from the house or garden.

caution essential lemon oil can often be heavily contaminated with pesticides unless it is produced from organically grown fruit; use organically grown or unwaxed fresh lemons wherever possible.

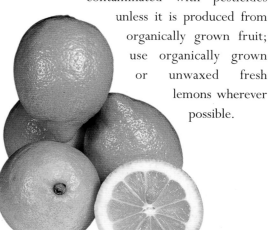

➤ Coffee *Coffea arabica*

coffee *Coffea arabica*

Originally grown in Ethiopia, coffee spread throughout the Arab world, reached Western Europe in the 17th century and was finally introduced into South America by settlers. It is now one of the world's most important cash crops; millions drink cups every day and an entire industry has emerged producing the necessary equipment – percolators, cafetières and filters – to process it.

using coffee

Coffee's best known medicinal action is as a stimulant, thanks to its high caffeine content (three parts in 1,000). This alkaloid stimulates the central nervous system and increases heart rate (which in turn speeds blood flow through the kidneys, so has a mild diuretic action as well). Coffee is also anti-narcotic and is used in narcotic poisoning to prevent sleep. Palpitations are a common side-effect of too much coffee-drinking. Individual tolerances vary – try not to drink more than a maximum of four cups (not four mugs) a day.

Coffee also helps to counter nausea and vomiting (much appreciated by hangover sufferers) and in folk medicine the powdered beans have also been used as an emergency application to burns and scalds to control inflammation. In homoeopathic doses, coffee has the opposite effect and is used for anxiety, insomnia, stress, nervous headaches and hyperactivity. As a home remedy coffee is worth remembering as a digestive stimulant which can increase gastro-intestinal activity and also for its anti-emetic effects.

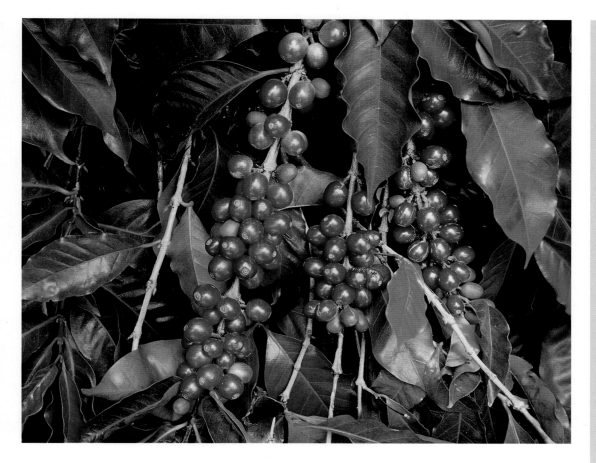

coffee

part used
beans

commercial products
available in
homoeopathic dosage
(Coffea 30X or 60X);
included in
anthroposophical
remedies used for
nervous stress and
excitability.

how to use
homoeopathic dosages
for insomnia, nervous
excitement and fainting –
one tablet or 1-2 drops
of tincture every 30-60
minutes.

cucumber *Cucumis sativus*

"Cool as a cucumber" reminds us that in Galenic medicine plants were classified as "cool" or "hot", "dry" or "moist", and that the classification largely dictated medicinal properties. John Gerard, writing in 1597, describes cucumbers as "cold and moist in the second degree they putrifie soone in the stomacke and yield unto the body a cold and moist nourishment, and that very little, and the same not good".

Later writers have been rather more encouraging – the French herbalist Jean Valnet considers cucumber as cleansing, diuretic and refreshing, helping to dissolve uric acid, so useful for gout and arthritis, where build-up of urates in the joints can contribute to inflammation; he suggests cucumber cooked in soups as a suitable remedy.

using cucumber

Cucumbers are around 95% water but do contain vitamins A, B-complex and C as well as manganese, sulphur and other minerals, so are reasonably nutritious. Slices of cucumber are useful as eye-pads for soothing tired and inflamed eyes, while internally they can – as Gerard noted – cool the stomach, so are a useful food to eat for gastric irritations and colic: lightly cooked cucumber is best for digestive problems.

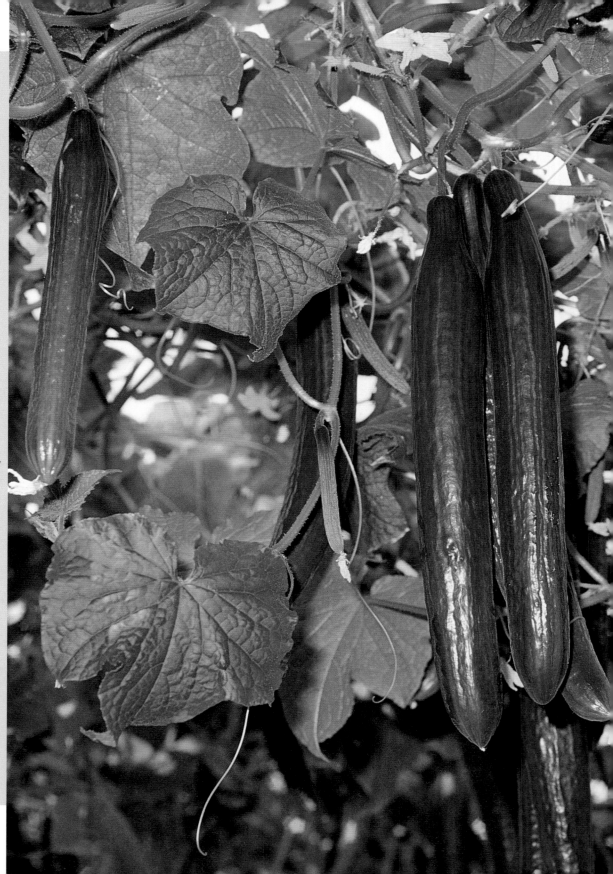

cucumber

part used

fruit

commercial products

not generally used in commercial medicinal products although fresh cucumber can be bought throughout the year.

how to use

freshly cut cucumber slices – to soothe tired eyes, insect bites or skin irritations;

lotion – make a skin lotion by combining 50g/2oz of shelled and peeled almonds and 250g/9oz of cucumber, peeled and deseeded in a food processor, add 250ml/9fl oz of alcohol (e.g. vodka) and 2 drops of rose oil and use for dry skin.

Cucumbers are also a favourite with beauticians as the basis for moisturisers and other skin products. They are ideal for relieving sunburn and minor skin irritations. Cucumber lotion or juice can also be helpful for enlarged pores, oily skins, wrinkles and skin blemishes and are soothing for insect stings, cold sores and prickly heat.

globe artichoke
Cynara cardunculus
(Scolymus Group)

Globe artichokes have been regarded as a delicacy since the days of Theophrastus in the fourth century BC: he tells us that the plant grew in Sicily and while good to eat, must be enjoyed fresh since – unlike many other vegetables – it could not be pickled in brine (a favourite Greek method of storing winter vegetables).

using artichoke
The edible part is actually the flower head and until recently this bitter-tasting vegetable was regarded as little more than a mild digestive stimulant. However, we now know that cynarin, found in the plant, can stimulate bile flow and also has a protective action on the liver, encouraging crème regeneration and repair. It is also considered a potent remedy for gall bladder problems, with artichoke juice used to ease the symptoms of nausea, pain and indigestion associated with poor gall bladder function. The plant's stimulating effect on the liver and gall bladder also makes it laxative – which explains

◄ Cucumber *Cucumis sativus*

why eating a large serving of artichokes can have a surprisingly stimulating effect on bowel function.

Researchers have also found that globe artichoke can help to lower blood cholesterol levels, possibly associated with the healing effect it has on fatty degeneration of the liver.

As well as these important actions, artichokes are diuretic and will encourage uric acid excretion, so may be supportive for gout sufferers; the flowerheads are also cleansing and energising. Eating artichokes can be helpful in convalescence, arthritic disorders and whenever there are liver or gall bladder problems.

The globe artichoke should not be confused with Jerusalem artichoke *(Helianthus tuberosus)*, a North American relative of the sunflower cultivated for its tuberous roots, which are eaten as a vegetable. The plant was brought to Europe at the end of the 16th century and was known as "potatoes of Canada". The tubers are rich in a starch called inulin, which does not break down in the digestive process to form glucose, so Jerusalem

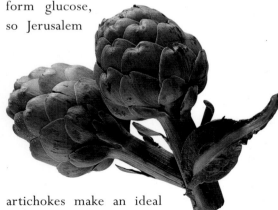

artichokes make an ideal food for diabetes sufferers. Although little used medicinally, Jerusalem artichokes can be helpful as a digestive stimulant and in constipation.

globe artichoke

part used
flower heads

commercial products
available as bottled juice or in capsules from health food shops; artichoke tincture is sold by specialist herbal suppliers; the herb is included in a number of over-the-counter products mainly sold as stimulating liver remedies.

how to use
juice – 10ml/2tsp, three times daily; *tincture* – up to 5ml/1tsp per dose, three times daily; *capsules* 300mg, three times daily.

jerusalem artichoke

part used
tubers

commercial products
not generally used although fresh tubers are sold as a seasonal vegetable in late autumn and winter.

how to use
cook in salted water for 25-30 minutes and mash with a little crème fraîche or yoghurt as a nutritious food in debility and convalescence or for constipation; alternatively allow to cool, then thinly slice the cooked tubers and serve with vinaigrette and chopped parsley.

carrot

Daucus carota subsp. *sativus*

The wild carrot *(D. carota),* also known as Queen Anne's lace, is a popular medicinal herb widely used as a diuretic and carminative and given for urinary stones, cystitis and gout. Wild carrot root is white and inedible but the more familiar orange vegetable also has valuable properties.

The carrot has been cultivated in most parts of Europe and North Africa since ancient times and, until the introduction of the potato from North America, it was widely eaten as a staple food. It is rich in a substance called *beta*-carotene, which is converted into vitamin A in the body, and is traditionally said to improve the eyesight – vitamin A is essential for good night vision. Carrots are also a good source of vitamins B and C, and of several minerals including iron, potassium and calcium.

using carrot

As well as being highly nutritious, carrots are believed to stimulate the immune system and in recent years have been regarded as an important addition to anti-cancer diets. Carrots and carrot juice are also recommended as a readily digestible food source in debility and convalescence and for anaemia, diarrhoea, chest problems (including chronic bronchitis), rheumatism, gout, constipation, intestinal worms and digestive upsets.

Externally they can be used for skin disorders – including eczema – and abscesses: both the juice and carrot oil are used. Research also suggests that *beta*-carotene can provide some protection from the sun's ultra-violet rays, so carrot is often suggested by beauticians as a useful supplement before sunbathing.

caution vitamin A is one of the few vitamins that can be extremely toxic in large doses, affecting the liver and turning the skin a yellow colour; however, *beta*-carotene is believed to be rather safer as most of the surplus is excreted.

fig *Ficus carica*

Fig syrup has been used as a household standby for constipation since the days of the Pharaohs. An ancient Egyptian papyrus dating from 1500 BC gives a recipe based on figs soaked overnight in "sweet beer" which had to be drunk "often". The Egyptians also regarded the fig as a heart remedy and recommended it to combat lung disease – possibly based on a Doctrine of Signatures theory as the rounded, ripe fig vaguely resembles these organs.

The fig originated in Asia Minor but has been grown in Western Europe since Roman times: the French king Charlemagne encouraged fig growing in the ninth century and the tree is still a common sight in rural French gardens.

using figs

The fruits have a laxative effect and are often used combined with senna *(Senna alexandrina).* Externally fig poultices were once applied to boils and varicose ulcers, and the fruit is also considered as a demulcent to soothe irritated tissues such as in sore throats, coughs and bronchial problems.

Eating fresh or dried figs for breakfast is a pleasant way to counter any tendency to habitual constipation.

➤ Fig *Ficus carica*

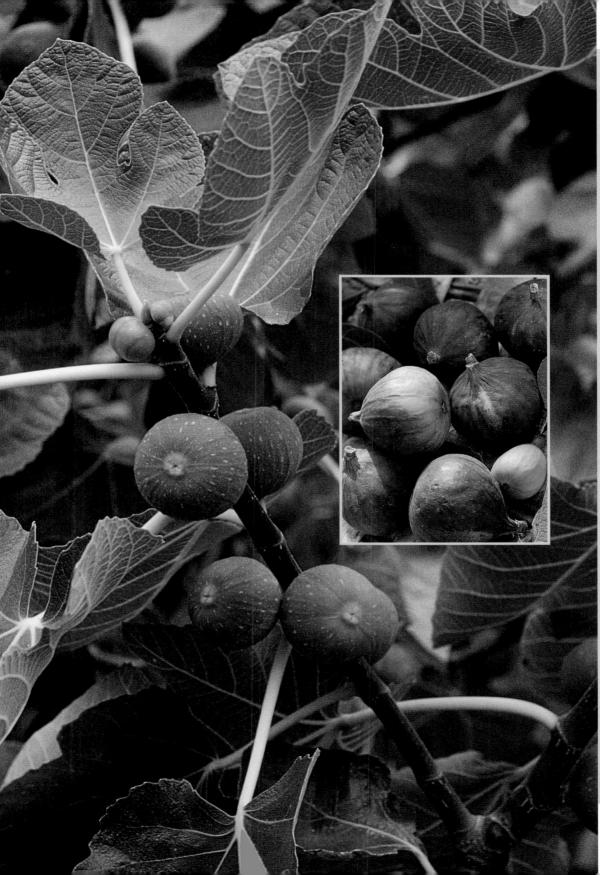

fig

part used

fruit

commercial products

bottled juice is sold in
health food shops; figs
and fig extracts are
included in various
proprietary remedies for
constipation and sluggish
digestion.

how to use

juice – 10ml/2tsp, three
times a day;
whole fruit – eat 1-2 fresh
or dried figs a day or add
to breakfast cereal; use
the fresh fruit pulped in
poultices for skin sores.

strawberry

parts used
fruit, leaves

commercial products
dried leaves available
from specialist herbal
suppliers; included in
some anthroposophical
remedies for stress and
nervous tension.

how to use
infusion - 25g/1oz of
dried leaves to
500ml/1pt of boiling
water taken in three
doses during the day for
digestive upsets;
fresh fruit - crushed in
poultices for skin irritations
or combined with an
equal volume of distilled
witch hazel in a food
processor to make a skin
lotion.

strawberry *Fragaria vesca*

In Galenic medicine strawberries were considered as very cooling: Gerard recommends them to "quench thirst, cooleth heate of the stomicke and inflammation of the liver". He did, however, warn against eating them in winter or on a "cold stomicke" as this would increase the

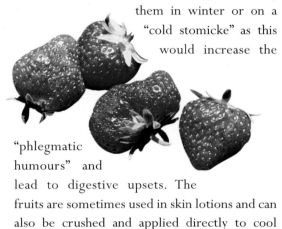

"phlegmatic humours" and lead to digestive upsets. The fruits are sometimes used in skin lotions and can also be crushed and applied directly to cool sunburn, skin irritations and minor wounds.

They contain vitamins B, C and E as well as high levels of iron, sodium, calcium and silica, so are extremely nutritious. Strawberries are, however, high in salicylates so those sensitive to aspirin often find that consumption leads to irritant skin rashes.

using strawberries

Strawberries have been cultivated in Britain since at least the 10th century and were valued as both a food and a healing remedy. The leaves are mildly astringent and diuretic and are often added to herbal tea blends: they can be helpful for diarrhoea and digestive upsets.

The root was once a popular household remedy for diarrhoea and the stalks were used for wounds – Culpeper declared it "singularly good for the healing of many ills".

The fruit has been used for various ailments in folk tradition and will help clear uric acid from the system, so can be helpful for gout, urinary stones and liver disorders. The juice also has some anti-bacterial action and was traditionally taken to combat typhoid. Furthermore, strawberries were supposed to encourage longevity and one French herbalist claimed that eating 500g/1lb of the fruit a day during the season was essential for a long life.

walnut *Juglans regia*

The Greeks believed that in some far-off Golden Age when the gods walked upon the earth they lived on walnuts – hence the name *Juglans* or *Jovis glans,* Jupiter's nuts. The tree probably originated in Persia but has been cultivated in Europe since ancient times: the Roman writer Varro (born 116 BC) records that walnuts were growing in Italy in his lifetime.

using walnut

Walnut leaves and bark have traditionally been used in Europe as a remedy for constipation and skin problems while the Chinese regarded the nuts as a tonic for the kidneys. A recent US study suggests that regular consumption of walnuts can also reduce cholesterol levels and lower the risk of heart attacks. Under the Doctrine of Signatures the nuts were taken to resemble the brain, so they were used for mental illness – one expects with little effect.

The oil, pressed from the seeds, was popular with the Romans and is still a favourite salad oil today. In recent years it has been found to contain essential fatty acids (*cis*-linoleic and

➤ Walnut *Juglans regia*

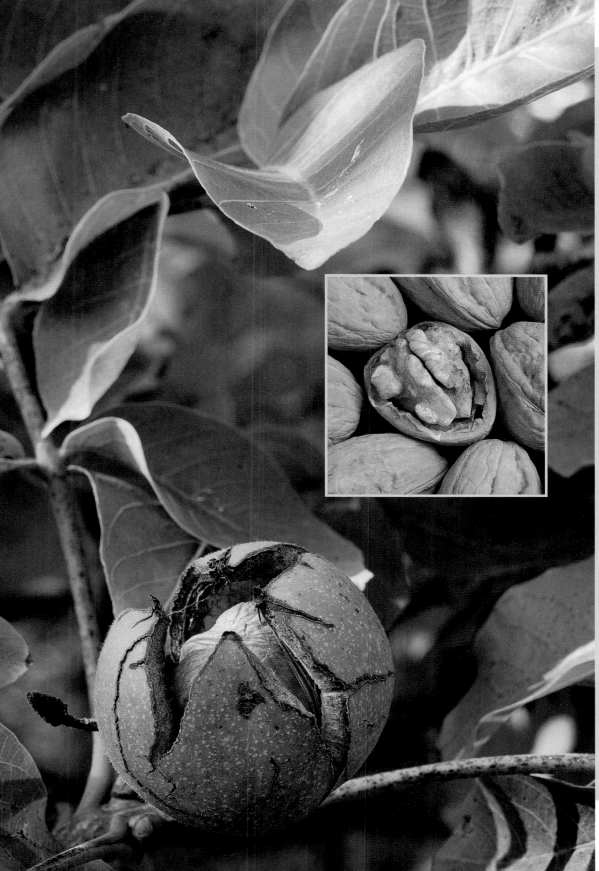

walnut

parts used

nut, inner bark, seed oil

commercial products

walnut extracts are included in some proprietary remedies for digestive problems; tincture (leaf) is available from specialist suppliers; walnut oil (cold pressed) is available from good-quality grocers.

how to use

infusion (leaves) – 25g/1oz of dried leaves to 500ml/1pt of boiling water taken in three doses daily;

tincture (bark) – up to 3ml/60 drops, 2-3 times daily as a laxative;

nuts – eat a serving, fresh, daily as a kidney tonic;

oil – take 5-10ml/1-2tsp daily in salad dressings or on vegetables.

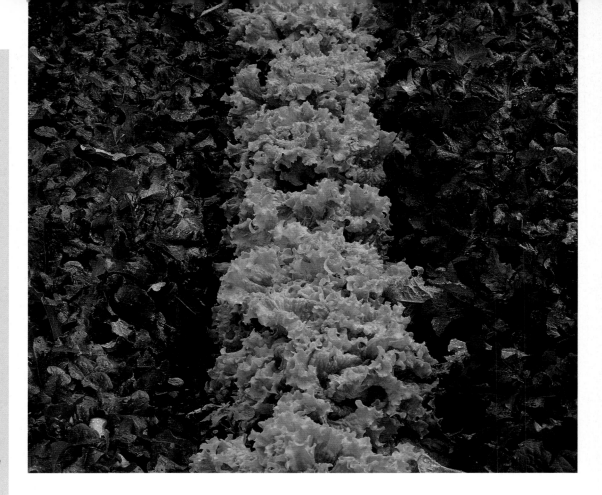

lettuce

parts used

aerial parts, dried juice

commercial products

wild lettuce leaf and juice extracts are included in numerous proprietary mixtures for insomnia and nervous tension sold by health food shops; tincture available from specialist suppliers.

how to use

fresh lettuce – eat at the start of a meal as a digestive stimulant; *decoction* – use 75g/2½oz to 750ml/1½pt of water in a decoction, simmered for 30 minutes and taken in wine glass doses after meals as a digestive remedy and mild sedative or externally as a lotion for acne; pulp a whole fresh lettuce in a food processor and take in 10ml/2tsp doses for period pains; *wild lettuce tincture* – up to 5ml/1tsp at night for insomnia or 1-2ml/20-40 drops, three times daily for nervous tension.

alpha-linolenic acids) which, like the more widely promoted *gamma*-linolenic acid from evening primrose oil (see page 153), are vital for normal bodily function. Thanks to its essential fatty acids, walnut oil makes an ideal and comparatively low-cost base for cold infused oils or massage rubs.

lettuce *Lactuca sativa*

Although the wild lettuce *(L. virosa)* is normally used in herbal medicine, as a potent sedative and painkiller, cultivated varieties have a long history of healing uses as well. The cos lettuce was cultivated in Ancient Egypt and held sacred to Min, the god of fertility – probably because its milky juice was thought to resemble semen. This latex was used by the Assyrians as a cough mixture and until the 1930s similar dried juice – extracted from the wild lettuce – was sold in British pharmacies as "lettuce opium" and applied in much the same way as the rather more potent drug.

Despite Egyptian preoccupations, lettuce latex is generally regarded as an anaphrodisiac and the herb was known as "the eunuch's plant" in ancient Greece.

using lettuce

The cultivated lettuce is milder in action than its wild cousin, but can also be used as a cleansing, mildly laxative and digestive stimulant. Serving lettuce as a first course can help stimulate the digestion for heavier instalments of the meal. As a cleansing remedy lettuce can be helpful for various arthritic problems and constipation. It has also been used for period pains, liver congestion and a variety of nervous disorders and over-excitement (including hyperactivity in children).

Externally the leaf decoction can be used as a lotion for acne, while the leaves steeped in olive oil have been recommended for boils and abscesses.

shiitake mushrooms
Lentinula edodes

Among the many exotic fruits and vegetables which have joined the supermarket shelves in recent years is the shiitake mushroom – favoured by many because it has a more exotic flavour than the familiar cultivated button and cap mushrooms *(Agaricus bisporus)*. It is also an important medicinal plant with an impressive list of actions now identified by modern research.

The plant is known to reduce cholesterol levels, protect the liver from toxins, stimulate the immune system and combat various viruses, including HIV, *Herpes simplex* and viruses responsible for polio, measles, mumps and encephalitis. Much of this activity is due to a chemical called lentinan which is sometimes sold as a specific extract. Shiitake has been used in Japan to help support patients undergoing chemotherapy and it has been shown to reduce

the growth rate of liver tumours; in the USA it has been used for AIDS sufferers and is believed to improve the immune and endocrine function in the elderly.

The mushroom has featured in traditional Chinese medicine for at least 2,000 years although shiitake is actually the Japanese name – the Chinese call it *Xiang Gu*. It was regarded as restoring and stimulating and used as a gentle tonic.

using shiitake mushrooms
Given their array of properties it is well worth making shiitake mushrooms part of a regular diet: they can be especially helpful in colds and influenza to help combat the viral infection and strengthen the immune system and they can also be useful in candidiasis (contrary to some advice to avoid eating fungi when suffering from yeast infections). Many nutritionists also consider them as a useful addition to anti-cancer diets.

In traditional Chinese medicine the typical dose was 6-16g/⅛-½oz of dried mushroom or 90g/3¼oz of fresh taken in a soup up to three times a day. That sort of quantity may be ideal for combating acute colds but for regular therapeutic use could well result in gastric upsets. A single daily serving would be more suitable for general use.

tomato
Lycopersicon esculentum

The familiar tomato originates from Peru and was introduced into Europe by the Spanish *conquistadors* in the 16th century. The first tomatoes to arrive were golden in colour – hence the Italian name *pomodoro*, golden apple. By the

---

shiitake mushrooms

part used
fruiting body

commercial products
fresh and dried mushrooms generally available from good supermarkets; tincture and capsules often sold by Chinese herbalists under the name *Xiang Gu*.

how to use
tincture – up to 5ml/1tsp, three times daily;
capsules – up to 600mg three times daily;
fresh mushrooms – up to 100g/3½oz per portion (or dried, up to 25g/1oz) in soup.

tomato

part used
fruit

commercial products
juice widely sold in
supermarkets as a soft
drink or as a therapeutic
extract in health food
shops; buy organically
grown extracts if possible.

how to use
eat at least 10 servings
(1tbsp as juice or pulped
extracts) each week; use
raw slices to ease skin
irritations.

apple

part used
fruit

commercial products
juice readily available;
powdered apple
available for use in teas.

how to use
stewed apple - eat a
serving (1tbsp) 1-2 times
per day for diarrhoea
and digestive upsets;
ripe apples - eat daily
for constipation or
mashed in poultices for
skin problems;
juice - use externally to
bathe eyes to ease
conjunctivitis.

time the fruit arrived in Britain in the 17th century, this had been corrupted, via France, to *pomme adorée* – hence the old name "love apples".

At first the fruits were grown purely as ornamentals and, like other members of the Solanaceae family, were considered as highly toxic. Eventually they found their way into the kitchen and are now an essential component of numerous recipes: cooking without tomatoes would be bland indeed.

using tomato

The fruits are rich in vitamins A, B_1, B_2, B_6, C, D, bioflavonoids and folic acid; they also include a number of trace elements and organic acids, so are highly nutritious. Tomatoes stimulate the digestion – particularly the pancreas – so tomato juice makes a good aperitif. It can improve the appetite and is ideal in debility and

▼ Tomato *Lycopersicon esculentum*

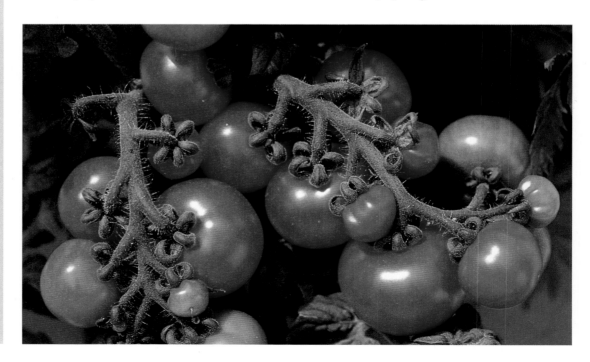

convalescence. As tomatoes also contain the flavonoid rutin, they can be helpful for strengthening the capillaries. Externally slices of raw tomato can ease insect bites and the juice makes an effective lotion for acne.

Recent reports from the USA suggest that men who eat at least 10 servings of tomatoes a week have a 45% reduction in the risk of prostate cancer, possibly due to the presence of lycopene, a type of carotene, which may be anti-tumour; studies also suggest that tomatoes could have a similar effect in reducing the risk of ovarian cancers.

apple *Malus communis*

Eating an apple a day to "keep the doctor away" is advice that many will remember from childhood. Today, research suggests that regular doses could play a significant role in anti-cancer

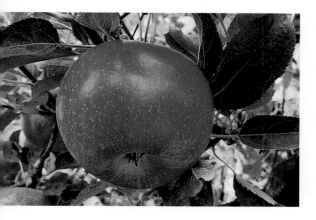

▲ Apple *Malus communis*

diets and have considerable therapeutic properties; apples have also been shown to help lower blood cholesterol levels, so can act as a preventative for heart and arterial disorders.

Our ancestors may have lacked scientific research but they certainly knew apples were good for them: the crab apple *(M. sylvestris)* is mentioned in the Anglo-Saxon poem, the *Lacnunga,* which tells of the nine herbs given as healing plants to the world by the god Woden. Cultivated apples *(M. communis)* have figured in the household medicine chest since at least Roman times.

using apple

Unripe apples can be eaten as an astringent remedy for diarrhoea, while ripe ones have a laxative effect. The Greeks regarded apple juice and apple teas as cooling and so prescribed them for fevers or used them externally on inflammations such as conjunctivitis.

Raw apples can also be mashed and used as a soothing poultice for skin inflammations. Cooked apples — like unripe ones — are a traditional remedy for diarrhoea and dysentery. They can be soothing in gastritis and ulcerative colitis.

watercress
Nasturtium officinalis

Watercress originates from Persia and was highly valued in the ancient world. The Greek writer Xenophon describes how the Persians would eat large amounts of watercress as an energy tonic when faced with heavy physical labour and they also, very sensibly, fed it to their children to encourage healthy development. Mediaeval herbalists appreciated its diuretic properties and recommended it for kidney stones and bladder disorders.

using watercress

The plant has an exceptionally high mineral and vitamin content, making it one of our most nutritious vegetables. The leaves contain four times as much vitamin C, weight for weight, as lettuce and more calcium than whole milk. It is also an excellent source of vitamin A and is very rich in manganese and iron, making it a valuable food in iron-deficient anaemia, debility and convalescence. It is also an ideal spring tonic — either eaten in salads or as freshly pressed juice.

Watercress can also help to reduce blood sugar so can be helpful in late-onset diabetes and its slight bitterness makes it a valuable digestive stimulant.

As a cleansing remedy it can be helpful for arthritis, rheumatism and skin disorders.

olive *Olea europaea*

Olive trees have been cultivated in Europe since well before 2500 BC and amphoras of olive oil have been found at such historic sites as the citadel at Mycenae — palace of Homer's

watercress

parts used
aerial parts

commercial products
included in few over-the-counter cleansing remedies for rheumatic and skin disorders or products to reduce blood pressure; bottled juice available from health food shops; tincture available from specialist suppliers.

how to use
tincture – up to 5ml/1tsp three times daily;
juice – 10ml/2tsp three times daily, home-made juice can be made by pulping a bunch in a food processor.

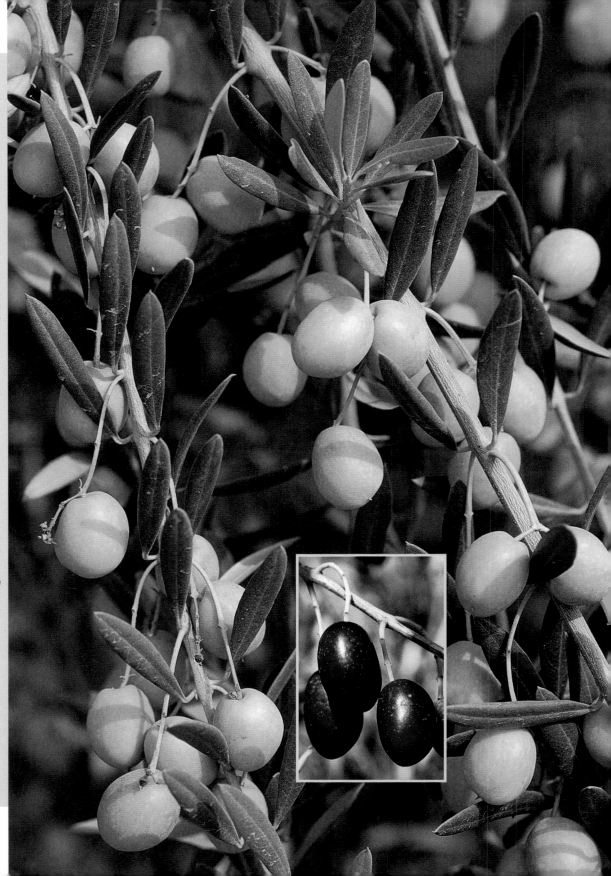

olive

parts used

fruit, oil

commercial products

good-quality olive oil is readily available in supermarkets although health food shops also sell capsules containing up to 300mg of olive oil either alone or in combination with other seed oils; dried leaves occasionally available from specialist herbal suppliers.

how to use

oil – 5ml/1tsp up to three times daily or use as a dressing on salads and vegetables; externally as a scalp massage and to ease aches and pains; *capsules* – up to 4 per dose, three times daily; *infusions* – 25g/1oz of dried leaves to 500ml/1pt of boiling water, the leaves are quite tough so need to be infused for at least 20 minutes, taken in three doses daily.

Agamemnon. In ancient Egypt, the oil was burned in lamps, used in cooking and formed the basis of scented oils. There is little evidence, however, that it was used medicinally. The Greeks also associated it with the goddess Athena – a symbol of wisdom.

using olive

Olive oil is still prized for cooking and today we know that it contains oleic acid (a mono-unsaturated fatty acid) and some *cis*-linoleic acid and is thus a good source of essential fatty acids and rather healthier than the saturated fats of butter and animal products. The oil can be taken in teaspoon doses for constipation or for treating pinworms in children; it also helps to reduce gastric secretions by coating the stomach lining and can thus be ideal for peptic ulcers, while a daily dessertspoonful of oil is believed to help protect against atherosclerosis.

In recent years olive oil has also figured in anti-candida diets and has been recommended by many to combat cancer and ageing, thanks to its anti-oxidant properties.

Traditionally olive oil has been massaged into the scalp to counter dandruff and improve hair quality or used as a rub for rheumatism. The oil is soothing and softening for the skin and can also be used in cosmetics preparations. Olive oil is a common ingredient in folk liniments for muscle strains and sprains and there are even anecdotal reports that swallowing a couple of olive stones can relieve back pain within hours.

The leaves are also used medicinally and are known to reduce blood sugar levels and – thanks to French research in the 1930s – lower

◄ Olive *Olea europaea*

blood pressure. They are antispasmodic, diuretic and will stimulate bile flow. Olive leaf tea can be helpful for reducing moderately high blood pressure and is used in Mediterranean countries for urinary tract infections.

apricot *Prunus armeniaca*

Apricots originate in China where the seeds, known as *Xing Ren*, are mainly used as a cough remedy for asthma and bronchitis. The trees spread gradually from the Middle East and arrived in England in Tudor times.

The Chinese bake apricot stones to reduce the amount of the chemical amygdalin they contain; this constituent has a sedative effect on the respiratory system and can be toxic in large quantities; the stones are then traditionally added to decoctions for coughs or ground into a powder and used in various remedies.

using apricot

The fruits are highly nutritious, being very rich in vitamins A, B-complex and C, and a good source of many essential minerals, including iron, calcium and manganese. Apricots are useful to counter iron-deficient anaemia and are often included in herbal "iron tonics".

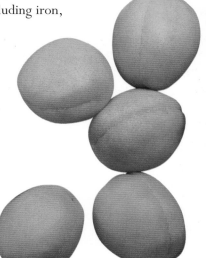

apricot

parts used
fruit, seeds, seed oil

commercial products
seeds are sold as *Xing Ren* by Chinese herbal suppliers and are sometimes found in tinctures; organically-grown dried apricots are readily available in supermarkets.

how to use
Xing Ren – usually up to 9g/¼oz per dose in traditional Chinese "*Tang*" or decoctions or 20-30 drops as tincture, three times per day;
tonic – make iron tonic by covering 500g/1lb of dried apricots with water, add 500g/1lb of sugar and simmer overnight in a slow cooker. remove stones and process in a blender, add 1 litre/ 1¾pt of red wine and mix well. Take 5-10ml/ 1-2tsp three times daily.

Dried apricots are laxative and eating an excess can often lead to diarrhoea; fresh apricots, however, are astringent and have an anti-diarrhoeal effect. The fruits are also strengthening for the immune system and both apricots and apricot jam have been variously used in European folk medicine as a nerve tonic, to combat insomnia and in convalescence.

Apricot oil can be used much as almond oil (see below) in cosmetics such as a skin softener.

almond *Prunus dulcis*

Almond trees have been a favourite in English gardens since Shakespeare's day and generally fruit well. The tree originates from the Middle East and its Hebrew name – *shakud* – means "hasty awakening", with the almond blossom seen as heralding the spring.

Almond oil has been produced from the nuts since the days of the ancient Greeks, while the Romans regarded eating almonds as the ideal means of countering the effects of alcohol. Gerard, writing in 1597, repeats the tradition telling us that "…five or six being taken fasting do keepe a man from being drunke". He also recommends eating almonds after childbirth to encourage expulsion of the placenta and suggests mixing almonds with barley water to produce a strengthening drink for "sicke and feeble persons". Rather more familiar to us today are his recommendations for using almond oil in hand creams and as a remedy for spots and pimples.

using almonds

Almonds are extremely rich in vitamin A and have a high calorie value, so are a useful nutrient; they are also considered a good nerve tonic and have some antiseptic properties helping to cleanse the digestive system. Externally almond oil makes an excellent base for many skin remedies, including eczema and acne, and is widely used in cosmetics. The oil can be used as a base for massage rubs for aches, pains and other ailments. Traditionally almond oil was rubbed into the scalp and left overnight, before shampooing, as a hair tonic and conditioner.

Almond milk is made by pounding almonds with a little water and has a long tradition of use as a restorative drink in convalescence. It can also be mixed with barley water and drunk to help pass kidney and bladder stones.

pear *Pyrus communis*

Like many fruits, pears were regarded in Galenic medicine as "colde" with a "binding quality". William Turner recommended a broth of dried pears as a remedy for diarrhoea, while the juice was reckoned to be "good for the biting of venomous beasts". Turner also added that "pears are good for the stomach and quench thirst if they be taken in meat".

We tend to consider pears as more suitable for constipation, but as with apples much depends on ripeness and how the fruit has been prepared, as the properties can vary significantly. To quote from Turner again: "Raw pears burden the stomach, but roasted or sodden relieve and lighten the stomach." Unripe fruit tends to be more astringent and suitable for diarrhoea, while the ripe or stewed fruits have a more laxative effect.

using pear

The pear's cleansing characteristics make it especially suitable in rheumatism and arthritis and the fruit is also rich in vitamins and minerals (including iron, phosphorus and calcium), so can be helpful in debility, convalescence or iron-deficient anaemia. Hildegard of Bingen recommended pears and honey as a cleansing remedy for any toxic problem as well as for migraine.

Gerard recommended hot perry (a pear-based alternative to cider) for stomach chills, while in France pear juice before meals is believed to help the digestion. The fruits are also mildly sedative which explains why they are used in some European cough mixtures. Try warm pear juice for stomach upsets or eat two or three fresh pears a day for habitual constipation.

potato *Solanum tuberosum*

Potatoes belong to the same family as deadly nightshade and henbane and, like these highly toxic herbs, contain poisonous alkaloids. Solanine, found in potato skin, has the same sort of antispasmodic properties as atropine (found in deadly nightshade) and in large quantities would be equally fatal. Indeed, as mentioned in the introduction, if the potato was discovered today scientists would probably condemn it as not safe for human consumption. Fortunately

potatoes were introduced into Europe in a more adventurous age: they were brought to Spain from Peru around 1530 and Sir Walter Raleigh is credited with planting the first potatoes in Britain during the days of Elizabeth I. It took around 200 years for the potato to supplant bread, barley and carrots as the main staple in our diet – partly because of its association with the nightshade family. Tomatoes – another close relative – suffered a similar fate and were regarded as toxic and purely ornamental until well into the 18th century.

Today, potatoes are possibly the most important source of vitamin C in the average British diet. They are also rich in B-complex vitamins (including B_1, B_5, B_6 and folic acid) and contain several minerals, including iron, calcium, manganese, magnesium and phosphorus.

using potato

In the days when every housewife knew how to make a poultice, mashed potato, which is also a mild painkiller, was the preferred choice of many of them and was widely applied to just about every ache, pain and inflammation. Externally raw potato can also be used to soothe skin inflammations. It has long been regarded as a folk remedy for burns and scalds (try grated potato mixed with vegetable oil), but the tradition is now being adopted by orthodox medicine thanks to some pioneering work by burns specialists in India using potato peelings.

As well as being an important food source, potato juice is a useful addition to the medicine chest. It can be helpful for relieving digestive problems associated with excessive stomach acid – including indigestion, gastritis and peptic ulcers – and is a good liver remedy, helpful for bile stones and gall bladder problems.

potato

part used
tuber

commercial products
bottled juice is sold in some health food shops.

how to use
juice - 10ml/2tsp, three times daily;
cooked mashed potato - as a poultice for painful joints;
slices of raw fresh potato - to ease burns and skin irritations.

wheat

parts used
seeds, aerial parts

commercial products
not generally used in
commercial medicinal
products.

how to use
wheatgerm - add 1-2tsp
to breakfast cereals;
bread - use as the basis
of poultices for drawing
boils and splinters.

bilberry

parts used
leaves, fruit

commercial products
included in some over-the-
counter remedies mainly
used as old-age tonics,
for infections or late-onset
diabetes; dried leaf sold
in capsules and available
loose from specialist
herbal suppliers; fruits
available in season from
greengrocers.

how to use
fresh berries - use in fruit
toppings and puddings
as a digestive remedy;
leaf infusion - 5g/⅙oz
to 500ml/1pt of boiling
water to help normalise
blood sugar levels.

wheat *Triticum* spp.

Wheat is one of our oldest cereal crops, cultivated in Mesopotamia more than 10,000 years ago and still the major staple for millions of Europeans. It is highly nutritious and the whole grains are rich in vitamins A, B-complex, D and E while wheatgerm oil is an even better source of vitamin E than the grain and contains a number of essential fatty acids. Commercial over-processing means that many of these nutrients are lost from the bread we eat and are often artificially added at the production stage – using wholemeal and organic flours is always advisable.

using wheat

Although primarily regarded as a nutrient, wheat has its medicinal uses as well. Wheat bran is irritant on the gut and can be helpful for constipation – although excessive use can lead to long-term damage and increase the risk of diverticular disease. Wheatgerm, because of its vitamin E component, is a good anti-oxidant, so can counter the effect of ageing on the body's cells. It can also be helpful for menstrual problems and can increase fertility.

Externally wheat bran can be used like oatmeal as a facial scrub, while bread poultices have long been a favourite folk remedy for drawing splinters and boils and also reducing swellings and inflammation.

Wheatgrass can be made by sprouting wheat grains on blotting paper in the kitchen and is a good source of chlorophyll and many enzymes. Cut the grass after three or four days, when it is around 5cm/2in high, and add it to salads as a good source of trace elements.

bilberry *Vaccinium myrtillus*

Although bilberries – and their close relatives cowberries (*V. vitis-idaea*), cranberries (*V. oxycoccos*) and farkleberries (*V. arboreum*) – were once regularly used as medicinal herbs, they – like many other traditional folk remedies – have fallen from favour in recent years because of more readily available products on the market. Fruits of all four plants are rich in vitamin C, highly astringent – due to their tannin content – and anti-bacterial. These culinary berries are closely related to bearberry (*Arctostaphylos uva-ursi*), an important urinary antiseptic, and recent work has highlighted the use of sizable doses of cranberry juice as an effective remedy for recurrent cystitis.

using bilberry

Elizabethan apothecaries used to make a syrup of bilberries with honey, called "rob", which was used as a remedy for diarrhoea. In large quantities, however, the berries have a laxative effect, so make an extremely palatable remedy for constipation. They can be eaten stewed or fresh: the German herbalist, Dr Rudolf Weiss, recommended cooked bilberry topping on cheesecake made with soft white cheese as a particularly palatable remedy for diarrhoea and gastric upsets.

Externally bilberries have been used in salves and ointments for piles, burns and skin complaints. Recent research has shown that the leaves, taken internally, will also reduce blood-sugar levels, so they make a useful support for late-onset diabetes that is under dietary control. There have also been some suggestions that bilberry leaves can encourage insulin production.

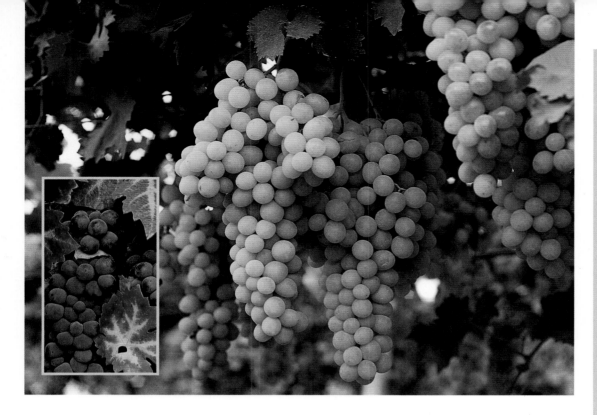

grape *Vitis vinifera*

▲ Grape *Vitis vinifera*

Both vine leaves and grapes have been used in herbal medicine, while there is also increasing evidence that wine can have a beneficial effect on the heart and circulation – something the French have argued for years.

using grape

Vine leaves have been used to improve circulation and control bleeding. Ointments made from vine leaves can still be used to relieve the discomfort of varicose veins and vine leaf tea can be used as a gargle for sore throats and a mouth wash for inflamed gums.

Although little used as orthodox medicines, grapes are credited with numerous medicinal properties. They can reduce inflammation, increase urination and bowel movement, improve muscle tone and help to stimulate bile flow and cleanse the liver. Grapes are also regarded as a good tonic food, helping to raise energy levels – hence their popularity with hospital visitors and in convalescence. Grape juice is often recommended as a key component in detoxification programmes and in chronic illness, including cancer and severe arthritis, while eating grapes (fresh, or dried as raisins and sultanas) can be helpful for constipation and a sluggish digestion.

Once fermented as wine, grape extracts – in moderation – are now known to help reduce cholesterol levels and provide some protection from heart disease. Some French enthusiasts carry wine remedies to even greater lengths suggesting various types of wine for just about every ailment from acidosis (try Pouilly-Fuissé) to urticaria (a Médoc or Côtes de Ventoux).

grape

parts used
fruit, leaves

commercial products
not generally used; grape juice, grapes and whole vine leaves widely available from supermarkets; crushed dried vine leaves sometimes sold by specialist herbal suppliers.

how to use
vine leaf infusion – 25g/1oz to 500ml/1pt of boiling water taken in three wine-glass doses or used as a gargle or mouth wash; *juice* – 1-2 glasses a day as a general cleansing remedy.

over-the-counter remedies

From being a rather esoteric curiosity, herbs have moved firmly into mainstream health care in recent years. Where once they were only available in limited assortments from specialist suppliers, an enormous number of herbal remedies is now sold in both health food shops and pharmacies. Herbal medicine is a multi-million pound business with well over 1,000 different products on offer.

Many of these are what are known as "simples"— products containing a single herb; others use combinations of plants that are often based on traditional brews or derive from the North American physiomedical tradition which became popular in the UK during the 19th century. Adding to these traditional European and North American remedies are a growing number of herbs from the Far East and South America. Sometimes these herbs are very similar in action to more familiar European varieties but from the supplier's point of view they do have the advantage of novelty and limited availability so, in marketing terms, are far more attractive than using herbs which can be found in any hedgerow or garden.

The choice of over-the-counter (OTC) products is steadily growing and has become increasingly bewildering. Fifty years ago devil's claw, which originates from the Kalahari Desert in Southern Africa, was virtually unknown in Europe; today it has been extensively researched and is one of the more popular products for arthritis. More recent arrivals on British shelves include *Dang Gui*, *amachazuru* and Peruvian cat's claw, an Amazonian tonic discovered in the 1970s and now becoming a fashionable cure-all.

In the UK many of these newcomers are sold as "food supplements" rather than licensed medicines, largely because acceptable evidence of efficacy or any tradition of use is not available (see page 232). This can lead to problems when buying OTC remedies due to the limited information which suppliers can legally put on their pots or in accompanying leaflets. In-depth knowledge of the actions of some of these newer remedies is not always readily accessible so a degree of caution is essential when choosing lesser known herbs for regular use.

The quality of OTC herbal products has been a problem in the past and there are several well-documented cases where quite the wrong herb has been put on sale – tubs of sea mayweed, for example, labelled as feverfew. Regulation, however, is improving and standardised extracts offering a consistent concentration of significant constituents are becoming more common. This is especially true for German herbal remedies which are widely prescribed by orthodox physicians.

From the many hundreds of herbs that could have been included, the plants in this section have been limited to those that are most readily available from health food shops or pharmacies, or are among the most widely used in proprietary OTC remedies.

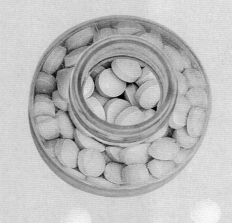

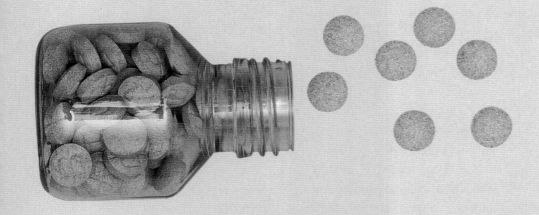

buchu

part used

leaves

commercial products

included in many
remedies sold for urinary
disorders; tincture
available from specialist
suppliers.

how to use

infusion – 15g/½oz of
dried herb to 500ml/1pt
of boiling water taken in
three equal doses per
day;

tincture – up to 2ml/40
drops per dose, three
times a day.

aloe

parts used

leaves, sap

commercial products

generally sold as a
simple containing juice or
sap extract in liquid or
powdered form; leaf
tinctures also available
from specialist suppliers;
whole leaf extracts are
commonly included in
commercial laxative
products.

how to use

juice – generally 10-
20ml/2-4tsp, three times
daily;

capsules – up to 1.5g
daily;

tincture (purgative) – up
to 2ml/40 drops per
dose, three times a day.

buchu *Agathosma betulina*

The buchu bush originates in South Africa and was first introduced into Europe at the end of the 18th century. The name comes from an African word meaning "dusting powder" and the plant was traditionally used externally as an insect deterrent and has some anti-bacterial and anti-inflammatory activity.

using buchu

By the 1920s it was established in the British pharmacopoeia as a remedy for urinary gravel and cystitis – much as it is used today – although in parts of the Cape it was recommended as an internal remedy for digestive problems and rheumatic disorders.

The name is applied to a number of closely related South African shrubs. "Oval", "long" and "round" forms of buchu are known, with the names descriptive of leaf shapes, although all have identical medicinal uses. The herb contains a volatile oil with a smell reminiscent of blackcurrants, which helps to make it one of the more palatable herbs in the repertoire, as such it is sometimes included as a flavouring. Buchu has a stimulant effect and is tonic and warming for the kidneys. Its taste makes it particularly palatable in teas for home use.

aloe *Aloe* spp.

Aloe is a tropical African plant which has been used medicinally since ancient Greek and Roman times. The plant reached the West Indies with the slave trade in the 16th century and has

➤ Aloe *Aloe vera*

been widely cultivated there ever since – hence such common names as Barbados or Curaçao aloes. In the West, the juice has traditionally been regarded as a soothing wound herb, although in Ayurvedic medicine it is treated as a restorative tonic.

using aloe

The whole leaf is a bitter purgative and digestive stimulant and a common remedy in OTC products for constipation: an extract "bitter aloes" was once standard on pharmacists' shelves as a laxative and is generally made from a combination of various species of aloe. The same liquid was popularly painted on children's fingers to stop them sucking or biting nails.

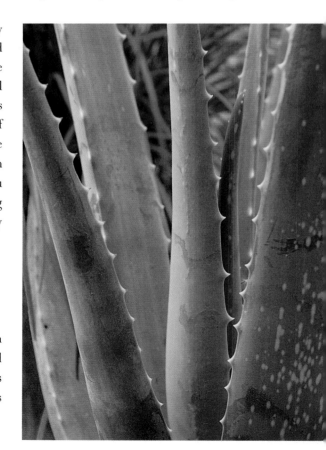

"Aloe vera" is the name commonly given to the mucilaginous sap obtained from such species as *A. barbadensis* and this was largely used externally in the West as a wound healer and to relieve burns and skin inflammations including eczema and thrush. This gel, usually cold-pressed from the leaves is now also made into a variety of popular tonic remedies promoted as energy restoratives and pick-me-ups. In Ayurvedic tradition, the sap is used as a restorative for the female reproductive system and as a tonic for the liver. It is more palatable if mixed with apple juice or water.

Aloe grows well in the UK as a house plant but will generally not survive out of doors for long. Although it looks like a succulent, it is more closely related to the lily family so needs plenty of water. The gel is easy to collect by simply breaking open a leaf and scraping out the sap; alternatively fresh leaves can be split and applied directly to wounds and inflammations. It can usefully be grown on a kitchen windowsill as a convenient first-aid standby for minor burns. The sap can also be used on eczema and can help with fungal infections such as ringworm and thrush.

cautions avoid in pregnancy as it is strongly purgative; high doses of leaf extracts may cause vomiting. Commercial sap extracts are often contaminated with leaf so may also cause nausea and digestive upsets.

dang gui
Angelica polyphorma var. *sinensis*

Chinese angelica is one of the East's most important tonic remedies, regarded by many as second only to Korean ginseng and an important woman's energy tonic helping to restore and invigorate the reproductive system.

The herb's Chinese name, *Dang Gui* literally means "expected to be back home" and it was said that if anyone missed their relatives they should send a piece of the root to the person who, on receiving it, would immediately return. Other names sometimes given in the West are *tang kwai*, from an older system of transliterating Chinese characters, or *dong quai* which is a phonetic rendering of its *pinyin* name popular in the USA and health food trade.

using *dang gui*

Traditionally *Dang Gui* is said to "nourish the blood" and is used as a blood tonic for anaemia, menstrual problems and at the menopause. In folk medicine it is cooked in a stew with chicken or lamb as a tonic food following childbirth. The herb is also a mild laxative and is generally prescribed for the elderly where digestive energies may be weak

Although usually recommended for women, *Dang Gui* also makes an effective liver tonic for men. The plant also has some action as a circulatory stimulant and is mildly anti-bacterial.

caution avoid in pregnancy.

arnica *Arnica montana*

Also known as leopard's bane, this daisy-like alpine flower has a long history of use in central Europe as a remedy for bruises and sprains. It was also once popular in folk medicine for the heart condition angina pectoris. It is still used in

---

dang gui

part used
rhizome

commercial products
included in numerous traditional Chinese formulations sold by specialist herb shops and a few Western-style proprietary mixtures mainly for menstrual and menopausal problems; capsules and tincture available from health food shops.

how to use
tincture – up to 5ml/1tsp per dose, three times daily;
decoction – up to 35g1¼oz to 750ml/1½pt of water taken in three equal doses;
capsules – up to 600mg daily.

arnica

part used
flowers

commercial products
used in many creams and ointments for external use and also available in homoeopathic preparations (6X, 30X).

how to use
take only homoeopathic doses internally - one tablet every 30-60 minutes; use externally only on unbroken skin.

huang qi

parts used
root

commercial products
included in numerous traditional Chinese formulations and a growing number of Western proprietary mixtures generally for immune-related problems; capsules and tincture available from health food shops.

how to use
tincture – up to 3ml/60 drops, three times a day;
decoction – up to 45g/1½oz in 750ml/1½pt of water taken in three equal doses;
capsules – up to 600mg a day;
fried root – traditionally chewed as a snack.

Germany for heart problems, although it is extremely toxic and its internal use is restricted in many countries (including the UK).

using arnica

The plant is astringent, anti-bacterial and will reduce inflammation; it is most often used in creams and ointments for injuries, such as strains and bruises, and inflammations such as chilblains or painful varicose veins. It encourages the circulation to promote healing and tissue repair, while recent work suggests that it may have immune-stimulant properties.

As an internal remedy, arnica is most often used in homoeopathic doses for shock, traumatic injury and to encourage healing after surgery or childbirth. Homoeopathic medicines are stronger at higher dilutions: both Arnica 6X tablets, suitable for general use, and Arnica 30X, preferable after surgery or childbirth, are readily available.

cautions arnica should not be used on open wounds and can cause contact dermatitis. It should only be used externally: taken internally it can lead to palpitations, muscle paralysis and breathing problems; in rare cases it may be fatal.

shatavari

Asparagus racemosus
see page 109.

huang qi

Astragalus membranaceus

Huang Qi is an important energy tonic traditionally used in China for younger people while Korean ginseng is considered better for the over-40s. The two herbs are also frequently used together as a general tonic. The name translates literally as "yellow leader" reflecting both the colour of the root and the plant's importance as a major tonic remedy. The herb is included in the famous herbal attributed to Shen Nong – the legendary founder of Chinese herbal medicine – and is listed among the "superior" remedies. The plant is known in the West as milk vetch and can occasionally be found in health food shops under this name although it is more commonly labelled as "astragalus".

using *huang qi*

Huang Qi is believed to strengthen defence energy (*Wei Qi*) which in Chinese tradition is the body's protection from external "evils". Modern research has confirmed that the plant is an important anti-bacterial and immune stimulant and it has been used in AIDS treatments and also as an immune tonic in cancer patients undergoing chemotherapy. Because of its strong immune-stimulating action astragalus is often promoted as a cancer preventative and can be useful for those suffering from recurrent infections.

The plant is also used as a heart tonic to combat heart disease and stimulate the blood circulation. It will reduce blood pressure and lower blood sugar levels.

As well as its energy stimulating action, *Huang Qi* is regarded as a blood tonic and is sometimes used in China with *Dang Gui* in blood deficiency associated with prolonged bleeding – as in heavy menstrual bleeding. The herb also acts as a nerve and digestion stimulant.

gotu kola *Centella asiatica*

Indian pennywort or gotu kola is known as *brahmi* in Sanskrit as it increases knowledge of *Brahman*, the supreme reality. It is one of the most important rejuvenative remedies *(rasayana karma)* in Ayurveda.

These types of tonics are believed to help combat ageing and senility and to improve the memory. They are also believed to enhance mental clarity and spiritual awareness helping to revitalise the brain and nervous system. Gotu kola is a specific tonic for the *pitta* (fire/bile) humour while clearing excess *vata* (air/wind) and *kapha* (damp/phlegm) so is calming and an important aid for spiritual renewal.

using gotu kola

In the West it has been variously used for skin problems, poor circulation and rheumatic disorders. It was once used for severe conditions such as leprosy and syphilis and is a powerful blood cleanser to clear toxins from the system. Gotu kola is also used for nervous problems and depression and is sometimes given to help strengthen the nervous system in Parkinson's disease. It is known to be anti-inflammatory and will also stimulate the immune system so is a useful herb for infections.

Research in the 1990s suggests that the plant could reduce fertility so is best avoided by those hoping to conceive. In India fresh leaves are given to children to combat digestive disorders, including dysentery, and it is mixed with oil as a scalp rub to stimulate hair growth. Gotu kola is traditionally taken in a milk decoction or can be mixed with *ghee* (clarified butter) as a revitalising remedy for the spirit. It is also used with basil as a cooling remedy in fevers and food poisoning.

cautions avoid high doses in pregnancy and completely in epilepsy.

black cohosh
Cimicifuga racemosus

Black cohosh – also known as black snakeroot or squaw root – was very widely used by Native Americans for rheumatism, yellow fever, snakebite, and kidney problems, as well as an impressive list of gynaecological problems. It was used for smallpox by the early settlers and by the beginning of the 19th century had joined the European repertoire. Primarily, though, black cohosh was regarded as a remedy for rheumatism and as such it was a "favourite remedy" of the 19th-century American eclectic physician John King (1813–1893) who used it for both acute and chronic cases of rheumatism and for other inflammatory conditions including respiratory problems and neuralgia.

using black cohosh

As well as its use as a rheumatic remedy, more recent studies have focused on its gynaecological action and several have confirmed that it effectively relieves menopausal symptoms. Researchers currently disagree as to its actual action with some suggesting that it has oestrogenic-like activity while others maintain it is non-hormonal. Whatever its action, the herb has been shown in trials to relieve all sorts of menopausal discomforts including hot flushes, sweating, sleep disturbances, emotional upsets and

---

gotu kola

parts used
aerial parts

commercial products
included in a number of OTC tonic mixtures; capsules and tinctures available from health food shops.

how to use
powder/capsules – up to 500mg per dose, three times daily;
dried herb – infusions made from 20g/¾oz of herb to 500ml/1pt of water taken in three equal daily doses;
tincture – up to 4ml/80drops per dose, three times daily;
paste made of the powder is used externally for eczema and skin sores.

black cohosh

part used
rhizome

commercial products
included in a number of proprietary remedies for both menstrual problems and rheumatic disorders; capsules and tinctures available from health food shops.

how to use
tincture – up to 2 ml/40 drops of tincture per dose, three times a day;
capsules – up to 200mg per dose.

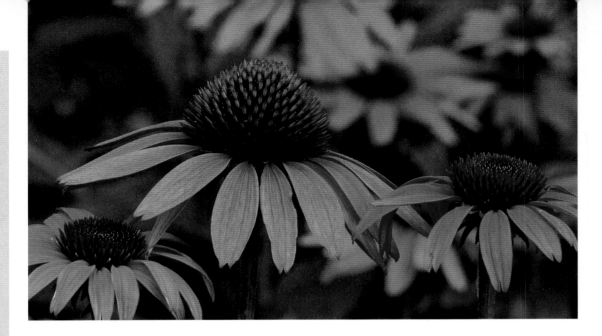

echinacea

parts used

root, aerial parts

commercial products

very widely available in proprietary remedies for colds, catarrh, and immune stimulating mixtures; capsules, tinctures and juice available from health food shops.

how to use

tincture – up to 25ml/1fl oz daily for up to four days in acute conditions; *capsules* – up to 1.5g in capsules daily for up to four days in acute conditions or 200mg daily as a low-dose preventative for mild infections; *decoction* – 25g/1oz of root to 750ml/1½pt of water taken in three equal doses during the day; *infusion* – 25g/1oz of leaves to 500ml/1pt of water taken in three equal doses.

depression. As a result, it is rapidly becoming a popular OTC remedy for menopausal problems, although it can also be helpful for breast discomfort associated with pre-menstrual syndrome. Traditionally the herb was used to prevent threatened miscarriage, although such use requires skill and experience and is not an area for home remedies.

Black cohosh is still popular for aches and pains and is included in many OTC remedies for arthritis and rheumatism: it is also recommended for cramps, sciatica, back pain, facial neuralgia and aches and pains following strenuous exercise. Studies suggest that it will also reduce blood pressure and blood sugar levels and is mildly sedating.

Several Oriental species (usually *C. foetida* or *C. dahurica)* are used in Chinese medicine as *Sheng Ma* – primarily regarded as a remedy for colds and measles.

cautions excess can cause nausea and vomiting and the herb should be avoided in pregnancy.

echinacea *Echinacea* spp.

Echinacea, or purple cone flower, was one of the most important herbs used by Native American healers. According to one 19th-century source it was used as a "remedy for more ailments than any other plant". The herb was treated as a universal antidote to snake bite, the juice was used to bathe burns and pieces of root were chewed for toothache.

By the 1850s echinacea was already widely used by European settlers, largely as an aromatic and carminative for digestive problems. Interest in the plant spread and by the 1930s research in Germany had highlighted its potent antibiotic actions.

The plant is anti-bacterial, anti-viral and anti-fungal and is used for a broad spectrum of infections. Today it is widely cultivated and regarded as one of the most useful herbs in the repertoire.

The roots of both *E. purpurea* and *E. angustifolia* are generally used medicinally, although German studies suggest that the aerial

◄ Echinacea *Echinacea* spp

parts of *E. purpurea* are more efficacious than its root; *E. pallida* is occasionally used but it is harder to cultivate commercially and wild-crafting (the collection of the plant from the wild) is leading to severe shortages of the plant in its native habitat. Harvesting aerial parts of home-grown *E. purpurea* – often sold as an ornamental in garden centres – makes the herb a more practical alternative in the herb garden.

using echinacea

Attitudes to dosage of echinacea vary, with some authorities suggesting that it should be taken in short sharp bursts only in acute infections, while others happily feed low dosages to school-age children on a long-term basis, successfully preventing the usual round of childhood ills.

As well as treating colds, kidney and urinary infections, echinacea can also be used for wound-healing and septicaemia. It is often sold as a licensed remedy for "minor skin problems", although it is really more suited to those associated with infection, such as acne, boils and carbuncles, rather than disorders like eczema which may have a more complex cause.

siberian ginseng
Eleutherococcus senticosus

Siberian ginseng belongs to one of the oldest known plant families, the Araliaceae, and has been used in Chinese medicine for around 2,000 years. It was traditionally regarded as a warming herb to strengthen the sinews and bones and to improve energy and blood flows,

especially in the elderly. Its Chinese name, *Wu Jia Pi,* means "bark of five additions" – reminding us that the Chinese used only the root bark, not the whole root as in the West.

The plant was "discovered" by Western scientists in the 1930s in Russia and subsequently extensively used by Soviet athletes to increase stamina and enhance performance. It has since been extensively researched and is known to stimulate the immune and circulatory systems and also help regulate blood pressure and lower blood sugar levels.

using siberian ginseng

As the Soviet researchers discovered back in the 1930s, it is good at increasing stamina and helping the body cope more efficiently with both physical and mental stresses. It is ideal to take, normally as a tincture or in capsules, whenever extra energy is needed – before a particularly busy period at work, during exams or before long-distance air travel, for example. It can help reduce the effects of jet lag and is an ideal all-round energy tonic, considered to be rather gentler than Korean ginseng (see Ginseng, page 153) and more suitable for women.

eucalyptus
Eucalyptus globulus

The majority of eucalyptus species originate from Australia where the plant was widely used in Aboriginal medicine to treat fevers, dysentery and sores. In the 19th century, Baron Ferdinand von Müller, director of the Melbourne Botanical Gardens from 1857 to 1873, brought the plant to Europe and

siberian ginseng

part used
root

commercial products
included in a number of proprietary tonic remedies; capsules and tinctures available from health food shops.

how to use
tincture – up to 5ml/1tsp three times a day; *capsules* – up to 600mg a day.

eucalyptus

parts used
leaves, essential oil

commercial product:
included in both internal and external OTC products mainly in lozenges for sore throats, rubbing ointments for aches and pains or nasal sprays to ease congestion; capsules of dried leaf and the essential oil are both available from health food shops.

how to use
generally the essential oil is used in external treatments although the leaves can be taken in infusions (15g/½oz to 500ml/1pt of water) or in capsules (up to 250mg daily).

parts used
whole plant (thalli)

commercial products
included in a very wide assortment of OTC products used for menstrual and urinary problems as well as promoted as slimming aids; capsules and tinctures available from health food shops.

how to use
tincture - up to 20ml/¾fl oz daily;
capsules or tablets - up to 1g daily;
hot infused bladderwrack oil, made from 500g/1lb of herb in 500ml/1pt of sunflower oil (see page 224), can be used to ease arthritic and rheumatic aches and pains.

cultivation spread in southern Europe and North America. The tree is a greedy drinker and widespread cultivation in parts of Italy has since had a dramatic and adverse effect on local water-table levels.

using eucalyptus

Eucalyptus is highly antiseptic and stimulating; it encourages coughing and will also ease spasmodic pains – hence its use in many cough remedies.

The essential oil (extracted by steam distillation) is mainly used externally and is included in numerous rubs for muscle aches, steam inhalations for catarrh and colds, or added in small quantities to throat pastilles.

Various species are used medicinally, some of them with slightly different actions: Australian peppermint (*E. dives*) is largely used for chest rubs, sciatica and arthritis; lemon-scented eucalyptus (*E. citriodora*) has a more anti-fungal action and is used for athlete's foot and candidiasis. Russian research has suggested that some species are effective against the flu virus, others are anti-malarial or combat a wide range of bacteria.

caution excess may cause headache and delirium.

kelp *Fucus* spp., *Ascophyllum* sp. *and* *Macrocysris* sp.

Several species of seaweed are marketed as kelp; including bladderwrack (*F. vesiculosis*) and its relative *F. serratus* as well as *Ascophyllum nodosum*, *Macrocysris pyrfera* and others. All are salty, tonic and rich in iodine and trace metals. The iodine content stimulates the thyroid gland and thus speeds up body metabolism.

Stimulating the metabolism can help to burn off extra calories so kelp is often promoted as a slimming aid. However, it is really only effective if a sluggish thyroid is part of the problem and excessive use can lead to thyrotoxicosis (over-active thyroid).

using kelp

Kelp is highly nutritious and a good source of sodium, manganese, sulphur, silicon, zinc and copper, so it makes a good general metabolic tonic especially in debility and convalescence. Studies also suggest it can reduce the risk of atherosclerosis by helping to maintain the elasticity of blood vessel walls.

Externally bladderwrack extracts and infused oils are used for rheumatism and arthritis.

caution bladderwrack will concentrate toxic waste metals such as cadmium and strontium which pollute our oceans and the plant should not be collected in a contaminated area.

ginkgo *Ginkgo biloba*

Ginkgo is something of a botanical anachronism – a rare, prehistoric deciduous conifer, unchanged since before the evolution of mammals. It owes its survival to preservation as a sacred plant in Japanese temple gardens and was introduced into Europe in 1727 when it became popular as a botanical garden ornamental. Some of Europe's oldest ginkgo trees – also known as maidenhair trees – can be found in the Chelsea Physic Garden in London and the Jardin des Plantes in Paris.

using ginkgo

Although the Chinese have prescribed the seeds (known as *Bai Guo*) for asthma and urinary problems for many centuries, it is only in the past few years that the herb has been used medicinally in the West. Research in the past decade has highlighted its action as a platelet-activating factor (PAF) which counters the allergic response – reinforcing its traditional use as an anti-asthmatic. More significantly, ginkgo leaf extract has been shown to improve cerebral circulation. In Germany gingko has been tested on patients after brain surgery following strokes, and been found to improve recovery rates dramatically. Its action in strengthening the cerebral circulation has led many to regard it as an anti-ageing remedy,

▼ Ginkgo *Ginkgo biloba*

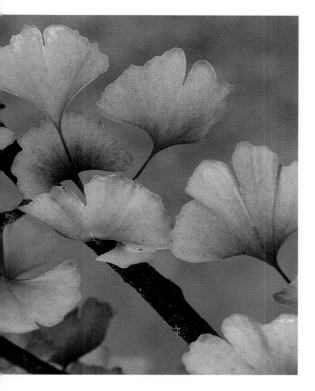

since hardening of the arteries in the brain is a common cause of apparent confusion in the elderly. It is generally beneficial for many circulatory ailments (including, according to some researchers, varicose veins) and its effect on cerebral circulation has also led to its use in the treatment of Ménières disease and tinnitus.

Ginkgo is widely sold as a food supplement and can be usefully taken by the elderly or those with chronic circulatory disorders.

maitake *Grifolia frondosa*

Maitake means "dancing mushrooms" in Japanese. Some say this is because the fruiting body of this fungus resembles a butterfly while others attribute the name more prosaically to the fact that collectors could exchange the mushrooms for their weight in silver and thus danced for joy on finding them.

The mushrooms are known as "hen of the woods" in English and are a type of bracket fungus occasionally found growing at the base of oak or beech trees. They are now commercially cultivated both for the culinary and medicinal markets.

using maitake

Over the past 20 years the mushrooms have been extensively researched, mainly for their anti-cancer and immune-stimulating properties. The mushrooms are now known to be rich in a number of potent chemicals, including unsaturated fatty acids, and have been shown to reduce raised blood pressure, combat hepatitis, and reduce blood sugar levels as well as their very significant action in stimulating the immune function and demonstrating some anti-tumour activity in animal studies. More recent studies in the 1990s also suggested that the fungus can be effective in AIDs.

Maitake is one of a number of fashionable "food supplements" often expensively marketed in health food shops. Fresh "hen of the woods" mushrooms are currently available from specialist suppliers as the fungus has yet to achieve the supermarket status of shiitake mushrooms which have similar properties.

gurmari *Gymnema sylvestre*

Gurmari, also known as *merasinghi* and *padapatri* in India, is a traditional folk remedy for digestive problems. The root is largely used for stomach pains while the leaf is also a traditional treatment for diabetes and high blood sugar levels. In southern China the plant is traditionally used for snake bites while fresh leaves are used in poultices for wounds.

using gurmari

Studies in the early 1990s confirmed its efficacy as a diabetes treatment and the leaves are believed to contain chemicals which can increase insulin secretions and normalise blood sugar levels in severe diabetics. Clinical trials have shown that the plant can help reduce the dosage of insulin required in insulin-dependent diabetics and can also normalise blood sugar levels in late-onset diabetics who are not insulin dependent.

The herb is believed to anaesthetise the sweet taste buds as well as limit the absorption of glucose. This has resulted in it being promoted as a weight-control aid as it can reduce cravings for sugar and other sweet – and

fattening – foods, thus *Gymnema* is increasingly sold in health food shops as a weight-loss agent. Studies also suggest that it can reduce cholesterol levels.

caution avoid in pregnancy.

amachazuru *Gynostemma pentaphyllum*

Sometimes known as "gospel herb" or "sweet tea vine" in English, *Amachazuru* – the Japanese name – is a member of the pumpkin family, and is well established in China as a folk cure for bronchitis, liver problems and stomach ulcers. During the 1980s Japanese researchers identified anti-cancer activity in the plant and it has also been found to be protective for the liver in helping to combat infections such as hepatitis.

using amachazuru

Amachazuru is rich in minerals and vitamins and contains similar steroidal compounds to those found in ginseng. Trials in China suggest that it can improve cell activity and strengthen the immune system as well as increase metabolism, reduce blood sugar and cholesterol levels. The plant also helps to improve heart function and stimulates the blood supply to the brain – rather like ginkgo.

In Japan and China it is used as an anti-ageing remedy to combat fatigue and as a cancer preventative. More prosaically it is also taken to combat hair loss and greying hair and is included in popular beauty treatments. In the 1990s *Amachazuru* was rated as among the 10 most important tonic remedies at an international conference in Beijing.

witch hazel

Hamamelis virginiana

The witch hazel tree was used for numerous ills by several Native American tribes: the Menomees in Wisconsin rubbed decoctions on their legs during sports to keep the muscles supple, while a maceration of the twigs was recommended for back ache. The Potawatomis preferred the twigs in steam baths for sore muscles, while a Dr Colden, writing to a colleague in Leyden in 1744, describes how the Mohawks used steam from witch hazel decoctions to treat eye injuries and records a case of "almost total blindness occasioned by a blow" cured by this method.

The plant has been growing in Europe since the 17th century and its botanical name derives from a Greek word suggesting a resemblance to the apple tree. It is a small, shrub-like tree growing to around 5m/16ft in height and with yellow flowers in spring.

using witch hazel

The bark is steam distilled to produce the familiar, clear "distilled witch hazel" available from any pharmacy. It can be used as a first-aid remedy for bruises, sprains, nosebleeds, cuts and grazes, can soothe spots and blemishes, and is helpful to ease varicose veins and piles. It is ideal for all sorts of minor household injuries and essential standby in the first aid box. The tincture of the bark, well diluted, can be used much as commercially made generic distilled witch hazel.

Taken internally, the leaf tincture or an infusion of the leaves is effective for treating diarrhoea, colitis, excessive menstruation and haemorrhage.

devil's claw

Harpagophytum procumbens

Devil's claw has been known in the West for less than a century, although the plant has long been used in folk medicine by the Bushmen of the Kalahari Desert in southern Africa where it grows wild. The herb takes its common name from its large thorny seed pods which are a hazard for animals when they become entangled in fur – its botanical name is derived from the Greek *harpago*, meaning "a grappling hook".

The story of devil's claw's discovery by Western medicine exists in several versions: the plant was variously spotted by a Boer farmer or German doctor, being variously used by local people or a tribal witch doctor to cure digestive upsets or rheumatism, and was subsequently despatched to Germany for investigation. Certainly by the late 1950s its anti-inflammatory and anti-rheumatic properties were well established. Researchers have also found that constant use of the herb for at least six weeks significantly improved the movement of arthritic joints and reduced swelling.

Some 40 constituents have been identified and research now suggests that the key active constituent is a chemical called harpagoside. Standardised mixtures giving a constant concentration of this substance are now produced in Germany.

using devil's claw

The plant produces simple roots and secondary storage roots or tubers. These tubers, rather than the whole root structure are used medicinally, although some commercial preparations combine the entire root mix thus diluting the overall therapeutic effect.

---

witch hazel

part used
bark, leaves

commercial products
widely available from chemists as distilled witch hazel; included in many proprietary ointments for varicose veins, piles and skin problems; powdered herb sold in capsules; tincture of both bark and leaves available from health food shops.

how to use
distilled witch hazel – apply as need be to minor injuries, bruises and varicose veins;
tincture – up to 3ml/60 drops, three times a day;
capsules – usually 200mg 2-3 times a day;
infusion – 20g/¾oz to 500ml/1pt of water taken in three equal doses.

devil's claw

part used

root

commercial products

included in some proprietary mixtures (for both internal and external use) for arthritis but mainly sold as a simple in capsules or tablets; tincture available from health food shops.

how to use

tincture – up to 5ml/1tsp, three times daily; *capsules* – 500mg per dose, three times daily. Doses are generally increased during acute phases of the arthritic illness.

golden seal

part used

root

commercial products

included in many proprietary mixtures mainly for digestive problems; capsules and tincture available from health food shops.

how to use

tincture – up to 4ml/80 drops, three times daily; *capsules* – up to 600mg daily.

Devil's claw is bitter and can be used as a digestive stimulant. Externally it can be used in creams and rubs for muscle and joint pains.

caution devil's claw is believed to stimulate uterine contractions and should therefore be avoided in pregnancy.

golden seal
Hydrastis canadensis

Golden seal originates in North America where the root was used by the Cherokee people for digestive problems, skin inflammations and to make an insect-repellent ointment. The Iroquois preferred it for whooping cough, liver disorders and – mixed with whisky – heart problems. It soon became popular among the settlers as a cure-all and was listed in the official US pharmacopoeia until 1936.

using golden seal

Golden seal has been used in Europe since the 1760s, although it is rarely found growing here and most is imported ready dried or powdered from the USA. The herb has a bitter taste, which helps to make it an effective digestive stimulant, it is mildly laxative and also helps to heal damaged mucous membranes in the digestive tract. It is largely used as a gastric remedy although it is also a very potent anti-microbial and tonic.

In addition, the herb can be useful for a range of menstrual and menopausal problems – it combines well with chaste-tree (see page 162) – and is particularly helpful for cooling hot flushes and night sweats. It has also been used to stop post-partum haemorrhage.

Golden seal is a difficult plant to grow in cultivation and it is now becoming rare in the wild, so many herbalists prefer to use alternative remedies. Its tonic and immune-stimulating properties are hard to match, but as a digestive remedy many choose to prescribe barberry (*Berberis vulgaris*) instead – this has very similar constituents and actions and is still plentiful.

cautions golden seal's anti-microbial action can damage beneficial gut flora, so it should not be taken for long periods without a break. The herb is best avoided in pregnancy.

st john's wort
Hypericum perforatum

Although a traditional wound herb and pain remedy, St John's wort is now becoming better known as an anti-depressant. In Germany it is one of the more popular remedies prescribed by orthodox physicians.

The plant is believed to take its name from the Knights of St John of Jerusalem who used it as a wound herb on Crusade battlefields – although others suggest that it is associated with the midsummer rites of St John's Day (24 June) and the blood-red extracts that can be obtained from the herb. It is a good example of the Doctrine of Signatures, since the herb is helpful for inflammations and wounds.

St John's wort was believed to ward off evil spirits and the insane would often drink an infusion in an attempt to cure their madness.

➤ St John's wort *Hypericum perforatum* (about 4 times actual size)

using st john's wort

Today we know that the herb is an effective anti-depressant which is believed to inhibit the enzyme monoamine oxidase (MAO), which itself inhibits neurotransmitters involved in stimulating the brain. MAO inhibitors are widely used in orthodox medicine and some researchers suggest St John's wort has similar action. The herb has been successfully used in seasonal affective disorder (SAD), for emotional upsets associated with the menopause and for mild cases of depression. The herb has long been regarded by herbalists as a restorative for the nervous system and it can ease pre-menstrual tension and some types of period pain.

It is now popular across Europe as an effective and non-addictive alternative to the drugs commonly prescribed as anti-depressants. Inevitably with popular herbs, the researchers also have fed large amounts to laboratory animals to find unpleasant side effects – in this case a possible risk of cataracts in extremely high doses. Many cautions as to its use have now been issued by regulators.

Research in recent years has also focused on its effect on the immune system and the herb has been used in AIDS treatments.

The plant produces bright yellow flowers in early to midsummer and these can be collected and infused in sunflower oil for two weeks (see page 224) to produce a red oil which is ideal for soothing minor burns and sunburn.

cautions excessively high doses and prolonged use have been linked to cataracts and nerve hypersensitivity; in rare cases prolonged use may increase the photosensitivity of the skin; current advice is to seek professional guidance before taking St John's wort while using prescription drugs.

tea tree
Melaleuca alternifolia

Extracts from the Australian tea tree were originally used by the Aboriginals as a wound remedy. The plant was first studied in Europe in the 1920s when French researchers found that tea tree oil, collected by steam distillation, was a more effective antiseptic than phenol. They also identified its impressive antibiotic properties and by the Second World War it was a regular component in field dressing kits among Australian troops.

The plant is anti-bacterial, anti-fungal and anti-viral and can be used to combat a great many infecting organisms.

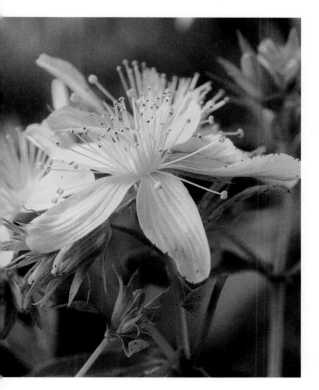

st john's wort

parts used
flowering tops, leaves

commercial products
included in a few proprietary remedies sold mainly for infections; used in many external wound and burn creams and lotions; many capsules and tablets are now marketed as anti-depressive remedies; also available as juice and tincture from health food shops.

how to use
tincture – 4ml/80 drops up to three times daily;
capsules – up to 250mg, three times daily;
infusion – 25g/1oz to 500ml/1pt of water taken in three equal doses.

tea tree

part used
essential oil

commercial products
mainly included in ointments or creams although occasionally found in throat lozenges; tea tree pessaries are sold for vaginal infections; essential oil widely available.

how to use
massage rubs - use ½-1ml/10-20 drops of oil to 5ml/1tsp of almond or wheatgerm oil; oil can be used directly on minor wounds or skin sores or applied to a tampon for use in vaginal thrush (see below).

noni

parts used
leaves, fruit, root

commercial products
mainly sold in capsules.

how to use
capsules - up to 600mg daily;
dried leaves - traditionally used in poultices for fevers and stomach pains.

using tea tree

In the past few years a thriving tea tree industry has grown up which has led to a number of highly adulterated oils appearing on the market. True tea tree oil is one of the few which does not usually irritate mucous membranes and it can be used neat on the skin.

A few drops added to a tampon make a topical treatment for vaginal thrush (insert and leave the tampon for no longer than four hours). Tea tree oil also stimulates the immune system and if taken internally (only under professional guidance) acts as an expectorant and diaphoretic, making it useful for chills and coughs.

Tea tree is readily available both as oil and in creams and is an essential household standby for use in antiseptic dressings for cuts and grazes, for acne and other skin infections, or for fungal infections such as thrush and athlete's foot.

A drop of tea tree oil can help prevent cold sores developing if applied as soon as the pricking sensation that heralds the sore starts, or it can help soothe them once they appear. It is also effective on warts, verrucas and insect bites. The oil, used neat on a comb or added to shampoos, can be used for head lice and nits in children.

noni *Morinda citrifolia*

Noni, or Indian mulberry, is a comparative newcomer to the Western herbal repertoire. The plant grows in various parts of Asia and Australia and has numerous folk uses throughout the South Pacific: in Fiji liquid from the young fruits (which are inedible) is inserted into the nostrils to counter bad breath and the plant is also used for mouth ulcers and piles

while in Samoa the leaves are used as a remedy for rheumatism, the flowers are a treatment for styes and the fruit chewed for toothache.

Noni is also important in many Pacific islands for treating "ghost sickness" — illnesses of unknown cause associated with spiritual possession. Juice from the fruits, which have a foul smell, is dropped into the eye, nose or mouth in the belief that the ghosts will be repelled by the plant's odour.

using noni

Its numerous traditional applications have encouraged recent research and *noni* has been extensively studied over the past few years, largely at the University of Hawaii. A number of active chemicals have been identified and isolated and the herb has been show to be antibiotic, anti-inflammatory and an effective painkiller. It can also help to normalise blood pressure and cholesterol levels and shows some anti-cancer activity.

The leaves are rich in carotene (pro-vitamin A) which helps to combat cell damage and is needed for various body functions including night vision. Of particular significance is the chemical proxeronine which is rarely found in plants. This is converted in the body into xeronine which is used to repair cell damage. Our ability to produce xeronine diminishes with age, in illness or when under stress so the herb can be an effective tonic remedy to counter some of the effects of ageing and reduce the damage caused by stress. As such *noni* — the Hawaiian name for the plant — has become increasingly popular among the manufacturers of herbal products as a new and fashionable tonic remedy which is marketed as a general cure-all and restorative.

evening primrose

Oenothera biennis

A native of North America, evening primrose is now widely naturalised across Europe and is commonly found in hedgerows as a garden escape. The leaves were traditionally used for asthma and digestive disorders; however, during the 1970s researchers identified that the seeds are rich in an essential fatty acid called *gamma-linolenic acid* (GLA) that is vital for good health.

GLA is a building block for various prostaglandins – hormone-like chemicals vital for a number of bodily systems. A normal, healthy metabolism will convert commonly occurring *cis*-linoleic acid (found in leafy vegetables and seed oils) into GLA, but this process can be affected by poor diet and high cholesterol levels. Some individuals are also unable to complete this metabolic pathway – a failure that has been linked to disorders such as chronic psoriasis and rheumatoid arthritis. With evening primrose oil able to fill the gap, there has been a massive growth in sales and the plant has become a major cash crop in many parts of the world. Typically evening primrose oil contains around 9% GLA, although in recent years plant breeders have worked hard to develop strains that will yield even more.

using evening primrose

GLA is reputed to ease menstrual and menopausal problems, strengthen the circulatory system, combat certain sorts of eczema and boost the immune system. Research suggests that it can ease irritable bowel syndrome where symptoms are associated with the menstrual cycle. In clinical trials dosages of 3-5g a day have been commonplace, although for general use 500-1000mg is usually recommended. The oil can also be used neat on the skin for eczema and similar problems and, because the oil helps to normalise liver function, it can also be useful to counter the symptoms of a hangover on "the morning after".

Licensed evening primrose oil products are available and, in the UK, can be prescribed for skin problems and some gynaecological disorders under the NHS. In the 1980s GLA was also found in borage (see page 77) and blackcurrant seed oils.

ginseng *Panax ginseng*

Ginseng has been regarded as something of a "wonder drug" for at least 5,000 years. Originating in China, where it has long been used to strengthen the vital energy (*Qi*) of the body, ginseng was known to Arab physicians by the ninth century, mentioned by Marco Polo in the 13th and introduced into modern Europe in the 17th century when a delegation from the King of Siam visited Louis XIV at Versailles and presented him with a root of "gintz-æn".

Ginseng has always been an expensive and highly prized herb that had, ideally, to be gathered in the wild using roots that were several years old. Today all ginseng is cultivated and it is an important cash crop. The plant is rich in steroidal compounds which are very similar to human sex hormones – hence its reputation as an aphrodisiac.

using ginseng

The Chinese believe it is best suited to the elderly, preferring other energy tonics for those

---

evening primrose

part used
seed oil

commercial products
very widely available in capsules containing the simple oil or in combination with various fish oils and other additives.

how to use
capsules – up to 1g daily.

ginseng

part used
root

commercial products
included in many proprietary tonic remedies often with royal jelly or ginkgo; numerous capsules also sold in health food shops and chemists; tincture available from specialist suppliers.

how to use
capsules – usually 600mg daily;
tincture – up to 5ml/1tsp, three times daily.

parts used
aerial parts

commercial products
included in numerous proprietary mixtures mainly marketed as remedies for insomnia and nervous tension; capsules and tincture widely available.

how to use
take at night only for insomnia repeating if need be once during the night or three times daily for anxiety or nervous tension;
tincture – up to 3ml/60 drops per dose;
capsules – up to 250mg per dose;
infusion – 25g/1oz to 500ml/1pt of water taken in three equal doses during the day.

under 40, while many herbalists regard it as more suitable for men than women since it raises *yang* energy. The Chinese also believe it acts on the lungs and spleen and so can be helpful during recovery from chest problems – such as asthma – and digestive disorders.

As a general tonic it is ideally taken for a month in late autumn when the weather is changing from hot summer to cold winter and the body needs to adapt to the new environment, although the herb can, of course, be taken whenever there are problems due to tiredness and overwork. Ginseng will also reduce blood sugar and cholesterol levels and helps to stimulate the immune system.

c a u t i o n s ginseng is best avoided in pregnancy although it may be taken then in small quantities for short periods. Other herbal stimulants, such as caffeine-containing drinks and horseradish, should be avoided while taking ginseng.

passion flower
Passiflora incarnata

Passion flower takes its name not from any effect it may have on the emotions, but from the religious symbolism of its flowers: the three stigmas were taken to represent the nails of the Crucifixion, the five anthers were Christ's five wounds, while the ten petals represented the Apostles present at the time (Peter and Judas Iscariot having absented themselves).

The herb is known as maypop in North America and was traditionally used by the Houmas in Louisiana as a blood tonic, while the Mayans regarded the crushed plant as helpful for swellings and used the decoction for

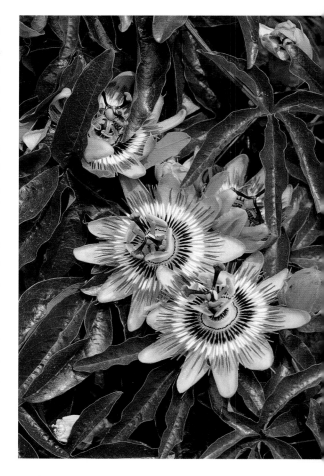

ringworm. It was first described by a European botanist in the 1780s and by the 19th century had joined the herbal repertoire, initially as a remedy for epilepsy and later as a cure for insomnia.

using passion flower
Today, it is considered as an effective but gentle sedative and painkiller which will also reduce blood pressure. Passion flower is widely used in OTC products for anxiety and nervous tension and is often combined with valerian or hops. An infusion of the dried herb can also be helpful for period pain or tension headaches, and can be supportive for a number of other nervous

conditions such as irritable bowel syndrome and irregular heartbeats. The plant is slightly bitter and cooling so can also be helpful in feverish conditions.

caution avoid high doses in pregnancy.

paratudo *Pfaffia paniculata*

Paratudo takes its name from *para todo* which is Portuguese meaning "for everything" reflecting its traditional use as a cure-all. The plant is also known as Brazilian ginseng while the alternative common name "suma" is a recent invention for the US health food market.

It was first described by the botanist Carl von Martius in 1891, but did not really come to the attention of the West until 1975 when one of the new generation of ethnobotanists was introduced to the herb by a Xingu shaman. Since then research has shown that paratudo is rich in steroidal compounds and saponins (similar to Korean ginseng) while pfaffic acid derived from the plant has been patented as an anti-tumour drug.

using paratudo

Traditionally paratudo was used as an aphrodisiac, wound herb, for diabetes and in cancer treatments. Since the 1970s the herb has been used effectively for chronic fatigue syndrome, arthritis, gout, to control cholesterol levels as a preventative for heart disease, to reverse arterial damage caused by arteriosclerosis as well as for some cancers. Studies have also shown that it is rich in stigmasterol which is a natural precursor for oestrogen and recent studies suggest it can be an effective treatment for menopausal problems or even a natural alternative to hormone replacement therapy.

kava *Piper methysticum*

Kava is of great ritual significance in the South Sea Islands – offered in ceremonies to honoured guests, used in rituals and recommended for an impressive list of ailments. The plant smells slightly of lilac with a pungent taste. Since the early 1990s kava has become increasingly popular in the USA and Europe as a calming remedy for stress and anxiety. Although the herb is very effective and is prescribed by many professional practitioners, it has also become associated with recreational drug use, popular with some for the relaxed state of *bonhomie* that it can induce. Inevitably this has led to abuse and high doses have been associated with cases of liver failure, including some fatalities. The result is that kava has been banned – or its use severely restricted – in a number of countries.

Its loss is unfortunate, as kava can be very effective at combating anxiety disorders. It is also antiseptic, will ease spasmodic cramps and encourages urination so is helpful for urinary tract problems, such as cystitis.

Traditionally, ritual drinks were made from the macerated root and root stump as a calming potion to increase mental awareness. The plant was chewed to a pulp, and this fermented the kava with saliva before it was infused in cold water. Nowadays mechanical grinding is more common and regarded as more hygienic. After infusion the chewed

paratudo

part used
root

commercial products
sold singly in capsules

how to use
capsules – up to 4g daily

kava

parts used
root, leaves and stump

commercial products
included in some proprietary mixtures for bladder problems or fluid retention; tincture and root available from specialist suppliers; sale of capsules and other over-the-counter products is restricted in some countries (including the UK and Germany).

how to use
capsules/powdered root – up to 150 mg daily; tincture – 10-20 drops daily.

ispaghula

parts used
seeds, seed husks

commercial products
included in some
proprietary remedies for
constipation and
digestive problems but
mainly sold as a simple
either in capsules or
processed into powders
or granules.

how to use
capsules – usually up to
1g daily;
dried seeds/husks – 1tsp
to a cup of boiling water,
infused until it is cool
enough to drink and then
both the seeds, and
mucilaginous gel they
produce with water,
should be swallowed.

guarana

part used
seeds

commercial products
included in some tonic
preparations with herbs
such as ginseng and gotu
kola but mainly sold as a
simple in capsules.

how to use
capsules – up to 2g daily

residue was removed, the mixture strained and then served in half coconut shells.

using kava

Because of concerns over safety, keep doses of kava to a minimum. Most OTC preparations will detail the amount of kavalactones (the active ingredient) they contain. The maximum dose should be 30 mg kavalactones per day.

As well as its use in anxiety and tension, the root extract can be used for urinary and genital infections, menstrual syndromes, headaches, general debility, colds and chills, chest pains, rheumatic pains, digestive upsets, obesity, asthma, chest infections, as a poultice for skin diseases and as a restorative tonic. Kava is traditionally taken before the evening meal, as a full stomach can reduce appreciation of its psychoactive properties. It is also an appetite suppressant and is always followed by a small meal, as over-eating after kava can lead to nausea.

cautions never exceed 30 mg kavalactones a day or take kava for longer than one month without a break; avoid entirely in pregnancy.

ispaghula *Plantago* spp.

Popularly sold under a variety of brand names, black psyllium or flea seeds (*P. psyllium*) and pinkish-brown ispaghula (*P. ovata*) are among the most popular of prescription and OTC bulking laxatives which will encourage bowel movement and lubricate the bowel.

using ispaghula

Many find the glutinous mixture produced by soaking the seeds in water rather hard to take, hence the large number of proprietary capsules

which are swallowed with plenty of water so that the seeds swell and become mucilaginous in the stomach instead. Large amounts of water need to be taken with such capsules to prevent over-absorption of gut fluids by the seeds as they expand. Alternatively the seeds can be mixed with breakfast cereal or flavoured with fruit juice.

Although primarily used for constipation, the bulky mass of ispaghula can help to soothe diarrhoea and is sometimes recommended in irritable bowel syndrome and, since it also creates a feeling of fullness, promoted as a slimming aid by discouraging over-eating. The plant is also anti-bacterial, anti-inflammatory and soothing and softening for the skin so externally the seeds can be used in healing poultices for wounds and skin infections.

guarana *Paullinia cupana*

Guarana has been known in the West as an energy elixir since the 17th century when missionaries reported that members of the Maués-Sateres tribe used the seeds as currency (much as the Aztecs did with cocoa beans) and carried them on journeys to take for hunger, fatigue, fevers, headaches and muscle cramps.

using guarana

It is still a popular everyday drink in Brazil – much preferred to coffee – and is believed to stimulate the nervous system, improve concentration, and speed recovery after illness. It is also used to encourage urination in cystitis and other urinary tract disorders, as a painkiller for menstrual problems, and to relieve the discomfort of extreme heat.

Guarana contains a caffeine-like compound

called guaranine, which is slower to metabolise so gives a gentler, more sustained stimulating effect than the artificial high of strong coffee.

The herb is usually promoted in the West as an energy-giving tonic. It can be helpful in chronic fatigue syndrome and is sometimes suggested for seasonal affective disorder (SAD) – a condition characterised by tiredness and depression in the winter months.

caution avoid in cases of high blood pressure and heart disease.

he shou wu
Polygonum multiflorum

He Shou Wu is one of the great Taoist longevity tonics – according to tradition one sage, Li Ching Yuen, born in 1678, reputedly lived to be 252 years old on a daily brew of *He Shou Wu* and ginseng. He died in 1930, reportedly after a banquet given in his honour by the government, was married 14 times and lived through 11 generations of his own descendants.

In Chinese theory, kidney energy reduces with age and this is the cause of many problems of ageing such as deafness, tinnitus and greying hair. Kidney energy is also associated with the reproductive system so the menopause is often linked to weakeness here.

using he shou wu
He Shou Wu (also known in the West as *Fo Ti* from its Cantonese name) is regarded in Chinese tradition as an important blood tonic which also helps kidney and liver energy. The root is the part mainly used although the plant stems (called *Ye Jiao Teng* in China) are also used as a

heart and liver tonic to calm the nerves and improve blood circulation.

He Shou Wu is included in a number of remedies for menopausal and ageing problems and is also used with ginseng and *Dang Gui* for chronic debility. It is a good heart tonic and helps to reduce blood cholesterol levels; the plant is also an effective anti-bacterial and is used to clear abscesses and boils.

caution avoid if suffering from diarrhoea.

saw palmetto
Serenoa repens

Saw palmetto originates in the south-eastern states of the USA and the berries were a popular food among Native Americans and early settlers, highly valued for their tonic effect and taken as a strengthening remedy in debility and convalescence.

using saw palmetto
The herb was traditionally used for cystitis and prostate problems and in recent years researchers have demonstrated that saw palmetto actually prevents the conversion of the male hormone testosterone into dihydrotestosterone (DHT) – a chemical now blamed for the excessive cell multiplication which leads to the enlargement of the prostate. Saw palmetto also encourages breakdown of any DHT that may have formed, so helping both to prevent and cure the problem, rather than simply superficially relieving it. Clinical trials involving the plant have demonstrated a significant reduction in the symptoms of prostate problems, and although quite high

he shou wu

parts used
root, stems

commercial products
included in numerous traditional formulations sold by Chinese herb shops; tincture and powdered herb available from specialist suppliers.

how to use
tincture – up to 5ml/1tsp, three times daily;
capsules – up to 600mg daily;
decoction – up to 25g/1oz per dose used in traditional remedies equivalent to 75g/3oz decocted with 750ml/1½pt of water for three daily doses although 25g/1oz per 750ml/1½pt would be more usual.

doses have been used in these experiments – up to 10g/⅓oz of the berries twice a day – herbalists often find much lower doses bring about a similar improvement.

Saw palmetto is often included in OTC products aimed at improving male libido as well as a number of general tonic preparations, usually targeted at older men. It can be useful in debility and convalescence helping to increase weight and strength. It is also believed to help encourage breast development so is sometimes promoted as a bust enhancer.

pau d'arco
Tabebuia impetiginosa

Pau d'arco, also known as lapacho or ipê-roxa, is an exotic Brazilian tree, which has carnivorous purple flowers to protect it from fungal attack, parasites and pests. It has been recognised as an important anti-cancer and anti-microbial remedy since the 1860s and is traditionally used by Amazonian tribes for treating asthma, diabetes, bronchitis, cancer, rabies, stomach ulcers, syphilis and various infections.

Pau d'arco is generally *T.impetiginosa* (syn. *T. avellenedae*) although, as always with wild-crafted South American herbs, numerous varieties of *Tabebuia* can end up in the mix. Research in the early 1990s confirmed that pau d'arco extracts are effective for both cancer and candida (yeast) infections while Japanese studies suggest that it can be effective against leukaemia and stomach cancer. Studies at the University of São Paulo have identified potent anti-bacterial, anti-inflammatory and anti-fungal components and the herb has also been used in treating breast and prostate cancers.

using pau d'arco

In the West pau d'arco is generally marketed as an anti-candida remedy but is also known to be effective for colds, flu and fevers. High doses have been used in experimental cancer treatment and it is often used for ulcers, rheumatism, high blood pressure, skin infections, urinary inflammations and pelvic inflammatory disease.

Traditionally the decoction is preferred although studies suggest that finely powdered bark is more effective.

feverfew
Tanacetum parthenium

Like comfrey, feverfew has hit the media headlines in recent years – this time as a major "cure" and prophylactic for migraine and some types of arthritis. Since the 1970s, the plant has been extensively researched and is known to contain chemicals called parthenolides which are believed to account for its action in easing the symptoms of both migraine and chronic arthritis. The herb is anti-inflammatory and will relieve spasmodic pains so can be helpful for period pain and is useful for minor fevers. The name feverfew refers less to its use as a fever remedy but is a corruption of featherfew – a description of its finely divided leaves.

Although there is some tradition of using feverfew for headaches, this was largely in external applications – writing in 1640, the herbalist John Parkinson suggested that the leaves were too bitter and unpleasant to eat: so in order to treat headaches, he recommended that they should be made into a poultice and placed on the crown of the head.

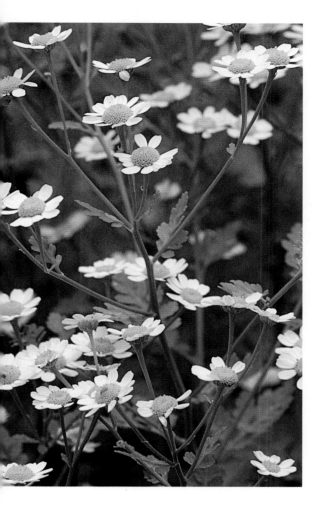

◄ Feverfew *Tanacetum parthenium*

size capsules which could be more liable to side-effects. Feverfew also reduces the blood's ability to clot, so should not be taken by those on blood-thinning drugs.

cautions not to be taken by those prescribed warfarin, heparin and similar drugs. Migraine sufferers should stop taking regular doses of feverfew if side-effects (skin rashes or mouth ulceration) occur. Avoid in pregnancy.

damiana
Turnera diffusa var. aphrodisiaca

Damiana is a popular stimulant and aphrodisiac used to combat fatigue and give energy. It is an aromatic shrub largely found in Central and South America and acts as a restorative tonic for the nervous system. The leaves are used as a substitute for tea in Mexico and the plant is also used to flavour various South American liqueurs.

using feverfew

Today, rightly or wrongly, the leaves are one of the most popular OTC herbs for treating migraines – although the bitter substances they contain do have a tendency to cause mouth ulcers in a significant number of users. Feverfew poultices are still sometimes used to relieve muscular aches and pains.

Clinical trials have well demonstrated its efficacy as a migraine remedy and many sufferers happily eat a couple of leaves a day as a prophylactic; two large leaves contain about as much parthenolide as in 125mg capsules although many companies market much larger

using damiana

The plant has been poorly researched and although it is a popular nerve tonic and appears to strengthen male hormones there is very little understanding of its action or constituents. Damiana has long been used for impotence, loss of libido and premature ejaculation but it is also a strengthening tonic for the female reproductive system and is often given for painful or delayed periods.

It can be helpful in convalescence and general debility, both as a tonic and to encourage the appetite. It is mildly anti-

---

feverfew

part used
leaves

commercial products
mainly sold as a simple in capsules or tablets (150mg-500mg); tincture available from health food shops.

how to use
tincture – up to 1ml/20 drops per dose, three times daily;
capsules – up to 200mg daily;
fresh leaves – one or two large leaves daily.

damiana

part used
leaves

commercial products
included in a number of proprietary tonic and aphrodisiac mixtures; capsules and tinctures available from health food shops.

how to use
tincture – up to 3ml/60 drops, per dose, three times daily;
infusion – 20g/¾oz to 500ml/1pt of water taken in three equal doses during the day;
capsules – up to 600g daily.

slippery elm

part used
bark

commercial products
included in many
proprietary digestive
remedies and some
external ointments for
minor wounds or skin
infections; capsules and
tablets available from
health food shops;
powder sold by specialist
herb suppliers.

how to use
capsules - up to 400mg
per dose; *powder* - used
in poultices or made into
a gruel by mixing 1/2tsp
with a little water to form
a paste and then adding
enough boiling water or
milk to make up to a cup.

depressant and is generally labelled as "thymoleptic" which means "mood enhancing" – positively uplifting. Damiana is also a urinary antiseptic and will encourage urination so can also be be used for treating conditions such as cystitis and other urinary tract problems.

It is often combined with saw palmetto for male sexual problems, with oats and vervain for depression, or with raspberry leaf and St John's wort for menstrual discomfort and irregularity.

slippery elm *Ulmus rubra*

The bark of the slippery or red elm was one of the most widely used of Native American medicines. The Ozark people took it for colds and bowel complaints, the Houmas used it for dysentery and the Missouri valley tribes used a decoction as a laxative. The bark is mucilaginous, providing a protective coating for the stomach, so it is ideal for soothing the mucous membranes in cases of stomach inflammation (gastritis), ulceration and heartburn.

using slippery elm

As well as being extremely soothing and demulcent, slippery elm is also highly nutritious and is a useful dietary supplement in debility and convalescence. It can be made into a gruel (see panel, left) which can be flavoured with honey and a little cinnamon to make it more palatable. The powder can also be added to porridge or muesli.

Native Americans used a tea of the root to help with difficult labour in childbirth and the strips of bark were once popular as a mechanical abortifacient. Today slippery elm is

always sold in powdered form to prevent this potential misuse.

Slippery elm tablets are worth keeping in the household medicine chest as a useful remedy for indigestion and they can be taken before a journey to combat travel sickness. A couple of tablets before the party starts can also reduce the likelihood of a hangover as the herb provides a coating for the stomach lining which will help to reduce alcohol absorption. Slippery elm will also encourage the coughing response to clear phlegm so can be useful for some respiratory complaints.

Externally slippery elm will soothe wounds and burns; the powder can be made into a poultice or added to creams and it is also available in ointments (sometimes combined with marshmallow) as a drawing remedy for splinters and boils.

peruvian cat's claw
Uncaria tomentosa

Credit for "discovering" Peruvian cat's claw is variously awarded to Dr Klaus Keplinger, who found the plant in the Peruvian rain forests in the 1970s, or a Bavarian school teacher called Arturo Brell who used it to cure his cousin's breast cancer in 1965. By 1994 the World Health Organisation had organised the first international conference devoted to "*uña de gato*" and by 1995 products containing the herb were becoming readily available on Western health food shelves.

Cat's claw – so called because the woody vine-like plant is covered with thorns resembling the claws of a cat – had been used for centuries by the Ashaninka tribe in Peru.

Two species are used: *U. tomentosa* and *U. guianensis* which grow in different parts of South America. They share many common properties, although there are some differences: *U. guianensis* is said to be more specific for cancer of the female urinary tract and more suitable for digestive problems, while *U. tomentosa* is better for gynaecological problems (including use as a post-childbirth tonic) and to combat the side-effects of chemotherapy.

using peruvian cat's claw

Extracts of both species have been variously used for AIDS, genital herpes, chronic fatigue syndrome, asthma, diabetes and circulatory problems. Traditionally the remedy is also believed helpful for arthritis, digestive problems such as gastritis (stomach inflammations), sexually transmitted diseases, and cirrhosis of the liver. It is used by some native peoples as a contraceptive. In the West

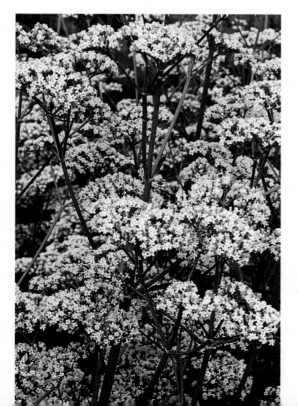

cat's claw is generally promoted as a preventative for cancer, an immune stimulant and general tonic.

caution cat's claw is a traditional contraceptive so is best avoided by women trying to conceive.

valerian *Valeriana officinalis*

Valerian is sometimes described as nature's tranquilliser — a calming nervine without the side-effects of comparable orthodox drugs: it is one of the few sedatives that can be safely taken to steady the nerves before driving tests. It has a distinctive, rather unpleasant smell and was aptly called *phu* by Galen; cats, however, love it and will roll ecstatically in the growing plants.

Valerian is identified by some as the "spikenard" referred to in the Bible. It has been very well researched over the past few years and found to contain chemicals such as valerenic acid (also found in other sedative herbs) and valepotriates — which develop in the dried herb: these seem to have a depressant effect on the nervous system while the fresh plant is more sedating. The valepotriates are a complex group of chemicals that also show anti-tumour activity but are only present in dried plant material.

using valerian

Valerian is probably the most widely used OTC herbal sedative, featuring in numerous remedies for insomnia and anxiety. It is often used to reduce high blood pressure and is prescribed by herbalists for a variety of heart conditions. It is

◄ Valerian *Valeriana officinalis*

peruvian cat's claw

parts used
inner bark, although roots and leaves are also used in folk medicine.

commercial products
increasingly available in capsules and tinctures from health food shops.

how to use
research and traditional use suggest that finely powdered bark or root needs to be decocted for at least 45 minutes to extract the active chemicals with a typical effective dose of 20g/¾oz of the herb to 1 litre/1¾pt of water taken in 60ml/2¼fl oz doses daily;
capsules – up to 1g daily;
tincture – up to 5ml/1tsp per dose, three times daily.

valerian

part used

root

commercial products

included in a great many proprietary mixtures recommended for stress, nervous tension, insomnia, digestive problems and heart and circulatory disorders; available as a simple in capsules (150-500mg); juice and tincture available in health food shops.

how to use

capsules - up to 400mg three times daily;

tincture - up to 4ml/80 drops per dose, three times daily;

maceration - soak 25g/1oz in 500ml/1pt of cold water overnight and take in three equal doses.

chaste-tree

part used

fruit

commercial products

mainly sold as a simple in capsules, tablets and tincture.

how to use

capsules - up to 250mg daily; *tincture* - usually ½-1ml/10-20 drops in a single dose. Chaste-tree is best taken in the morning as it affects the pituitary gland which is at its most active at that time.

popular in proprietary remedies targeted at menopausal women and also for anxiety associated with pre-menstrual syndrome and period pain. The herb also shows some anti-bacterial action, it will help to clear gas from the digestive track and ease spasmodic cramps.

Drink valerian tea for nervous irritability, tension headaches, menopausal problems or to relieve bronchial spasm and smoker's cough. A strong maceration of the fresh root can be added to bath water to make a relaxing bath when suffering from nervous exhaustion — although the smell is not to everyone's taste.

chaste-tree
Vitex agnus-castus

In recent years *Vitex agnus-castus* has become one of the most popular herbs for a wide range of gynaecological problems. It acts on the pituitary gland to increase the production of female sex hormones, especially progesterone. These control ovulation and the menstrual cycle so the herb can be very helpful for a wide range of gynaecological problems.

The herb is known as chaste-tree and grows wild in Mediterranean areas including Greece and Turkey, where it is regarded in folk medicine as a potent female aphrodisiac. Some argue that the common name is derived from its pure white flowers, although an equally likely explanation derives from its use as a male anaphrodisiac in mediaeval times. Then, it was taken by celibate monks to reduce libido and lascivious thoughts — hence its alternative country name of monk's pepper. It is still sometimes prescribed for problems with premature ejaculation.

using chaste-tree

Chaste-tree can be used to regulate the menstrual cycle, to stabilise hormone production at the menopause, improve fertility in those trying to conceive or to encourage milk production in nursing mothers.

For women, it is considered best to take chaste-tree in the early morning when the pituitary gland is believed to be most active and low doses are generally preferred. In higher doses it sometimes has the side-effects of "formication" – a sensation generally described as ants crawling over the skin.

ashwagandha
Withania somnifera

Known in English as winter cherry, *Withania somnifera* is becoming more familiar under its Sanskrit name, *ashwagandha*, which translates as "that which has the smell of a horse" as the plant was believed to endow any who took it with the strength, vitality and sexual energy of a horse. It is one of Ayurvedic medicine's most important tonic herbs and has been studied extensively in recent years showing significant anti-tumour activity in laboratory tests. The herb is sometimes called "Indian ginseng".

using ashwagandha

It is a traditional remedy in India to encourage healthy growth in children and to combat emaciation caused by famine. It can increase vigour and energy in the elderly and — in one clinical trial — improved sexual performance in more than 70% of the over-50s men involved. Studies have also shown that the herb can help increase body weight, slow the development of lung cancers in laboratory animals, and combat iron-deficient anaemia. The plant also shows strong anti-inflammatory activity similar in action to human steroidal hormones.

Although the root is mainly used, the leaves are taken in India in teas to encourage sleep if suffering from exhaustion and fevers, while the seeds have been shown to help protect against aspirin- and stress-induced ulcers, although they are traditionally avoided in Ayurvedic medicine as toxic.

yucca *Yucca* spp.

Although the yucca is mentioned in John Gerard's herbal of 1597 as a "hot and dry" plant and he was clearly impressed by its novelty, he does not have any suggestions as to its use.

The plants, also known as Joshua tree or soap tree, originate in North America and found many uses among the native peoples. Several species were used as a source of fibres for rope making while the flower buds of others were roasted as food. The Navajo used extracts for cataracts while the leaves – which are rich in substances called saponins – were used like soap for washing. Leaves of *Y. filimentosa* are known in the USA as Adam's needles and are mainly used for liver and gall bladder problems. The roots of several varieties have similarly been used as a detergent while these same saponins also make the herb strongly purgative.

using yucca
Saponins are steroidal so yucca is tending to be regarded as a natural source of progesterone-like chemicals which may be

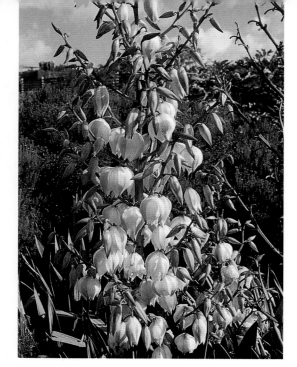

▲ Yucca *Yucca* spp.

helpful for various gynaecological problems and menopausal disorders.

Some reports also suggest that the plant can have an action on the gut flora helping to absorb bacterial toxins and improve function, while other studies suggest that yucca extracts may be able to shrink tumours.

Recent research in Dublin has highlighted yucca's ability to extract nitrogen-containing compounds from the air as a source of nutrients. Kept in a lavatory the plants will thus absorb urine smells. The leaves are also added to commercial pig feed to reduce the ammonia content of excreted material while, according to some experts, the saponin-rich faeces are easier to hose down in pig units.

cautions the high saponin content in *Yucca* spp. may lead to vomiting and nausea if taken in excess.

ashwagandha
parts used
root, leaves, seed
commercial products
included in several traditional Ayurvedic remedies; increasingly available in health food shops in capsules and occasionally as tincture.
how to use
capsules – up to 2g daily;
tincture – up to 5ml/1tsp per dose, three times daily.

yucca
parts used
root, leaves
commercial products
increasingly available in capsules and tinctures in health food shops.
how to use
capsules – up to 500mg daily;
tincture – up to 2ml/40 drops per dose, three times daily.

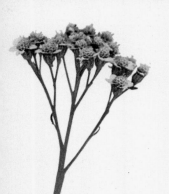

wildflower remedies

The sight of the village "herb wife" gathering her medicines from fields and hedges to brew into healing potions over the cottage fire is an image which probably stopped being commonplace in Britain more than 150 years ago. The Industrial Revolution and Enclosure Acts, which restricted access to common land, changed rural life dramatically and many of the old healing skills were lost. When Dr William Withering began experimenting with Mrs Hutton's cure for dropsy in 1775 – work which eventually led to the discovery of the heart drug digitoxin – Mrs Hutton was already an anachronism.

Today, many people are convinced that gathering a few sprigs from a hedgerow or garden and using them to make something to drink is likely to result in the creation of some highly toxic brew. Their concerns can sometimes be justified – excessive use of chemical sprays in agriculture can produce many poisonous residues on otherwise perfectly safe leaves.

This same over-enthusiasm for weed killers and pesticides, combined with vigorous roadside trimming, means that many of our once-common field and woodland flowers are now rare and it can be extremely difficult to find a natural source of herbs such as marsh woundwort and bear's breech. Others, such as yarrow, chickweed, and shepherd's purse do remain extremely common, and these plants can provide valuable emergency first-aid treatments when far from home. Fresh crushed leaves, rinsed in fresh water (if there is any nearby) to remove dust and soil, can be ideal to stop bleeding or use as a makeshift poultice.

In recent years attempts to reduce over-production of certain food crops and falling food prices have encouraged farmers to leave their land fallow, allowing the fastest growing weeds to prosper once more. These areas can be a good source of plants such as yellow dock, agrimony and common mallow. Many other roadside herbs can be grown in gardens, and wild flower seeds are readily available. Although these are native European plants, for historical reasons they have also been widely cultivated in other parts of the world, notably Australia and New Zealand. Several of the plants listed in this section can be invasive weeds (especially when grown outside Europe), so take care if you plan to introduce them into the garden!

Correct identification is, of course, important – especially where toxic plants are concerned. Foxglove when not in flower can easily be mistaken for comfrey, for example. It is always much easier to identify plants when they are flowering and since most can be collected then, this reduces the risk of error. Several plants can be difficult to find at certain times of the year: it is useful, for example, to note any coltsfoot plants in summer when the leaves are obvious so that the flowers – which are more difficult to spot – can be collected the following spring. When gathering plants in the wild try to choose specimens away from busy roads to limit pollution from petrol and diesel fumes and avoid areas close to farmland where chemical sprays may have been used.

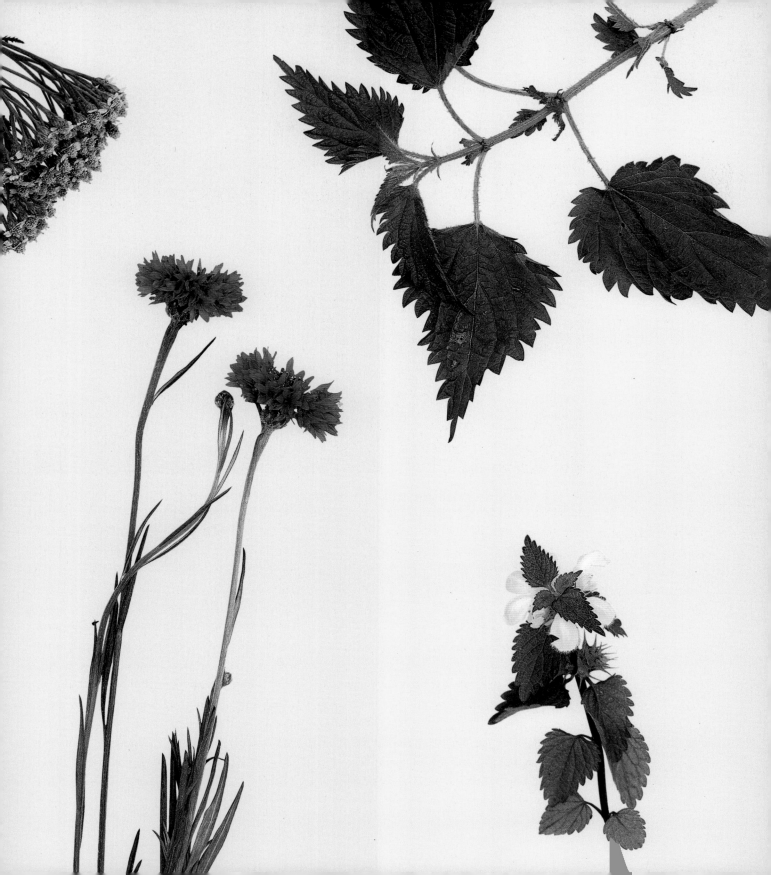

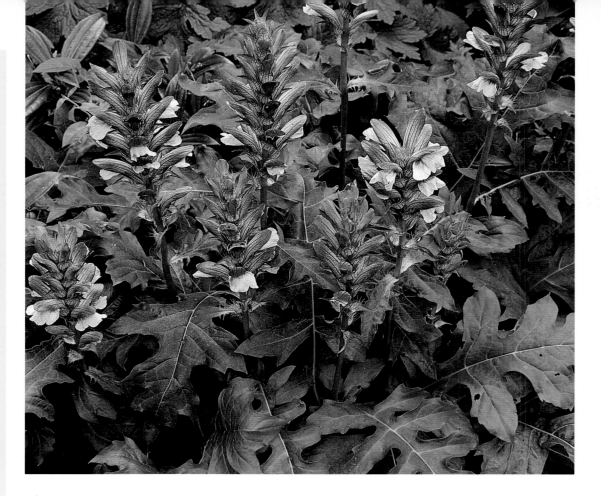

bear's breech

parts used
leaves, gathered before flowering

commercial products
not generally available

how to use
infusion - 25g/1oz of dried leaves to 500ml/1pt of water taken in three equal doses during the day; *fresh leaves* - crushed for poultices applied to minor injuries or inflamed joints.

bear's breech
Acanthus mollis

A hardy perennial growing to 1.5m/5ft with striking broad glossy, dark-green, pinnate leaves. The flower spikes bear white, pale blue or pale purple tube-shaped flowers with a three-lobed lip, appearing in late summer and lasting until early autumn.

Bear's breech originates from the Steppes of Asia but has long been grown in Mediterranean areas and was introduced into Britain in the Middle Ages. It was once common in the West Country, although it is now comparatively rare in the wild but is sometimes grown as a garden plant. Its botanical name comes from the Greek *akanthos*, "thorn flowers", and acanthus leaves are a common motif in ancient Greek sculpture and decoration – they are the inspiration for the classic design of Corinthian columns.

using bear's breech
The herb is rich in mucilage and tannins and was traditionally used as a soothing wound herb. Crushed leaves, soaked in cold water, were made into poultices for gout or used to ease minor burns and injuries. As a mild laxative and bile stimulant, the juice was traditionally used as a digestive tonic to improve appetite and cleanse the liver. "Acanthus tea" was also once recommended for bladder inflammations.

yarrow *Achillea millefolium*

A perennial herb with distinctive feathery leaves and tiny white flowers in clusters appearing throughout summer and autumn.

Yarrow was once used in divination and folk rituals still associate it with prediction (generally by identifying future husbands). The same tradition persists in China where yarrow stalks are used with the *I Ching*. In Germany and Nordic countries yarrow was once used instead of hops in beer making.

A common meadow herb, yarrow's folk name of nosebleed confirms its traditional use as an emergency styptic: a couple of feathery fresh leaves inserted into the nostril provide an ideal encouragement for clotting.

using yarrow

Yarrow relaxes the peripheral blood vessels, so can help to reduce high blood pressure and it is also cooling in fevers. Like chamomile flowers, yarrow flowers contain anti-allergenic compounds which are activated by hot water or steam, so are found only in infusions and the distilled essential oil, not in the tincture or fresh plant. The oil is available commercially, and is also anti-inflammatory. It can be used in steam inhalations for hay fever and chest rubs for colds and catarrh.

Yarrow tea can be helpful for colds, influenza, hay fever and catarrh. The herb also increases urination and is antiseptic for the urinary tract so is worth adding to mixtures for problems such as cystitis and fluid retention. It is slightly bitter to stimulate the digestion and also helps to clear wind and indigestion.

cautions yarrow should be avoided in high doses in pregnancy as it is a uterine stimulant. The fresh herb can sometimes cause contact dermatitis and, in rare cases, prolonged use may increase the skin's photosensitivity.

◀ Bear's breech *Acanthus mollis*

▼ Yarrow *Achillea millefolium*

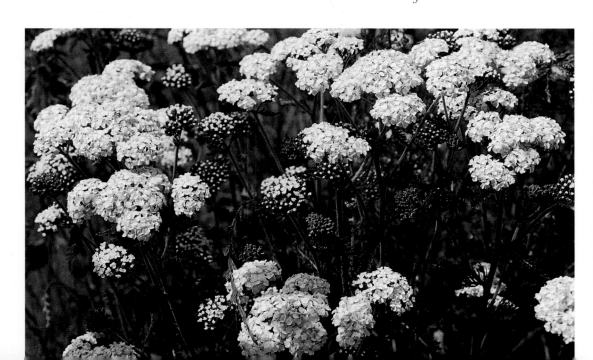

yarrow

parts used

leaves collected throughout the growing season; flowers gathered when in full bloom.

commercial products

included in several proprietary mixtures sold for colds, catarrh, rheumatic pains, digestive problems or menstrual irregularities; juice and tincture available from health food shops; essential oil sold by specialist suppliers.

how to use

juice – up to 10ml/2tsp, three times daily;
tincture – 3ml/60 drops, per dose, three times daily;
infusion – 25g/1oz of dried herb to 500ml/1pt of water taken in three equal doses;
fresh leaves – used in the nostrils to stop nose bleeds or as poultices to stop bleeding from minor wounds.

agrimony
Agrimonia eupatoria

An erect perennial herb growing to 60cm/24in in height with downy, serrated leaves in three to five pairs, larger at the base (where they may be 20cm/8in long) and getting smaller further up the stem. Five-petalled yellow flowers grow on tall flower spikes flowering from the bottom of the stem upwards, throughout the summer.

The tall yellow flower spikes of agrimony can still be seen at roadsides in high summer, giving the plant its old common name of "church steeples". The herb, like all members of the rose family, is strongly astringent so contracts blood vessels and tissues to stop bleeding and secretions. Writing in the second century AD, Dioscorides recommended it as a wound herb and for dysentery.

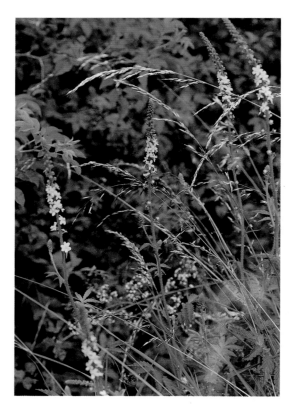

The *eupatoria* part of the plant's name is reputedly derived from Mithridates Eupator, an ancient king of Pontus and renowned herbalist. Since Saxon times agrimony has been used as a wound herb and, in the 15th century, was the prime ingredient of arquebasade water – a battlefield remedy for early gunshot wounds.

using agrimony

It is still used for the treatment of diarrhoea and is suitably gentle for children and babies – nursing mothers can take it as a means of dosing their babies via breast milk. Drink a cup of a weak infusion – 15g/½oz of herb to 500ml/1pt of water – two hours before feeds up to four times a day.

Agrimony is a bitter herb that will stimulate bile flow and has a tonic effect on the digestion. It can be useful for those prone to food allergies, helping food absorption while repairing damage to the gut caused by allergens. It also has a high silica content – hence its action as a tissue healer. Agrimony increases urination so is sometimes included in remedies for cystitis and other urinary problems and combines well with imported herbs such as buchu (see page 140).

jack-by-the-hedge
Alliaria petiolata

A biennial with a distinctive garlic smell, bright green rounded leaves and small white flowers in spring and summer. Grows up to 1.2m/4ft in height.

◀ Agrimony *Agrimonia eupatoria*

Garlic mustard is an alternative and very apt name for this common hedgerow plant which is characterised by the garlic smell obtained when the leaves are crushed. It makes a useful spicy addition to salads and can also be cooked to produce a mild garlic-flavoured sauce.

The plant has a long medical history and was once known as *Alliaria officinalis* – suggesting that it was once listed in official pharmacopoeia. Like garlic it contains various sulphur compounds as well as sinigrin, found in other members of the cabbage family, which account for its smell.

using jack-by-the-hedge
Poultices of Jack-by-the-hedge were once used for skin sores and cuts, applied hot to rheumatic aches and pains, or for neuralgia. The plant is slightly antiseptic and anti-inflammatory so makes an effective wound herb; it was also traditionally used for digestive problems and will increase urination.

William Turner included it as "saucealone" in the third part of his *New Herball*, published in 1568, suggesting that it was "hot in the second degree after the rules of Galen" and recommending it for "them that have a cold stomach ... but not good for them that ... have hot blood or be disposed to the headache".

As well as using the plant to spice up seasonal salads, it is well worth trying as a tea for colds and chills; it can also make a warming drink (or be used in sauces) for rheumatic sufferers.

▼ Jack-by-the-hedge *Alliaria petiolata*

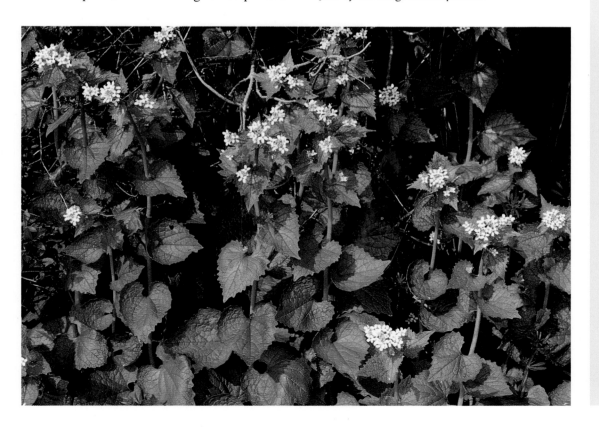

jack-by-the-hedge

part used
leaves, collected during flowering

commercial products
not generally available

how to use
fresh leaves – add to salads and sauces or use in poultices for minor injuries and muscle pains;
infusion – 25g/1oz of dried leaves to 500ml/1pt of water taken in three equal doses per day.

parts used
whole plant gathered
while flowering, or leaves
collected after flowering.

commercial products
occasionally found in
European remedies for
heart problems; juice and
tincture available from
health food shops.

how to use
juice – up to 10ml/2tsp,
three times daily;
tincture – up to 5ml/1tsp,
three times daily;
fresh leaves – chop and
add to salads.

ramsons *Allium ursinum*

A garlic-scented perennial growing from a white bulb with elliptical leaves up to 30cm/12in long and clusters of white, six-petalled, star-like flowers in early to midsummer.

Ramsons grow wild throughout Europe adding a wonderful garlicky scent to spring woodlands. The plant has been used in folk medicine since Greek times much as cultivated garlic has been – as a remedy for infections, chest complaints and digestive disorders, as well as being used as a blood purifier and spring tonic. The common name derives from *hramson* which was Old English for "wild garlic" and the plant is also known as bear's garlic or broad-leaved garlic.

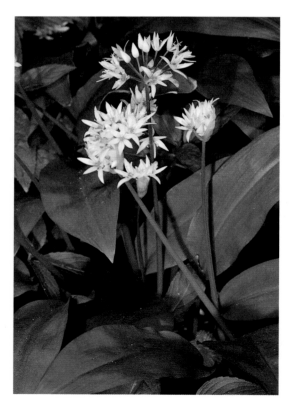

using ramsons

Like garlic, it helps reduce blood cholesterol levels and has been used to treat high blood pressure associated with hardening of the arteries (atherosclerosis). As a strongly anti-bacterial and anti-fungal plant, it is also used to treat yeast-related infections helping to normalise the gut flora.

Ramsons are rather milder in flavour than ordinary garlic and may be better tolerated by those with sensitive stomachs. The leaves can be chopped and added to salads.

marshmallow
Althaea officinalis

An erect, sturdy perennial with soft, downy, round to ovate leaves and large, pale pink flowers in the axils in summer. The plant grows to around 1.2m/4ft in height and prefers damp, marshy places.

Marshmallow grows in damp, sunny places and is a close relative of the garden hollyhock. It produces a sweet-tasting, highly mucilaginous root that is rich in sugars and is eaten as a foodstuff in many parts of the world – writing in the 1930s, the herbalist Maud Grieve recommended them boiled first and then fried with onions and butter.

The sugars help to make marshmallow very soothing and demulcent (softening) and the plant is widely used to calm inflamed mucous membranes especially of the lungs and digestive system – so it can be helpful for stomach inflammation (gastritis), heartburn and other similar problems.

◄ Ramsons *Allium ursinum*

using marshmallow

The botanical name comes from a Greek word, *altho,* meaning "to heal" and the plants have certainly been used medicinally since ancient Egyptian times. The leaves and flowers are also used medicinally and at one time the flowers were collected separately and made into cough syrups, although these days commercial cultivation means that all the aerial parts tend to be combined. The leaves can also be cooked as a vegetable while the young tips can be added to salads. Marshmallow root and leaves encourage urination, so both make a soothing addition to cystitis remedies.

Externally the plant is equally valuable and healing. It can be made into ointments for various sores and skin problems and, combined with slippery elm, it makes a good drawing ointment for splinters and boils. The root or leaves are soothing for irritating coughs and can easily be made into a syrup, providing a valuable and pleasant-tasting standby for winter coughs.

burdock *Arctium lappa*

A tall biennial herb growing to 2m/6½ft with large dock-like leaves, ovate to heart-shaped, with round purple flowers from early summer to early autumn. The seed heads form characteristic burrs with hooked tips.

It is still possible to find traditional "dandelion and burdock" cordials on supermarket shelves – although nowadays the product is likely to be promoted as a pleasant drink rather than a cleansing herbal remedy for skin problems and arthritis.

The herb commonly grows wild in Europe and parts of Asia and is familiar for its hooked burrs which get caught in clothing and animal fur – a property reflected in the botanical name, derived from the Greek words *arctium* meaning "bear", suggesting rough-coated fruits, and *lappa,* which means "to seize".

using burdock

As one might expect from a traditional cleansing herb, it is a mild laxative and increases urination, encourages perspiration and is useful where a sluggish digestion is contributing to a build-up of toxins.

Although not used in the West, the seeds are a traditional Chinese remedy for feverish colds – an action which modern research confirms

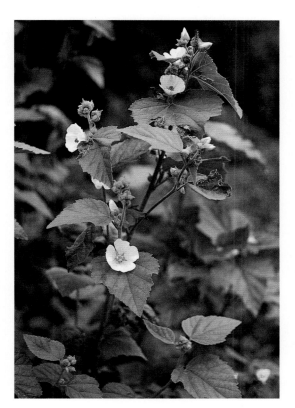

◀ Marshmallow *Althaea officinalis*

marshmallow

parts used
leaves collected before flowering, root collected in the autumn and flowers when in bloom.

commercial products
included in numerous proprietary mixtures mainly sold for digestive problems or coughs; tincture available.

how to use
tincture (root or leaf) – up to 5ml/1tsp three times daily;
infusion (leaves) – 25g/1oz of dried herb to 500ml/1pt of water taken in three equal doses during the day;
maceration (root) – soak 25g/1oz of dried root in 500ml/1pt of water overnight, taken in three equal doses during the day.

burdock

parts used

leaves collected during the flowering season, second-year roots lifted in autumn.

commercial products

included in a number of proprietary mixtures mainly sold for rheumatic and skin problems; capsules and tinctures available from health food shops; seeds sold by Chinese herbal suppliers as *Niu Bang Zi*.

how to use

tincture – up to 4ml/80 drops per dose, three times a day;

capsules – up to 500mg per dose, three times a day;

decoction – 25g/1oz of seeds or root in 750ml/1½pt of water taken in three equal doses; decoction up to 10g/⅓oz per dose;

infusion – 25g/1oz of dried leaves to 500ml/1pt of water, taken in three equal doses a day.

with the identification of strong anti-microbial activity in the seeds. They will also help to lower blood sugar levels, so could be useful in the management of late-onset diabetes.

Burdock produces a long tap root in its second year: this is cultivated as a vegetable (known as *gobo*) in Japan. Western herbalists tend to regard the root as more potent than the leaf and it is used in a number of OTC remedies, largely for skin and rheumatic complaints. Burdock is often combined with yellow dock in skin remedies.

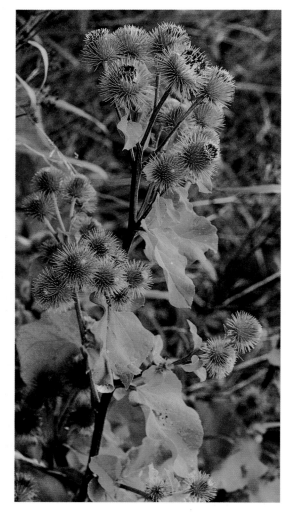

mugwort *Artemisia vulgaris*

Erect perennial with grooved stems, tinted with reddish-purple, reaching 1.75m/6ft; leaves 2.5-5cm/1-2in long, dark green above, whitish and downy on the underside, feathery and divided. Flowers are small, brownish-green to red and appear in tufts in late summer and autumn. The plant has a bitter smell when crushed.

To the Anglo-Saxons mugwort, as one of the "nine sacred herbs" given to the world by the god Woden, was described in the ninth-century poem the *Lacnunga* as: "...eldest of worts, thou has might for three and against thirty; for venom availest, for flying vile things; mighty gainst loathed ones that through the land rove...".

It was believed to be a potent totem against evil: surviving Anglo-Saxon herbals suggest hanging a root over the doorway of a house to prevent both it and its inhabitants coming to any harm, while sprigs were regularly worn to avert the evil eye. Even today sprigs of mugwort are worn on the opening day of the Isle of Man parliament – the UK's oldest civic gathering.

In the East, a local variety of mugwort leaf (*A. vulgaris*, var. *indicus* known as *Ai Ye* in Mandarin) is used as *moxa* – sticks or cones of dried herb that are burned at the end of acupuncture needles (moxibustion) for "cold" conditions such as arthritis.

More practically, the Romans are believed to have planted mugwort beside their roads so that they could line their sandals on a long journey to prevent aching feet. It is still commonly

◄ Burdock *Arctium lappa*
► Mugwort *Artemisia vulgaris*

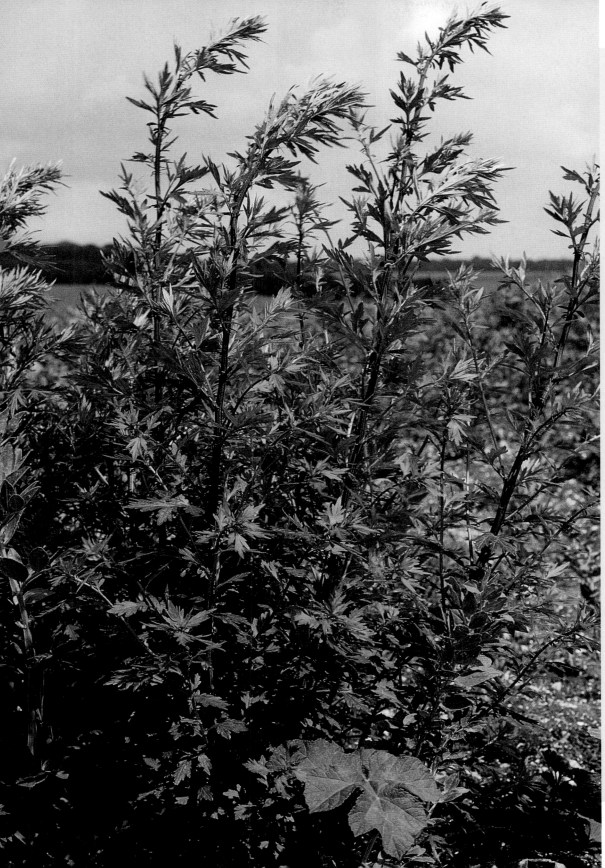

mugwort

part used
leaves

commercial products
not generally used in
proprietary medicinal
preparations; dried
leaves and tincture
available from specialist
herbal suppliers.

how to use
infusions – 15g/½oz of
dried herb to 500ml/1pt
of boiling water taken in
three equal doses;
tincture – up to 2ml/40
drops, three times a day.

daisy

parts used
aerial parts, gathered during flowering

commercial products
not generally available

how to use
fresh leaves – used in poultices for bruises, muscular pains and minor injuries;
infusion - 25g/1oz of dried leaves to 500ml/1pt of water, taken in three equal doses during the day.

---

found growing by old roads. The name mugwort reputedly derives from the Saxon "*mugga wort*" or midge plant as it will effectively repel insects.

using mugwort

Like its relative wormwood, mugwort is a bitter digestive stimulant. It is occasionally still used in cooking in stuffings for fatty meats such as goose. Mugwort is also a mild sedative and can help regulate menstruation so is often used by medical herbalists for gynaecological problems. It combines well with sage in teas for menopausal problems or can help normalise irregular menstrual activity.

caution avoid mugwort in pregnancy.

daisy *Bellis perennis*

A low-growing perennial with a basal rosette of oval leaves and numerous white and yellow flowers, often with a pink tinge to the petals. It blooms from spring to late autumn.

One of the old names for daisy was bruisewort – a reference to its popular use in ointments and poultices for bruises. The botanical name comes from the Latin *bellus* – pretty – and its English name is a corruption of "day's eye" as daisy flowers open only in sunshine and will tuck their heads away as dusk falls.

using daisy

The herb was once popular for wounds, while the leaves were used in poultices or made into an infusion to drink for lumbago, stiff neck or other aches and pains. Gerard suggests pounding fresh daisies with unsalted butter as a simple ointment for all sorts of pains, adding that "…they worke more effectually if mallowes be added thereto". He also suggests putting drops of daisy juice into the nostrils to clear catarrh and migraine while "the same given to little dogs with milke, keepeth them from growing great" – which provides an interesting insight into how Elizabethans regarded their pets.

A decoction of the root was used as a cleansing remedy for skin problems and could

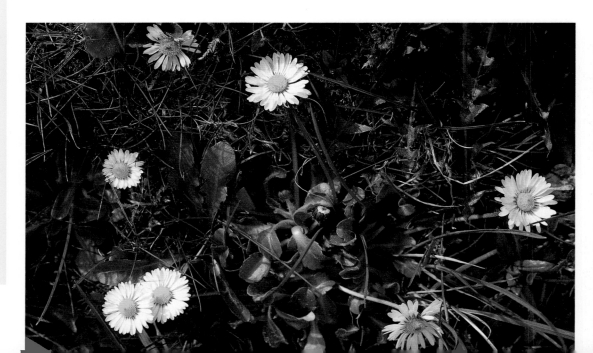

also be taken for respiratory complaints and liver disorders, while chewing fresh leaves is a traditional folk cure for mouth ulcers. The leaves contain saponins and have been used in cough remedies, and some anti-viral activity has been identified in the plant.

birch *Betula pendula*

A slender, short-lived tree, with drooping branches and silvery-white bark which tends to peel off easily. Male and female catkins appear in spring with winged nutlets in autumn.

Birch is highly regarded as a medicinal plant in many areas of Northern Europe – especially Russia and Scandinavia where it is a favourite for treating rheumatism, gout and arthritis. The tree contains salicylates, which accounts for its anti-inflammatory and anti-rheumatic action.

using birch
Both leaves and bark can be used in teas to relieve aches and pains and are also suitably astringent for use in mouth washes and gargles for sore gums, mouth ulcers and sore throats. The plant increases urination and can also be helpful in cystitis; it is often used with stinging nettles as a general cleanser and detoxificant for chronic conditions.

The sap can be collected as it falls back in the autumn by "tapping" the tree: make a hole through the bark and collect the large amounts of sap it produces in a bucket. Remember to block up the hole after taking out the sap, to prevent the tree from bleeding

◄ Daisy *Bellis perennis*

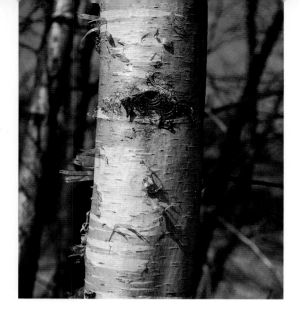

▲ Birch *Betula pendula*

to death. This sap can then be added to internal remedies for rheumatism or used to make birch wine.

An oil, distilled from the bark and known as birch tar oil, is used in ointments or lotions for psoriasis and eczema. Oils extracted from the North American sweet (*B. lenta*) and yellow (*B. alleghaniensis*) birch trees are around 98% methyl salicylate. In aromatherapy these are sometimes used in massage mixtures for muscular pains and as cleansing remedies to help eliminate toxins. These oils can also help remove uric acid from joints so can be valuable in gouty conditions.

cautions methyl salicylate derived from American birch oil is extremely toxic in large doses and can cause blistering of the skin; it should be used in a very weak dilution (around 2%) in massage therapy. Like all salicylate-containing remedies, birch should be avoided by those taking warfarin and similar blood-thinning drugs.

birch
parts used
leaves, collected in summer; bark and sap collected in autumn.

commercial products
included in proprietary mixtures often produced in Germany and Switzerland for rheumatic problems; tincture and essential oil available from specialist suppliers.

how to use
tincture – up to 5ml/1tsp per dose three times a day;
infusion – 25g/1oz of leaves to 500ml/1pt of water, taken in three equal doses during the day.

shepherd's purse

parts used
aerial parts collected
throughout the year

commercial products
sometimes included in
proprietary remedies for
urinary tract problems;
tincture available from
health food shops.

how to use
infusion - 25g/1oz of
dried herb to 500ml/1pt
of water, taken in three
equal doses during the
day;
tincture - up to 5ml/1tsp
per dose, three times
daily.

shepherd's purse
Capsella bursa-pastoris

*An annual or biennial with a basal rosette of feather-like
leaves and branched stems and tiny white flowers
throughout the year. The plant produces characteristic
heart-shaped seed pods, generally found on the stems
alongside the flowers. It is a common garden weed
growing to around 20cm/8in.*

Shepherd's purse takes its name from the heart-
shaped seed pods which were thought to
resemble the leather pouches once carried by
shepherds. These same seed pods account for
another of its country names, mother's hearts,
and the plant, like others with "mother's…" or
"lady's…" as part of their names, is a valuable
gynaecological remedy helpful for menstrual
irregularities and recommended as a tea in
childbirth to encourage contractions and ease
labour pains.

▼ Shepherd's purse *Capsella bursa-pastoris*

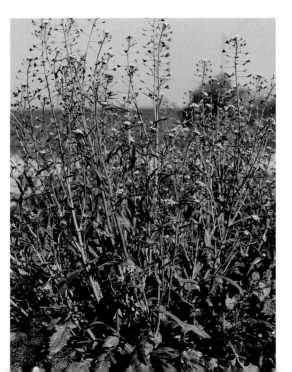

using shepherd's purse
Shepherd's purse has a pleasant, spicy flavour
and can be eaten in salads, added to sandwiches
and was once gathered and cooked as a spring
vegetable. Drinking shepherd's purse tea may
help relieve heavy periods, while its astringency
helps dry up secretions so it can also be helpful
for chronic diarrhoea and in colitis.

The herb will stop internal and external
bleeding, is an antiseptic for the urinary tract
and will increase urination, all of which makes
it very helpful in cystitis, especially in severe
cases where there is blood in the urine. It is used
in traditional Chinese medicine as a wound
healer, while the seeds are believed to help
improve eyesight. It has also been used to
reduce fevers in malaria.

caution shepherd's purse can cause
contractions of the uterus, so should be avoided
during pregnancy.

cornflower
Centaurea cyanus

*An annual with grey-green lanceolate (lance-shaped)
leaves and striking blue composite flowers in summer: some
varieties have white or purple flowers.*

The bright blue cornflower was once – like the
red corn poppy – commonly found in summer
cornfields across Europe. Increased use of
agricultural chemicals has long since rid the
farmer's acres of such attractive weeds and most
cornflowers found today are in gardens or
undisturbed wild areas.

➤ Cornflower *Centaurea cyanus*

using cornflower

In the Middle Ages the plant was known as bluebottle or blue bothem, but its wide use as a medicinal herb led to the adoption of the apothecaries' name – *flos frumenti* (which means literally "flower of the corn") – instead. Like its relative, centaury, cornflower contains a bitter compound (centaurine) which accounts for its use as a digestive stimulant. Cornflower tea made from the dried flowers is still used for indigestion in many parts of Europe and the bright blue flowers are often found in tisane mixtures in Austria and Hungary. They make a useful and revitalising addition to early morning teas.

An infusion of the flowers is also a traditional folk remedy for tired eyes – use a cool, dilute, well-strained infusion in an eye-bath. Under the Doctrine of Signatures theory, cornflower was regarded as better for blue eyes; brown-eyed people were advised to use plantain instead. The flowers have a mild tonic effect and will also reduce inflammation.

greater celandine
Chelidonium majus

A perennial with brittle stems which yield a brilliant deep yellow sap. The leaves are divided with oblong leaflets, while the four-petalled flowers appear in summer and are followed by long, linear seed pods.

Greater celandine is a member of the poppy family, completely unrelated to the lesser celandine or pilewort (see page 198), which belong to the buttercup group. It is notable for its brilliantly coloured sap which makes an ideal remedy for clearing warts – simply apply a little each morning and evening, taking care not to get too much of the juice on surrounding areas as it can be corrosive.

One of its old names is "swallow wort", which dates from an ancient Greek tradition, repeated by herbalists as late as the 17th century, that swallows fed the seeds to their

▼ Greater celandine *Chelidonium majus*

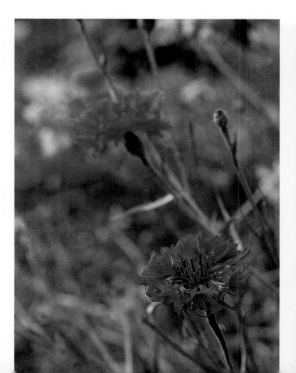

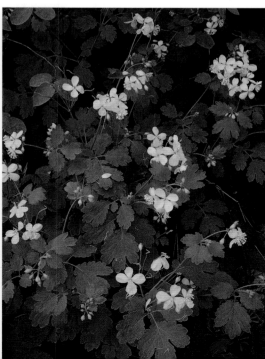

cornflower

parts used
flowers collected when just open

commercial products
sometimes included in tisane blends

how to use
infusion – 15g/½oz of dried herbs to 500ml/1pt of water (flowers are very light and the normal 25g/1oz amount is very bulky), taken in three equal doses during the day.

greater celandine

parts used
aerial parts collected when flowering; sap.

commercial products
occasionally found in proprietary liver and digestion tonics; tincture available in health food shops.

how to use
tincture – up to 2ml/40 drops three times a day; *infusion* 15g/½oz of dried herb to 500ml/1pt of water taken in three equal doses during the day; *fresh sap* – apply directly to warts up to two or three times a day.

177

hawthorn

parts used

flowering tops, collected in spring, and berries, collected when ripe in autumn.

commercial products

included in a number of proprietary mixtures for circulatory and heart problems; capsules, juice and tincture all sold in health food shops. Chinese hawthorn berries are old as *Shan Zha* in Chinese herbal medicine shops.

how to use

tincture - up to 2ml/40 drops per dose; *infusion* - 15g/½oz of dried flowers to 500ml/1pt of water taken in three equal doses during the day; *decoction* - 15g/½oz of dried berries to 750ml/1½pt of water taken in three equal doses during the day.

young to improve their eyesight. Certainly, it was widely recommended in the 17th century for eye complaints.

using greater celandine

Internally the herb is used as a liver remedy, cleansing the gall bladder and stimulating bile flow in liver disorders such as hepatitis and jaundice. It also increases urination and can be used as a cleansing remedy for skin conditions where liver stagnation is a contributing factor.

Greater celandine is a potent plant and its use is restricted in some countries, although as the recommended maximum dosage (200ml/7fl oz of tincture per week) is at least four times what would normally be prescribed, it can be considered as safe in normal dosages, although as a uterine stimulant it is best avoided in pregnancy.

cautions excess can cause skin irritation, dry mouth, dizziness and drowsiness; avoid in pregnancy.

hawthorn

Crataegus oxycantha

A common deciduous shrub or small tree, often used in hedging, with deeply lobed obvate leaves and pink or white scented flowers in late spring. Dark red oval fruits form in early autumn and are usually eaten by birds.

Like many members of the rose family, hawthorn is astringent and will help stop bleeding; as such it was largely used as a remedy for diarrhoea and heavy menstrual bleeding. Taking a Doctrine of Signatures approach, old

➤ Hawthorn *Crataegus oxycantha*

herbals also recommend the plant for drawing thorns and splinters. It has been used for centuries as a hedging plant to divide farms and fields and the name "haw" is actually an old word for a hedge – hence hedgethorn.

using hawthorn

Today we regard hawthorn primarily as a heart herb – a valuable tonic that will help normalise heart action and combat high blood pressure. This is, however, a comparatively recent use – apart from occasional mentions suggesting it as a remedy for dropsy (which can be related to blood pressure problems), there is little historical evidence linking hawthorn with heart disorders.

It helps to relax and dilate peripheral blood vessels, improving blood supply throughout the body, and has a relaxing effect on the

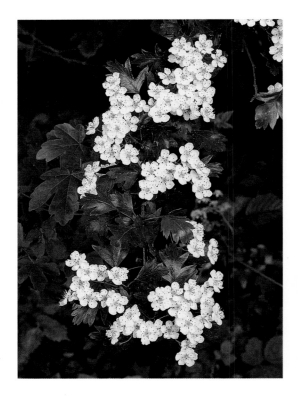

coronary blood vessels. Hawthorn also has a general tonic effect on heart action and contains chemicals called procyanadins which relax the central nervous system. It is used to reduce high blood pressure as well as counter the risk of angina attacks and helps to soften fatty deposits in the blood vessels which can lead to hardening of the arteries (atherosclerosis). Both flowering tops and berries are used in this way. The Chinese use only the berries of a closely related species (*C. pinnatifida*) and consider them primarily as a digestive remedy.

Hawthorn combined with linden flowers or yarrow makes a pleasant tea for those prone to high blood pressure. As an astringent, it is also worth remembering that hawthorn infusions can be used as a gargle for sore throats, a douche for vaginal discharges, and will be helpful for diarrhoea and other digestive upsets.

rose-bay willow herb

Epilobium angustifolium

A tall, dramatic wild flower growing to 2.5m/8ft in height with brilliant pink flower spikes and long, narrow, minutely toothed leaves.

In his classic book *The English Gardener,* William Cobbett, the 18th-century writer, recommends rose-bay willow herb as an ideal plant to grow at the back of a shrubbery – its bright pink flowers well worth adding to the garden. Today we tend to condemn the plant to the "weed" category and eradicate it ruthlessly. It is certainly one of our more attractive wild flowers – Gerard called it a "goodly and stately plant".

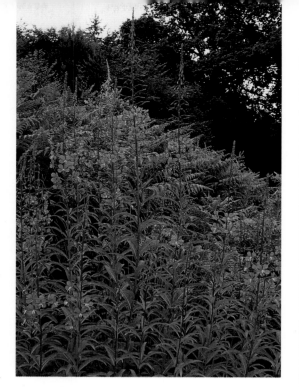

▲ Rose-bay willow herb *Epilobium angustifolium*

using rose-bay willow herb

Although little used in mainstream herbal medicine today, willow herb leaves were once dried and used as a substitute (and adulterant) for tea. Maud Grieve records that as late as the 1930s it was drunk regularly in Russia as kapoorie tea. The young shoots were also boiled and eaten as a vegetable. Medicinally, the root and leaves can be helpful for stomach upsets and gastroenteritis and can be ideal for diarrhoea in children.

As an astringent rose-bay willow herb is useful as a gargle for sore throats and mouth ulcers while compresses soaked in an infusion can be used to stop bleeding and soothe minor wounds; it was also once used in ointments for childhood eczema and shows some antibacterial activity reinforcing its traditional use as a wound remedy.

rose-bay willow herb

parts used
aerial parts collected before and during flowering, root collected in autumn.

commercial products
not generally available

how to use
infusion – 25g/1oz of dried aerial parts to 500ml/1pt water taken in three equal doses during the day;
decoction – 1tsp of chopped root to a cup of water, simmered for 15 minutes and taken three times daily.

horsetail

parts used
aerial parts

commercial products
included in several proprietary mixtures mainly for urinary tract problems; capsules, juice and tincture all available from health food shops.

how to use
juice - up to 10ml/2tsp per dose, three times a day;

tincture - up to 5ml/1tsp per dose, three times a day;

capsules - up to 2g per dose, three times a day;

decoction - simmer 25g/1oz fresh plant in 750ml/1½pt of water for 1-2 hours, adding more water if need be, as the stems are very tough and difficult to break down.

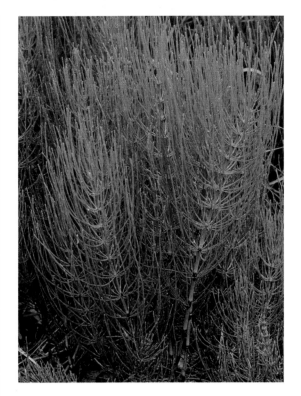

horsetail *Equisetum arvensis*

Upright, growing to 80cm/32in, often branched sterile stems with black-toothed sheaths and whorls of spreading green branches, the spores ripen in spring and the plant can be an invasive weed.

Horsetails grew on earth 270 million years ago in the Carboniferous period; their decayed remains helped form many of the world's coal seams. This primitive plant has neither leaves nor flowers, but spreads by spores and underground tubers.

Its hard stems made it effective for scouring in the days before sandpaper and wirewool: it was used by cabinet makers, tinsmiths, and even milkmaids who used it for polishing their pails. Its surviving country names, such as shave grass, bottlebrush and pewterwort, are reminders of this once-important application.

◄ Horsetail *Equisetum arvensis*

using horsetail

Horsetail's brittle-jointed stems are extremely rich in silica, which is very healing, and it is largely used for urinary tract problems, including prostate disorders, and deep-seated lung problems including chronic bronchitis, tuberculosis and emphysema. It is also very astringent and has been used as a wound herb since Greek times. It is helpful for a range of conditions including nosebleeds, heavy periods, or blood in the urine.

The plant is a good healing herb for the mucous membranes in the urinary tract and lungs and can be helpful in such diverse ailments as childhood bed-wetting and nasal catarrh.

cautions horsetail is rich in heavy minerals so it is best to stagger treatment with a week's break every fifth week to avoid straining the kidneys.

californian poppy
Eschscholzia californica

A hardy annual growing to 60cm/24in with numerous finely divided, blue-green leaves and bright orange four-petalled poppy-like flowers up to 7cm/2¾in in diameter, which appear throughout summer and early autumn, followed by a slender, ribbed seed capsule up to 10cm/4in long.

Californian poppies are a popular and easy-to-grow garden plant with cheerful bright orange flowers. Although a member of the poppy

➤ Californian poppy *Eschscholzia californica*

family, Californian poppy contains none of the alkaloids which depress the nervous system that its more potent relatives do. It is a mild sedative and sleep-inducing herb, suitable even for restless children. Californian poppy also encourages sweating so can be a useful cooling sedative in feverish illnesses.

using californian poppy

In North America, Californian poppy has the country name of "nightcap". It is an effective pain reliever and was used by Native Americans as an internal remedy for colic and gastric pains; it will also encourage urination. It is poorly researched, although anecdotal reports suggest that it can be helpful in the relief of some nervous conditions, bedwetting in children, bladder and urinary disorders and various painful conditions.

For home use it is easy to gather the whole herb during the flowering season, dry in small bunches and store for use as a night-time tea to combat insomnia.

hemp agrimony
Eupatorium cannabinum

A tall, sturdy plant with narrow leaves longer at the base and arranged in opposite pairs. The flowers form in dull pink clusters in late summer and early autumn.

An attractive wild plant generally found in damp places, hemp agrimony has been used since the days of Dioscorides as a laxative and to stimulate bile flow in liver stagnation and poor digestion. It was popular during the Middle Ages as a wound herb and the leaves were once used to wrap bread to prevent it from going mouldy.

using hemp agrimony

The plant is a useful remedy for colds and chills, helping both to reduce fevers and to ease coughs. Recent research suggests it may be antibiotic and immune-stimulating, and hemp agrimony has also been found to

californian poppy

parts used
aerial parts

commercial products
available in capsules (200-250mg)

how to use
capsules – 2-3 at night; *infusion* – 1-3tsp per cup of boiling water at night for insomnia for adults or ½-1tsp for children or 25g/1oz to 500ml/1pt of boiling water in three equal doses for general use.

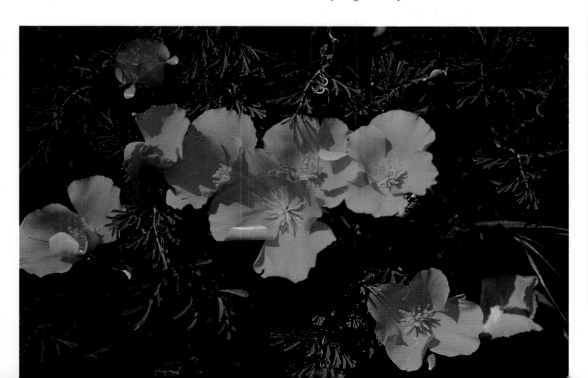

181

parts used
aerial parts, collected when flowering; roots collected in autumn.

commercial products
not generally available

how to use
infusion (aerial parts) – 25g/1oz to 500ml/1pt of water taken in three equal doses during the day;
decoction (root) – 25g/1oz to 750ml/ 1½pt of water taken in three equal doses during the day.

contain a substance called eupatoriopicrin, which is known to have anti-tumour properties.

Hemp agrimony is laxative and also increases urination so the plant can be useful for clearing toxins from the system in arthritis and chronic skin disorders. Poultices of the herb were once used on prurient skin sores, ulcers and infected wounds.

Hemp agrimony can be combined with elder flowers and yarrow to ease colds and chills, while a decoction of the root is a good remedy for coughs and also has a laxative action. An infusion of the flowers and/or leaves can be helpful for the relief of rheumatic pains. When fresh, the plant can be purgative so it needs to be used with caution.

caution high doses may cause nausea.

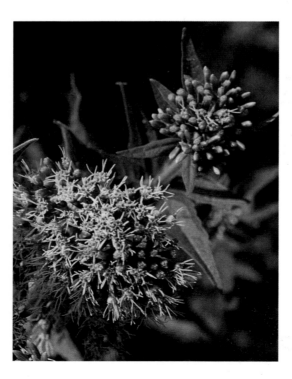

meadowsweet
Filipendula ulmaria

A hardy perennial growing to around 1.2m/4ft in height and generally found in damp ditches and hedgerows. The plant has irregular pinnate leaves and large, fluffy, creamy flower heads, which smell slightly of aspirin, appearing from midsummer to early autumn.

Meadowsweet's best-known claim to fame is as the herb which gave us the name "aspirin". In the 1830s chemists first identified a substance called salicylic acid, extracted from willow bark, as an anti-inflammatory and analgesic, and over the following years worked to produce a synthetic drug. By the 1890s, the pharmaceutical company Bayer had finally patented the result and since salicylates, extracted from meadowsweet, had been involved in the development work, they named the drug aspirin after the old botanical name for meadowsweet, *Spiraea ulmaria*.

using meadowsweet
Crushed meadowsweet flowers have an aspirin-like scent and the plant was used in Elizabethan times as a strewing herb to improve the smell of less than clean houses, as well as to flavour wine and ales. Meadowsweet has long been used in much the same way as the proprietary drug – for easing pains and feverish colds and as an anti-inflammatory for arthritic conditions.

Unlike aspirin, which can irritate the gastric lining and in prolonged use lead to ulceration, meadowsweet is extremely soothing and

◄ Hemp agrimony *Eupatorium cannabinum*
➤ Meadowsweet *Filipendula ulmaria* (and overleaf)
➤➤ Cleavers *Galium aparine*

calming for the digestive tract. It helps to reduce excess acidity and is ideal for gastritis (stomach inflammations), indigestion and heartburn and is sometimes even described as having anti-ulcer activity. Meadowsweet infusion is excellent for many minor stomach upsets and, taken after meals, is good to counter indigestion: for digestive problems it combines well with marshmallow and lemon balm. The tincture is ideal in holiday first aid kits for stomach upsets

Strong extracts of meadowsweet are used by professional herbalists in treating arthritis and rheumatism, although in mild cases a home-made infusion can be useful.

cautions meadowsweet is best avoided by those sensitive to salicylates and aspirin; avoid if taking blood-thinning remedies such as warfarin and heparin.

cleavers *Galium aparine*

A weedy, scrambling annual with whorls of up to nine elliptical leaves along the stem. Tiny green-white flowers appear beside these whorls in spring, followed by round purple-green fruits. The sticky stems will often spread for 3m/10ft or more among shrubs and climbing plants.

To most gardeners, cleavers – also known as sticky willy and sweetheart – is an irritating weed with a fondness for scrambling through shrubs and threatening to choke prize specimens. Cleavers is also known as goosegrass and is a favourite food for these birds.

using cleavers

The herb is particularly valued for its tonic effect on the lymphatic system, making it a popular cleansing herb for skin problems and glandular disorders including tonsillitis, benign

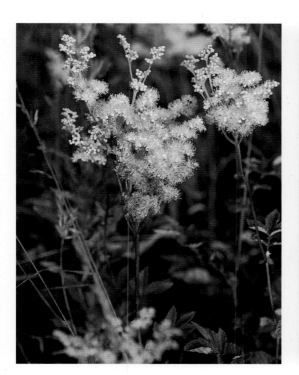

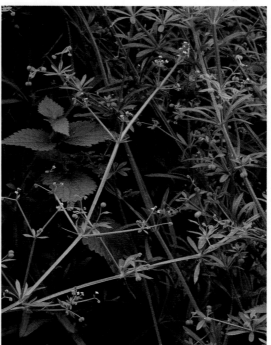

meadowsweet

parts used
all the aerial parts, collected when flowering.

commercial products
included in several proprietary remedies for digestive problems; tincture available from health food shops.

how to use
tincture – up to 5ml/1tsp, per dose, three times a day;
infusion – up to 60g/2oz to 500ml/1pt of water taken in three equal doses during the day.

cleavers

parts used
aerial parts, collected before fruiting

commercial products
used in numerous proprietary mixtures mainly for urinary tract disorders; tincture available from health food shops.

how to use
tincture – up to 5ml/1tsp per dose, three times daily;
fresh juice – make by pulping in a food processor – up to 50ml/2fl oz per dose, three times daily.

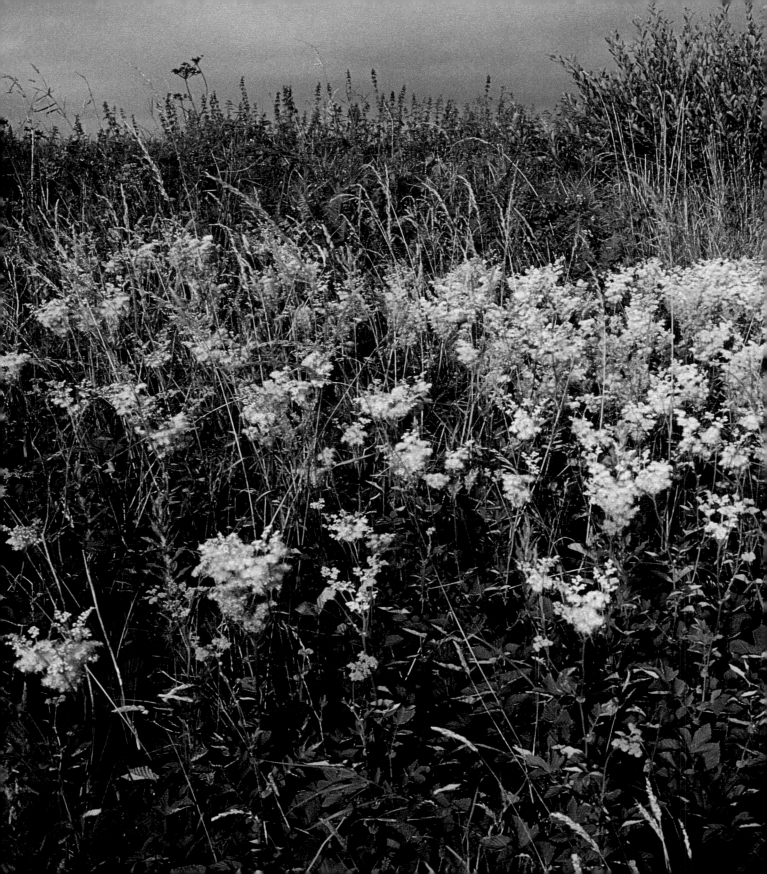

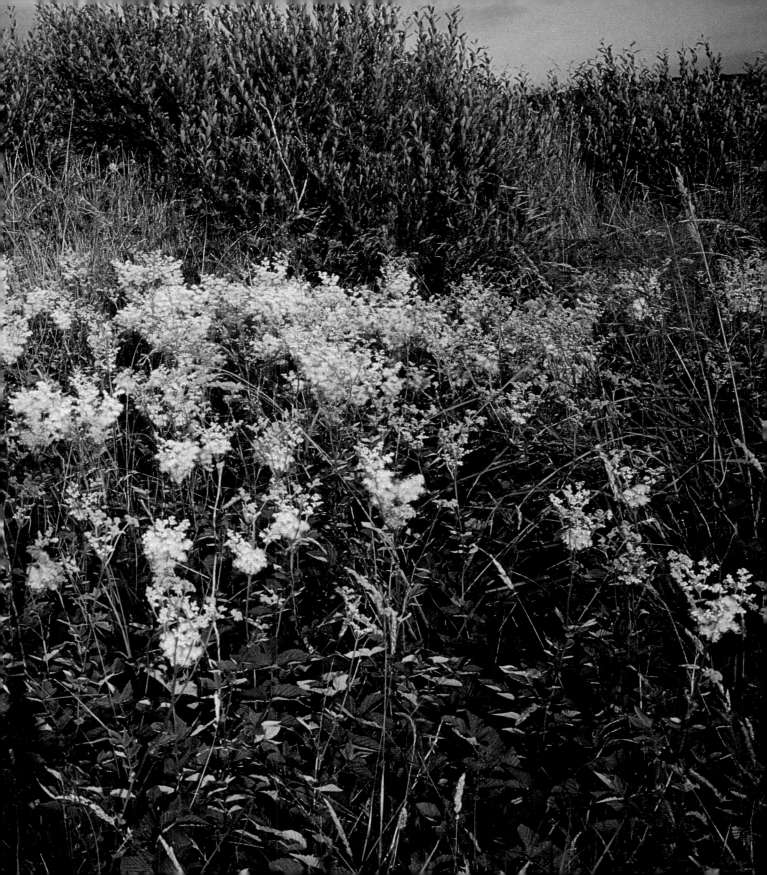

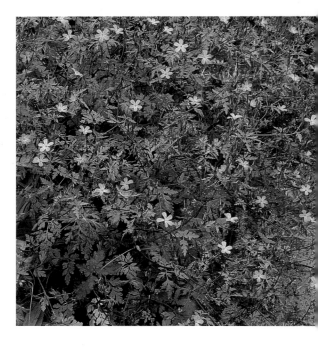

breast lumps, cysts, swollen lymph glands and glandular fever. It can also be made into creams and infused oils which will ease the symptoms of psoriasis.

The dried herb tends to display few diuretic properties (although it is popularly included in many OTC products), but when used fresh as a juice it can be extremely effective and can be useful for both urinary disorders and fluid-retention problems associated with heart disease. The young shoots gathered in the spring also make a valuable seasonal cleansing tonic — eat them either fresh in salads and sandwiches, pulped or in teas.

herb robert
Geranium robertianum

An annual or biennial with red-tinged stems and highly divided, palmate leaves. The plant has a foetid smell and bright pink five-petalled flowers from early summer until mid- to late autumn.

All members of the geranium family are astringent, wound-healing and styptic and although the American cranesbill (*G. maculatum*) is most widely used in commercial herbalism, the British herb Robert is equally effective. It makes useful ground cover in the shrubbery, although it can easily become invasive. Its leaves have a slightly foetid smell when crushed — effective at keeping insects away, so rubbing exposed skin with the leaves can help prevent insect bites.

Herb Robert is believed to take its name from a mediaeval St Rupert and was once known as *herba sanctii ruperti* and widely used in folk medicine. According to the Doctrine of Signatures theory, the plant's bright pink flowers and the reddish tinge to the stems suggested that it would be good for the blood and it was therefore once used for haemorrhages and diabetes. Modern research does suggest it has some action in lowering blood sugar levels, although it is rarely used in this way today.

using herb robert
Herb Robert tea is suitably astringent to counter diarrhoea and can also be used as a gargle and mouth wash for mouth ulcers and sore throats or in an eye bath (best if simmered for a few minutes to completely sterilise it) for conjunctivitis. The same infusion can also be used to bathe skin sores, minor cuts and grazes. Alternatively, the fresh leaves can be pounded to make a poultice for bruises and skin eruptions.

wood avens *Geum urbanum*

An upright perennial with slender stems and widely spaced pinnate leaves and small yellow flowers from early summer to mid-autumn. Purple-tinged fruits covered in hairy bristles appear in the autumn and the plant grows to around 60cm/24in. The root has a strong smell of cloves

Wood avens is also known as herb Bennet or Benedict's herb – a name derived from *herba benedicta* or *blessed herb*. In the Middle Ages its strong-smelling root was believed to ward off evil spirits and amulets of it were often worn or hung in homes to avert the evil eye. Although this belief in its potent effect on evil probably pre-dates Christianity, the plant is often seen in mediaeval illustration with the small trefoil-like stem leaves taken to symbolise the Trinity and the five-petalled flowers associated with the five wounds of Christ. The roots had symbolically to be collected on 25 March, Lady Day.

Its botanical name also focuses on this aromatic root: *geum* comes from a Greek word meaning "to produce a pleasant smell" – a smell which is easily lost when the root is dried, although fresh root can be used in cooking as an alternative to cloves and, like cloves, also helps stimulate the digestion.

using wood avens

Traditionally wood avens tea was taken for diarrhoea and to improve the appetite in debility and convalescence. It reduces inflammations and externally it has been used as a wound herb. Gargling with the infusion – as with many astringent herbs – was once a popular folk remedy for sore throats and gum disease. It helps to reduce fevers, is anti-microbial and can be useful as an anti-catarrhal, so is worth combining with herbs such as yarrow or elder for treating symptoms of the common cold.

elecampane *Inula helenium*

Tall, attractive perennial growing to 2-2.5m/6½-8ft with a long, thick tap root. Stems are hairy and erect, with large elliptical leaves up to 50cm/20in long, 20cm/8in wide, velvety beneath, rough and hairy above. The flowers are bright yellow, large – up to 10cm/4in in diameter – daisy-like with numerous long, slender ray florets and appear from mid-summer to autumn.

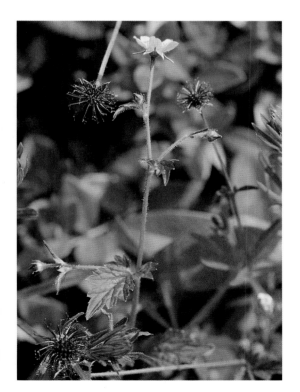

◄ Wood avens *Geum urbanum*

elecampane

parts used

root, flowers

commercial products

included in several proprietary cough and catarrh remedies; tincture is available from specialist suppliers; dried flowers (*Xuan Fu Hua*) are sold by Chinese herbal shops.

how to use

tincture – up to 5ml/1tsp, three times daily; *decoction* – 25g/1oz of root to 750ml/1½pt of water, simmered and taken in three equal doses, this can be converted to syrup by simmering with 500ml/1pt of honey and taken in 5ml/1tsp doses every 2-3 hours; *flowers* (*Xuan Fu Hua*) – used in complex Chinese decoctions usually 3-9g/⅛-⅓oz per dose.

white deadnettle

parts used

whole plant collected during flowering

commercial products

not generally available although the tincture is sold by specialist suppliers.

how to use

tincture – up to 5ml/1tsp per dose, three times a day;

infusion – 25g/1oz of dried herb to 500ml/1pt of water, taken in three equal doses during the day.

While today we regard elecampane as a cough remedy and tonic for chest problems, to the Anglo-Saxons it was the principal cure for "elf-shot" and averting the evil eye. Early writers mingle its medicinal action with magic and religion: it was not to be harvested until it was a man's height (just under 1.8m/6ft, believed to be the height of Christ at the crucifixion); the roots could not be dug with iron; and once it was collected it was best to lay it under an altar overnight and say plenty of Ave Marias and Pater Nosters.

While less preoccupied with elf-shot, the Greeks and Romans regarded elecampane as something of a cure-all for ailments as diverse as dropsy, menstrual disorders, digestive upsets and what Galen described as "passions of the hucklebone" (sciatica).

using elecampane

Today the plant's common names of elf-wort and elf-dock remind us of its magical history, although modern medicine, more prosaically, considers the herb as an important cough and catarrh remedy. It is also known to stimulate the immune system and, with its bitter taste, has a tonic effect on the digestive system. It is a very useful herb for the lingering coughs and debility that can follow bouts of influenza.

Although the root is used in Western herbalism, the Chinese use the flowers of a related species (*I. japonica*, called *Xuan Fu Hua* in Mandarin) in similar ways. Elecampane is easy to grow from seed, although it is a majestic plant that is best suited to large gardens. The roots should be collected in their second year: once dried they can be used in decoctions and syrups.

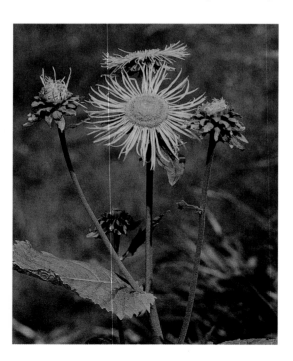

white deadnettle
Lamium album

A hairy perennial with leaves reminiscent of the stinging nettle and square stems, characteristic of the mint family, to which it belongs. The white tubular, two-lipped flowers appear in whorls in the spring and early summer. The plant grows to around 60cm/24in in height.

White deadnettle – so called because its leaves resemble those of the stinging nettle, although it does not sting – is a common wild plant often found growing as a weed in suburban gardens. It is no relation of the stinging nettle, but belongs to the mint family and takes its botanical name from the Greek word for throat, which was supposedly descriptive of the flowers.

◄ Elecampane *Inula helenium*
► White deadnettle *Lamium album*
►► Motherwort *Leonurus cardiaca*

using white deadnettle

These days the herb is mainly used for menstrual and urinary disorders: deadnettle tea can be helpful for cystitis and in prostatitis and it can speed recovery after surgery for enlarged prostate. It increases urination, has a soothing, anti-inflammatory action and will ease spasmodic cramps. Deadnettle can also be useful for heavy periods, can help regulate the menstrual cycle and is used as a douche for vaginal discharges.

White deadnettle also has some action on the bowel, helping to regulate function, so it can be useful for both constipation and diarrhoea. Externally, creams and ointments can be used on cuts and grazes and make a soothing, astringent lotion for piles and burns.

The plant can also be eaten – the young leaves and plant tips may be added raw to salads or cooked like spinach and served as a vegetable.

motherwort
Leonurus cardiaca

Erect perennial growing to 2m/6½ft with stout, square stems. Leaves are pale green beneath, darker above, usually three-lobed and heavily serrated. The flowers are small and pale pink to purple appearing in whorls in groups of 6-12 in the leaf axils in mid-summer to autumn. The plant is strong smelling.

Motherwort is mainly used today as a heart tonic and sedative. It reputedly takes its common name from a traditional use to calm anxiety in mothers during childbirth or as John Gerard put it in 1597: "for them that are in hard travell with childe". The *Leonurus* part of the botanical name comes from a Greek word meaning lion's tail and describes the shaggy shape of the leaves, while *cardiaca* reminds us that this has been an important heart herb since Roman times.

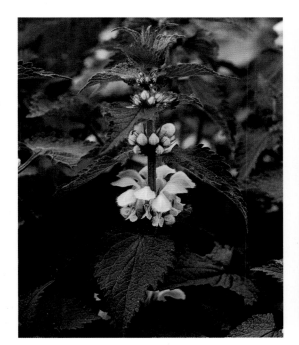

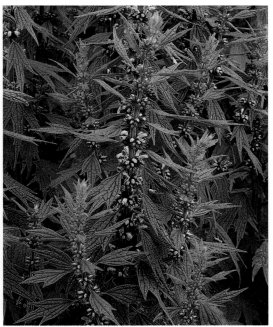

motherwort

parts used
flowers and seeds

commercial products
included in OTC remedies for gynaecological and blood pressure problems; tincture is available from specialist suppliers; *Chong Wei Zi* and *Yi Mu Cao* are available from Chinese herb shops.

how to use
infusion – 25g/1oz of dried herb to 500ml/1pt of boiling water taken in three equal doses; *tincture* – up to 5ml/1tsp, three times daily; *Chong Wei Zi* and *Yi Mu Cao* are generally used in complex Chinese decoctions (*Tang*) with a typical dosage of 4-10g/⅛-⅓oz and 10-25g/⅓-1oz respectively.

toadflax

parts used
whole plant collected just
before flowering

commercial products
not generally available

how to use
infusion - 25g/1oz of
dried herb to 500ml/1pt
of water taken in three
equal doses during the
day.

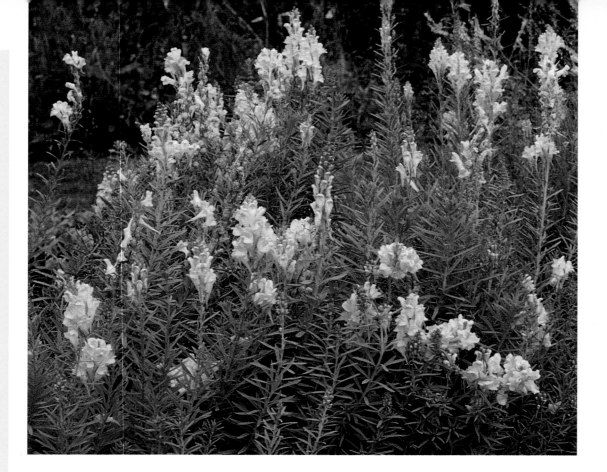

using motherwort

Motherwort can help to steady erratic heart beats and ease palpitations while more recent research also suggests that it can help prevent thromboses (blood clots). The herb can be helpful for menopausal upsets and is mildly sedative and calming: it works well in infusions in combination with sage or mugwort. As its traditional use in childbirth suggests it is also a uterine stimulant so can be helpful for some types of menstrual disorders and period pains.

The plant belongs to the mint family, and like others in the group motherwort is a rather drab plant with tiny pink flowers clustered at the axil where the leaves join the main stem. A related species, *L. heterophyllus* is used in China mainly for menstrual problems. The leaves are known as *Yi Mu Cao* and help to ease some types of eczema, while the seeds are called *Chong Wei Zi* and are also included in remedies for eye problems such as conjunctivitis.

caution avoid high doses in pregnancy.

toadflax *Linaria vulgaris*

A slender perennial with thin, pointed leaves and snapdragon-like flowers in yellow and orange. It grows to around 90cm/3ft and flowers throughout the summer.

Also known as "eggs and butter", the two-tone yellow flowers of toadflax not only provide the

◀ Toadflax *Linaria vulgaris*

country name but were also seen as a "signature" for its therapeutic properties: yellow signified jaundice and in the 17th century the plant was widely used as a remedy for liver disorders. The leaves are rather like those of flax – hence the botanical name (from *linum* meaning flax) – while the "toad" part comes from a tradition that toads sheltered under its stems.

using toadflax

The plant has a cleansing and stimulating effect on the liver and can still be used to treat hepatitis, gastroenteritis and gall bladder problems. Like many liver herbs, it has a role in treating skin disorders, including eczema and scrofula. Toadflax is mildly laxative and will also increase urination.

The herb is astringent so, externally, it can be used to bathe piles or be made into a healing ointment for wounds, sores and skin rashes. The infusion was once recommended for eye inflammations. Drink toadflax tea as a cleansing remedy for the digestion or to stimulate the liver.

creeping jenny
Lysimachia nummularia

A creeping perennial usually found in damp meadows. Leaves are rounded on square stems with bright yellow cup-like flowers growing singly in the leaf axils in summer. A gold-leaved cultivar is often sold in garden centres.

➤ Creeping Jenny *Lysimachia nummularia*

Once widely used as a wound herb, creeping Jenny is nowadays more likely to be found in an ornamental hanging basket than in the wild. Its botanical name comes from the Latin *nummulus* for money and refers to the round, coin-like leaves – hence its alternative common name of moneywort. The plant was originally found across Europe, from central Sweden to the Caucasus. In the garden it will meander happily through rockeries and around paving stones for 60cm/24in or more.

using creeping jenny

Gerard recommends the juice in wine for diarrhoea and blood in the stool, and adds that the plant boiled in wine with a little honey "prevaileth much against the cough in children" – a reference to its historic use as a specific for whooping cough. The leaves contain vitamin C and were once taken, dried and powdered by Dutch sailors as a preventative for scurvy. Ointment made from the fresh leaves was also once a favourite for cuts and sores, while an infusion of the fresh leaves was taken for internal bleeding.

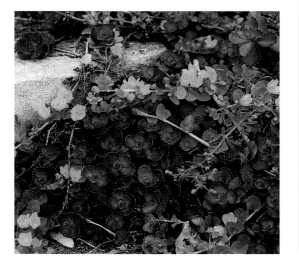

creeping jenny

part used
leaves, gathered before flowering

commercial products
occasionally found in creams for eczema.

how to use
infusion – 25g/1oz to 500ml/1pt of water taken in three equal doses during the day; *fresh herb* – add to creams for eczema or minor wounds.

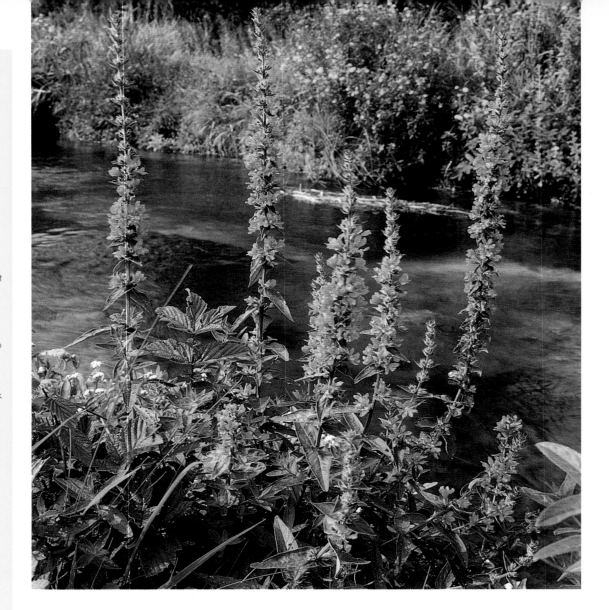

purple loosestrife

parts used

aerial parts, gathered as they are coming into flower

commercial products

occasionally found in digestive remedies for diarrhoea or stomach cramps.

how to use

infusion - 25g/1oz of dried herb to 500ml/1pt of water taken in three equal doses during the day;

decoction - 25g/1oz to 750ml/1½pt of water makes a strongly astringent mixture to drink for diarrhoea; or use 50g/2oz to 750ml/1½pt as a wash for skin sores and wounds.

purple loosestrife
Lythrum salicaria

A tall, upright perennial with bright purple flowers on whorled spikes from early summer to early autumn. The leaves resemble those of the willow and the plant will grow to around 1.5m/5ft in good growing conditions.

Usually found in damp, marshy areas, the tall flower spikes of purple loosestrife make an attractive addition to late summer country lanes. The plant has been used medicinally since Roman times – Pliny talks of the smoke from burning loosestrife as driving away serpents and adds that the "power is so great that, if placed on the yoke, when the beasts of burden are quarrelsome, it checks their bad temper".

The herb was once a popular European folk remedy for diarrhoea and dysentery and is still

◄ Purple loosestrife *Lythrum salicaria*

used like this in a few OTC products made in France and Switzerland. Research has shown that it can be effective against the amoeba which cause dysentery and can also combat the typhus bacilli.

using purple loosestrife

Purple loosestrife is both astringent and anti-bacterial so makes a valuable wound herb – use the infusion as a wash to clean cuts and grazes. Internally it can be helpful for heavy periods or in severe cystitis where there is blood in the urine. It also increases urination and can be used to stop nosebleeds (apply a cotton ball soaked in the infusion or insert crushed leaves in the nostril). The tea can be used as a douche for vaginal discharges; or a strong decoction may be used as a wash on eczema, skin sores and ulcers.

common mallow
Malva sylvestris

A vigorous, hardy perennial with round, lobed leaves and purple, five-petalled flowers, appearing throughout the summer and autumn. It will grow to 1.2m/4ft.

Common mallow with its lobed leaves and bright purple flowers is a not unattractive common garden "weed" and hedgerow plant: it will, however, self-seed enthusiastically, so needs treating with caution in the garden. The botanical name derives from both the Latin *malva* and the Greek *malake*, which mean "soft"

➤ Common mallow *Malva sylvestris*

– a reference to its medicinal property of softening skin and tissues (demulcent) rather than to any particular softness of its leaves.

using mallow

Mallow is closely related to both marshmallow and hollyhocks and all three have very similar medicinal properties: marshmallow (see page 170) is considered the strongest of the three and is the one normally chosen by medical herbalists, although common mallow makes a satisfactory alternative in an emergency.

In the 16th century mallow was known as *omnimorbia* or cure-all and Gerard's list of its uses is certainly comprehensive, ranging from wasp stings to digestive upsets, tumours and the rather unpleasant sounding "inward burstings".

The plant is rich in mucilage and is used as a soothing remedy for inflammations, irritation of the gastro-intestinal tract, coughs and bronchitis. It is mildly laxative and shows some anti-bacterial and immune-stimulating properties. The leaves and flowers are generally used; the root has similar actions but large doses can have a purgative effect. A poultice of mallow leaves is ideal for skin sores and inflammations.

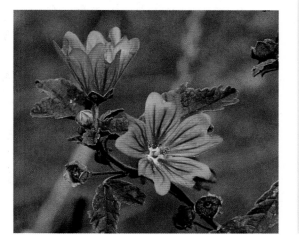

common mallow

parts used
aerial parts collected during flowering

commercial products
occasionally found in herbal cough sweets and lozenges.

how to use
infusion – 25g/1oz of dried herb to 500ml/1pt of water taken in three equal doses during the day;
fresh leaves – use externally in poultices or add to skin creams.

parts used

aerial parts

commercial products

not generally used although the tincture is available from specialist suppliers.

how to use

infusion – 25gl/1oz of dried herb to 500ml/1pt of water taken in three equal doses during the day;

tincture – up to 5ml/1tsp per dose, three times a day.

catmint *Nepeta cataria*

A strongly smelling, branching, erect perennial growing to 1m/3ft with coarsely serrate leaves, 3-7cm/ long, which are whitish beneath and green-grey above.White flowers dotted with purple appear in crowded terminal whorls and spiked axillary whorls from mid-summer to mid-autumn.

Catmint, as the name suggests, is a favourite with cats, who will roll in ecstasy in a bed of the plant and nibble it enthusiastically. The old rhyme: "If you set it, the cats will eat it/If you sow it, the cats don't know it" reminds us that cats only take to catmint once the leaves have been bruised, or are withering after being transplanted, but will ignore plants grown from seed.

using catmint

This is a gentle herb ideal for children and suitable for colic, feverish chills and hyperactivity. The herb encourages sweating, is a gentle nerve relaxant and eases spasmodic cramps so makes a very soothing drink in childhood illnesses or flu. Like other members of the mint family, it will expel gas from the digestive tract and ease the symptoms of indigestion but unlike peppermint, it does not contain irritant menthol so is quite safe in regular use or for children.

The plant can be used for flavouring in cooking and is still popular in France; in the 16th century, before tea was introduced from China, catmint infusions were a popular country drink.

Externally, catmint can be used in ointments or poultices for bruises and minor

➤ Catmint *Nepeta cataria*

wounds and the root was once ground with cloves and used for toothache. It was also once smoked for bronchitis but this can be mildly hallucinogenic.

The plant known as catmint or catnep commonly sold in garden centres is often a more ornamental variety (*N. mussini*) with pretty lilac flowers, which cats also quite like but which lacks the medicinal properties of true catmint.

butterbur *Petasites hybridus*

A dramatic plant growing to 2m/6½ft with leaves up to 90m/3ft across and generally found in damp, marshy places.The flowers appear in early spring – before the leaves – in dense reddish spikes of either male or female blooms; they may be bell-shaped or thread-like and vary from pinks to purple.

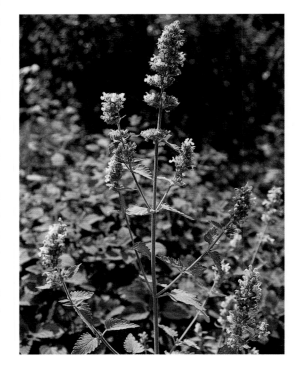

Butterbur's botanical name comes from the Greek word *petatos*, which was the term for a shepherd's felt hat and is descriptive of the large, soft leaves: butterbur leaves and stems make a useful parasol for sunny days. In the past the leaves were used to wrap butter – hence the common name.

Butterbur is a popular medicinal herb in mainland Europe and extracts are found in many Swiss and German OTC products, although there are some concerns about its toxicity as it contains traces of pyrrolizidine alkaloids (see comfrey, page 204).

The herb was traditionally used in European folk medicine as a cough remedy, while Gerard recommended it for the plague: "…because it provoketh sweat and driveth from the harte all venome and ill heat". He suggested that it "killeth wormes" and urged its use in ale for "pestilent and burning fevers".

using butterbur

While the traditional applications of butterbur have largely fallen into disuse, recent research has demonstrated that the plant has considerable anti-spasmodic and pain-relieving properties, making it suitable for tension headaches, migraine and period pain. Other researchers have shown that it can affect digestive function and is helpful for gastritis, gall bladder spasms and stomach upsets. The root, flowers and leaves have all been used medicinally in the past, although the root is generally regarded as the most effective and a decoction is ideal for home use.

It is best to collect butterbur from the wild rather than attempting to cultivate it in the garden: nothing will grow under its vast leaves and it can spread rapidly and prove very difficult to eradicate.

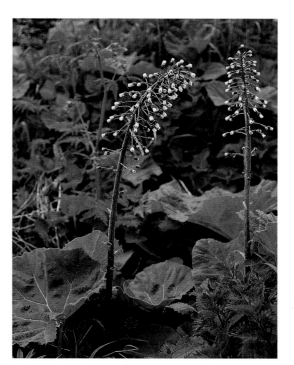

◄ Butterbur *Petasites hybridus*

butterbur

part used
roots collected in autumn

commercial products
included in some proprietary cough syrups and digestive remedies; capsules and tincture available from health food shops.

how to use
tincture – up to 4ml/80 drops, per dose, three times a day;
decoction – 25g/1oz to 750ml/1½pt of water taken in three equal doses during the day or made into syrup (see page 218) and taken in 5-10ml/1-2tsp doses every 2-3 hours.

plantain *Plantago* spp.

Common plantain (P. major) *is characterised by its rat's tail-like flower spikes and basal rosette of fleshy, rounded or ovate leaves. It grows to around 15cm/6in high and is commonly found in gardens and pavement cracks. Ribwort plantain* (P. lanceolata) *is taller, up to 75cm/30in, with more pointed, lance-shaped leaves with three to five prominent ribs. Its flowers are dark rust with clear white feathery stamens and appear from late spring to early autumn.*

Common plantain was known as "white man's foot" in North America as the native tribes watched it spread with the settlers. The plant is a familiar garden weed, often found filling

plantain

part used

leaves

commercial products

both ribwort plantain and common plantain are included in a few proprietary mixtures mainly for coughs, catarrh or winter colds; capsules, juice and tinctures are available from health food shops.

how to use

tincture – up to 4ml/80 drops per dose, three times a day;

infusion – 25g/1oz of dried herb to 500ml/1pt of water taken in three equal doses during the day;

fresh leaves (common plantain) – used on insect bites and stings.

---

the cracks in crazy paving and dominating lawns. To the Anglo-Saxons it was "waybread" – one of the nine sacred herbs given to mankind by Woden and listed in the ninth-century poem the *Lacnunga*. The plant has long been regarded as an important healing herb – Pliny even suggests that if several pieces of flesh are put in a pot with plantain they will join back together again.

using plantain

The plant is known to be soothing, anti-bacterial, anti-histamine and anti-allergenic and it is a good blood tonic and astringent so contracts tissues and blood vessels to stop secretions and bleeding.

Externally the leaves are a good emergency treatment for irritant insect bites, while internally common plantain tea – made from the leaves – can be helpful for gastric irritations, irritable bowel, haemorrhoids, cystitis or heavy periods. Plantain juice, mixed with honey, is a soothing remedy for cuts and minor wounds.

Common plantain's close relative, ribwort, is more likely to be found in the wild. It is a good anti-catarrh remedy used for colds, hay fever and allergic rhinitis, but also contains minerals and trace elements – particularly zinc, potassium and silica – so can act as a tissue healer and immune stimulant. The presence of aucubin, an antibiotic chemical, helps to make it healing and supportive for the immune system.

In addition, both common plantain and ribwort will encourage the coughing response and can be added to cough syrups and cold remedies.

bistort *Polygonum bistorta*

A perennial with thick, S-shape rhizomes growing up to 1m/3ft in height. Leaves are broadly ovate or lanceolate, lighter and hairy on the underside and up to 15cm/6in long; flowers are small, usually pale pink in dense solitary cylindrical spikes approximately 1cm/½in in diameter, appearing from mid-summer to early autumn.

Bistort is believed to be the plant the Saxons knew as *"atterlothe"* – one of the nine great healing herbs which the god Woden gave to the world. It is an extremely astringent plant largely used to stop bleeding – both internal and external – and for diarrhoea.

The plant was once cultivated as a vegetable with the leaves and young shoots known as Easter-

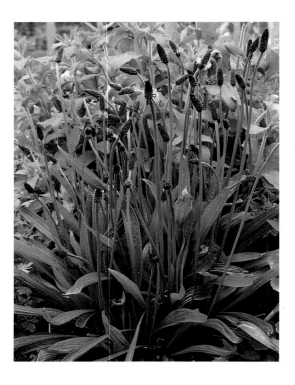

◄ Plantain *Plantago* spp

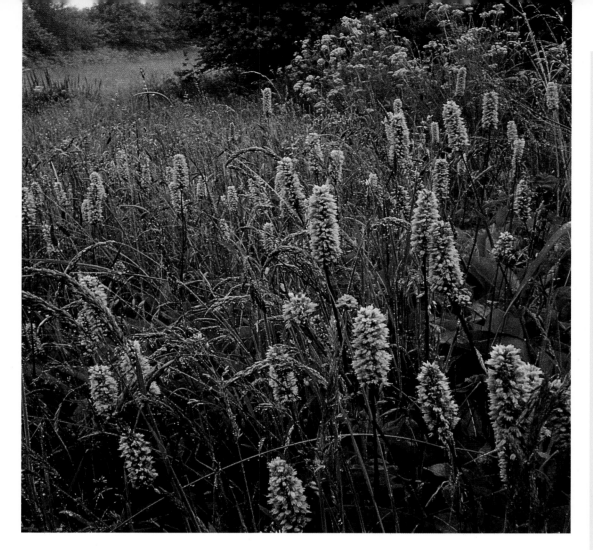

▲ Bistort *Polygonum bistorta*

bistort

parts used
root and rhizome
collected in the autumn;
leaves gathered in the
spring and early summer
before flowering.

commercial products
not generally used
although the tincture is
sold by specialist
suppliers.

how to use
tincture - up to 3ml/60
drops per dose, three
times daily;
decoction - 25g/1oz of
dried root to 500ml/1pt
of water taken in three
equal doses during the
day.

mangiant or passions. They were traditionally eaten in the North of England at Easter in a herb pudding made by cooking with nettles, barley and oatmeal and usually served with eggs.

The root, used medicinally, is long and twisting giving the plant the additional country names of snakeroot and adderwort – hence the link with the Saxon *atterlothe* – and the Doctrine of Signatures belief that it would cure snake bites, while the powdered leaves were used to clear parasitic worms in children.

using bistort

The herb is one of our strongest astringents so contracts blood vessels and tissues and in the past was used to harden spongy gums and correct loosening of the teeth. The Elizabethan herbalist, John Gerard suggests that the root "being holden in the mouth for a certaine space and at sundry times" will effectively tighten loose teeth.

Powdered bistort root can be used externally on bleeding wounds, piles or to stop nosebleeds, while the decoction is mainly used for diarrhoea.

self-heal *Prunella vulgaris*

An invasive, creeping perennial commonly found as a garden weed and one that readily invades lawns. It has ovate leaves and deep purple, lipped flowers produced in compact spikes, which ripen to produce brown spiked seed pods in autumn.

As its common name implies, self-heal is a well-established European wound herb, widely used to stop bleeding from "inward and outward wounds". The flower spikes were considered to resemble the throat and under the Doctrine of Signatures theory, it was also used for inflammations of the mouth and throat. In fact, the botanical name, *Prunella* – or so William Cole argued in 1657 – is derived from the German words *die Breuen*, meaning the mouth.

using self-heal

Self-heal is astringent and can be useful for all sorts of bleeding – including heavy periods where there is no known cause, and blood in the urine from severe cystitis. It will also increase urination and has some anti-bacterial action.

The same plant is used in Chinese medicine where it is known as *Xia Ku Cao* – which literally means "summer dry herb". In China

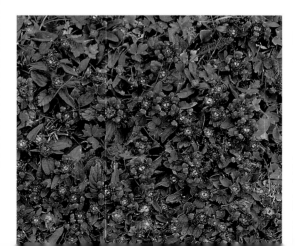

only the flower spikes are used and are considered especially cooling and tonifying for the liver and gall bladder. The herb is prescribed for any condition associated with what the Chinese term "liver fire" and generally characterised by irritability, anger, headaches and high blood pressure. The same remedy can also help calm hyperactive children – use it as an infusion up to four times a day.

Use an infusion of the whole herb as a wash for cuts and grazes or apply crushed, washed whole leaves as a poultice.

pilewort *Ranunculus ficaria*

Perennial with mainly prostrate-branched stem, heart-shaped leaves, on a slender stalk sheathed at the base, growing to 25cm/10in and yellow star-like flowers with 8-12 petals, up to 3cm/1¼in in diameter, appearing in early spring.

Pilewort, also known as lesser celandine, is an excellent example of the mediaeval Doctrine of Signatures, which reasoned that the appearance of plants indicated their actions. The roots of pilewort are full of tiny nodules which resemble a severe case of piles, so the plant was recommended as a remedy for haemorrhoids and given its common name. It is still used in this way and can be extremely effective. Pilewort flowers in early spring, but is low growing and soon dies back. Although it can be invasive, it is worth encouraging in the garden for the colour and ground cover it brings early in the year.

◄ Self-heal *Prunella vulgaris*
► Pilewort *Ranunculus ficaria*
►► Yellow dock *Rumex crispus*

using pilewort

Pilewort is highly astringent and contains chemicals called saponins which have an anti-haemorrhoidal action. The root can be taken in teas or combined with laxatives for piles associated with constipation. In folk medicine it was used to stop haemorrhages and taken internally for severe bruising. Creams and ointments made from leaves and root are widely available, or can be made at home (see page 222). As well as easing the discomfort and pain of piles, they can be used for perineal tears after childbirth.

caution pilewort contains a chemical called protoanemonin which is irritant but destroyed on drying, so the fresh plant should not be used.

yellow dock *Rumex crispus*

A biennial growing to around 1.5m/5ft in height with a robust tap root and long-stalked ovate leaves up to 50cm/20in long. The purple, thistle-like flowers appear from early summer to mid-autumn, followed by hooked fruits.

Yellow or curled dock is generally found in wild, grassy places, wasteland and along the road side. The plant is able to concentrate iron from the soil in its roots, thus making a valuable iron tonic for anaemia: in the past herbalists sprinkled iron filings around their yellow dock plants to produce iron-enriched specimens.

using yellow dock

Yellow dock is mainly used as a cleansing remedy for skin and rheumatic problems. It contains anthraquinone glycosides which encourage gut motions by irritating the mucous membrane lining, so the herb has a laxative effect. It is also useful for stimulating liver function, and for itching skin conditions and shingles.

In Galenic medicine, yellow dock was considered sufficiently cooling to purge the "choleric" humour or yellow bile associated with excess fire. Culpeper thought it more effective than its close relatives sorrel and red dock and also recommended the seeds – no longer commonly used in herbal medicine – as a remedy for diarrhoea and stomach upsets. In homoeopathy, yellow dock extracts are used in cough mixtures and to relieve irritated sore throats.

Use the root in decoctions for rheumatic pains, skin problems and digestive complaints. The leaves can be taken in infusion, but are significantly milder in action.

caution avoid in pregnancy or use only in moderation for short periods.

pilewort

parts used
dried leaves, root

commercial products
used in a number of proprietary remedies, both internal and external, for constipation and piles; tincture available from specialist suppliers.

how to use
creams/ointments – apply frequently to piles;
tincture – up to 5ml/1tsp per dose, three times a day;
decoction – 25g/1oz of dried herb to 750ml/1½pt of water used as a wash or taken internally in three equal doses during the day;
infusion – 25g/1oz of dried herb to 500ml/1pt of water used as a wash or taken internally in three equal doses during the day.

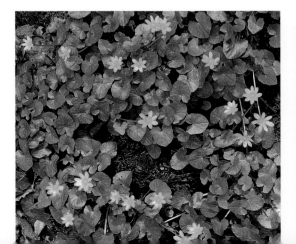

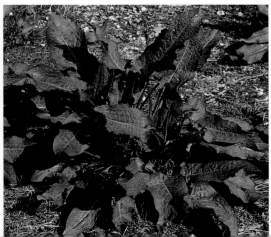

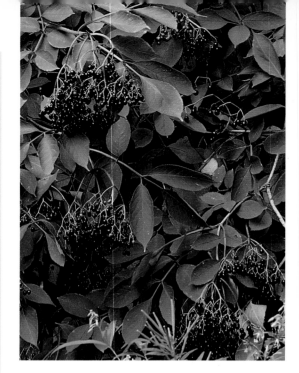

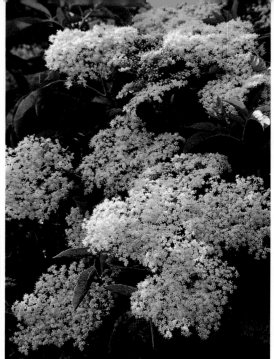

elder

parts used

flowers collected in spring and berries in autumn; the bark, leaves and root have all been used in the past – collect the leaves in summer after flowering.

commercial products

used in numerous proprietary mixtures for colds, catarrh and hay fever as well as in cough and throat lozenges; elder flower tincture and elder berry juice are available from health food shops; elder flower cordials widely available from supermarkets and food stores.

how to use

tincture – up to 5ml/1tsp per dose, three times daily;

juice – up to 10ml/2tsp per dose, three times daily;

infusion – 25g/1oz of dried flowers to 500ml/1pt of water taken in three equal doses during the day.

elder *Sambucus nigra*

A large shrubby tree with feather-like leaves and tiny, scented cream flowers borne in flat bunches in early summer. The purple berries ripen in late autumn.

In the Middle Ages, many people believed that the elder tree was inhabited by a spirit known as the "elder mother" whose permission was needed if ever the tree was to be pruned. The lady gave her consent by remaining silent but inevitably felling elders was considered to bring bad luck, although branches from the tree placed over doors and windows were believed to keep witches away and ward off the Evil Eye. According to Maud Grieve, author of the well-known *Modern Herbal* (1931), country people in the 1920s would still doff their hats when passing an elder tree as a salute to this otherwise forgotten sprite.

Such respect was understandable, since the elder was a complete medicine chest. The leaves formed the basis of a "green ointment" for sprains and strains, the inner bark is a strong purgative, the berries – a good source of vitamin C – provided protection against colds and infections, while the flowers are strongly anti-catarrhal.

using elder

Today we mainly use the flowers as a soothing anti-catarrhal remedy; they also encourage sweating so are cooling for feverish colds and flu. Used externally they are anti-inflammatory and softening so make a very effective hand cream: elderflower water (from distilling the flowers) was a favourite in the 18th century for whitening the skin and removing freckles.

Elder flowers also appear to strengthen the mucous membranes of the respiratory tract, so can increase resistance to irritant allergens. Drinking elderflower tea in early spring can help to reduce the symptoms of hay fever later in the year.

◄◄ Elder *Sambucus nigra*, with autumn berries
◄ Elder *Sambucus nigra*, with summer flowers

An infused oil of elder leaves also makes a useful alternative to the old "green ointment" to treat bruises and minor injuries.

caution avoid use of elder bark in pregnancy as it is a strong purgative.

skullcap
Scutellaria lateriflora

A perennial growing to about 75cm/30in with thin, oval, toothed leaves and small blue flowers produced on one side of the stem; characteristic skullcap-shaped seed pods appear from mid-summer onwards.

Virginian skullcap was first introduced into Europe in the 18th century and was used as a treatment for rabies – hence its alternative name of "mad dog". It was used by the Cherokee to encourage menstruation and also to treat diarrhoea and breast pains. Today it is mainly considered as a sedative and nervine by Western herbalists but may also be used to reduce fevers, calm the foetus and stimulate the digestion.

Like all skullcaps, the Virginian variety takes its name from the dish-shaped seed pods, while its botanical name is derived from the growing pattern of the flowers which appear on only one side of the stem. Virginian skullcap grows easily in British gardens and will self-seed enthusiastically – to the point where it can become invasive. European skullcap species

➤ Skullcap *Scutellaria lateriflora*

(such as *S. galericulata*) have very similar properties although there is little tradition of using them in herbal medicine.

using skullcap

As well as its sedating properties, skullcap is now also known to be anti-bacterial, to lower both blood pressure and blood cholesterol levels and to ease spasmodic pains. Drink skullcap tea to encourage relaxation and combat anxiety and nervous tension. Skullcap tea can also be useful to soothe pre-menstrual tension and menstrual cramps.

In China the root of *S. baicalensis (Huang Qin)* is regarded as a cooling remedy for the stomach and lungs and is used to clear "heat" which in Chinese theory may cause diarrhoea, jaundice and gastroenteritis. This variety of skullcap is also anti-bacterial, antispasmodic, diuretic and will stimulate bile flow.

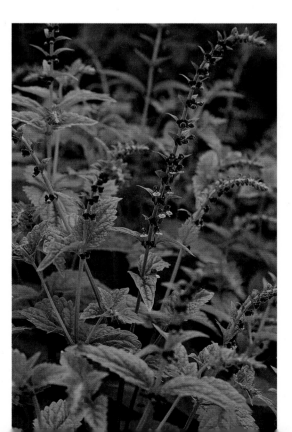

skullcap

parts used
aerial parts

commercial products
included in numerous proprietary remedies for nervous tension, anxiety and stress; capsules containing powdered herb and tincture are also sold in health food shops. *Huang Qin* is available from Chinese herb shops.

how to use
tincture – up to 4ml/80 drops, three times daily; *infusion* 25g/1oz to 500ml/1pt of boiling water taken in three equal doses daily.

wood betony

parts used
aerial parts

commercial products
not usually included in
proprietary remedies
although both tincture
and dried herb are
readily available from
specialist suppliers.

how to use
infusion - 25g/1oz of
dried herb to 500ml/1pt
of boiling water taken in
three equal doses during
the day;
tincture - up to 5ml/1tsp,
three times a day.

wood betony
Stachys officinalis

A low-growing perennial with small (2½cm/1in) oval, heavily veined, dark green leaves forming a basal rosette. The flowers are usually bright pink and carried on tall, slender stems in a dense terminal spike, up to 60cm/24in tall, in mid-summer to autumn.

Although wood betony tends to be rather neglected these days, it was one of the most important healing plants in the Anglo-Saxon repertoire: no fewer than 29 uses of it are known and as well as recommending it for a range of physical diseases, it was a popular amulet herb used well into the Middle Ages – tied on to the arm with red wool – to ward off evil or ill humours. As late as 1526 *The Grete Herball* was recommending it "for them that be ferful", while William Turner, in 1551, advises that it will heal "them that are mad" and John Gerard (1597) gives a very long list of applications concluding that "it maketh a man to pisse well".

using wood betony

The herb is an attractive one for the garden, prodcuing bright cerise flowers in late summer to autumn. It is mainly used these days as a nervine and sedative for headaches and nervous debility and makes a very pleasant-tasting tea. It is also a good anti-catarrhal herb and, taken in a tea or tincture, can help reduce the discomfort of sinusitis and severe nasal congestion. Betony is also slightly bitter so helps stimulate digestive function. In addition, it will help encourage blood flow to the brain so can be useful in the elderly where restricted cerebral circulation often leads to mental

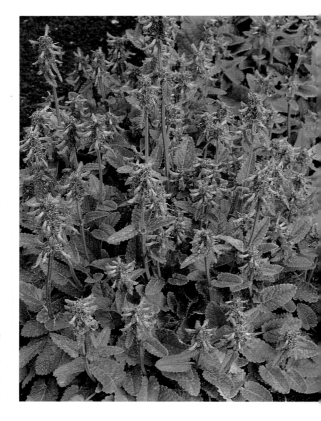

▲ Wood betony *Stachys officinalis*

confusion which can erroneously be interpreted as signs of dementia.

Culpeper, in 1653, stressed that it "preserves the liver and bodies of men from epidemical diseases and from witchcraft" and it certainly has an affinity with the liver – ideal for poor or sluggish digestion, and as a general stimulant. It can be especially helpful for menopausal problems and is ideal in childbirth to encourage contractions and relax the mother.

cautions although helpful during labour, wood betony should be avoided in pregnancy as it is a uterine stimulant.

➤ Marsh woundwort *Stachys palustris*

marsh woundwort
Stachys palustris

A hardy perennial with tuberous roots and hairy, lanceolate leaves. It has dark red or purple flowers in summer borne on tall spikes flowering from the base. It has an unpleasant smell when crushed.

Traditional country names often provide a clue to a plant's healing action and marsh woundwort is no exception. Gerard called it "clown's wound-wort" with the "clown" suggesting that the herb was widely used by the common people.

The leaves of marsh woundwort were once pounded with animal fats to make an ointment used on fresh wounds which was deemed so effective that the injury would apparently "heale in such short time and in such absolute manner that it is hard for any that hath not the experience thereof to believe". Gerard was a great enthusiast for the plant and his *Herball* details how he cured one Edmund Cartwright who had been badly injured in a duel – "thrust through the thorax" – with an ointment of marsh woundwort and a little rose oil.

using marsh woundwort
The herb grows in damp places but will thrive in most suburban gardens. As well as its healing actions, marsh woundwort eases muscle spasms and taken as a tea can be helpful for cramp. Folk tradition also suggests the aerial parts as a remedy for gout and vertigo.

chickweed *Stellaria media*

A common annual weed forming low-growing mats of slender stems with oval leaves and small, white, star-like flowers from early spring to early autumn.

marsh woundwort

parts used
aerial parts, collected while flowering

commercial products
not generally used

how to use
infusion – 25g/1oz of dried herb to 500ml/1pt of water used as a wash or taken internally in three equal doses during the day.

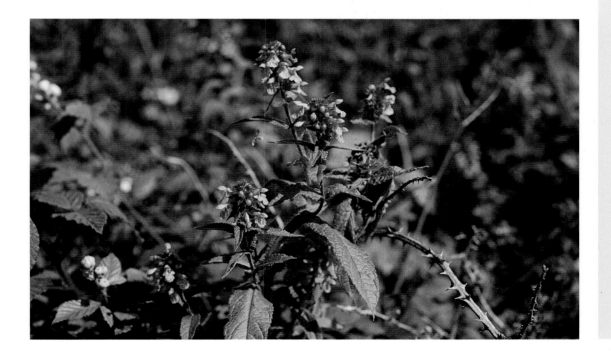

chickweed

parts used

aerial parts, gathered throughout the year whenever the plant appears

commercial products

included in several proprietary eczema ointments; tincture available from health food shops.

how to use

tincture – up to 5ml/1tsp per dose, three times daily;

infusion – 25g/1oz of dried herb to 500ml/1pt of water used as a wash or taken internally in three equal doses during the day; use in home-made creams (see page 222) as need be or infused oils (made by the hot method described on page 224) as a lotion, or add 10-20ml to a warm bath.

Chickweed, as the name suggests, is a favourite food for domestic fowl. In Elizabethan times it was fed to caged birds and in the Middle Ages was known as *morsus gallinae* or hen's bite. It is a common garden weed, once gathered as a vegetable to be cooked like spinach and tossed in butter, or else used as a salad herb.

using chickweed

Soothing and astringent, chickweed's main medicinal use is in creams and ointments for irritant skin rashes and eczema, or in the first-aid box for burns, boils and drawing splinters. Culpeper suggests combining chickweed with rose petals and adding various pig and sheep fats to create an extremely soothing ointment — it would certainly be a good combination, as rose petals have long been regarded as supportive for

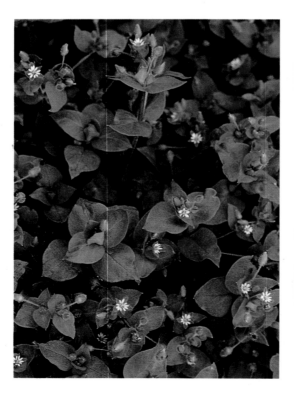

"the skin and the soul". The whole flowering chickweed plant can be made into infused oil and added to bath water to soothe skin problems. Chickweed poultices were once a favourite for rheumatic pains, gout and also varicose ulcers.

Although not so popular as an internal remedy, it is particularly cooling and can be added to mixtures for rheumatism and hot, irritant skin conditions. The leaves are also a useful source of vitamin C.

comfrey
Symphytum officinale

A robust, erect (up to 1.2m/4ft) perennial with thick, mucilaginous roots and large, ovate leaves. The funnel-shaped flowers appear in clusters in summer and can be white to purple.

Comfrey has been used for centuries as a wound healer and restorer of broken bones. Its country name is "knitbone" and the botanical name is derived from the Greek word *sympho* meaning to unite. It has had a more chequered history in recent years, veering from panacea to health hazard.

Its healing action is due to a chemical called allantoin which encourages growth of various tissue cells and so accelerates healing. Previous generations used comfrey poultices on pulled ligaments and minor fractures, while herbalists used it internally for stomach ulceration. The immense healing properties of the plant have been put to many diverse uses over the centuries: in the past comfrey baths

◄ Chickweed *Stellaria media*

➤ Comfrey *Symphytum officinale*

were popular with brides before marriage, in the belief that they would repair the hymen (the membrane covering the opening to the vagina) and thus create the appearance of virginity.

During the 1960s and 1970s the plant became over-hyped as a cure-all for arthritis and this inevitably focused research interest on its constituents. Scientists fed large amounts of the plant to rats which subsequently died of liver disease and comfrey's pyrrolizidine alkaloids were blamed. Comfrey supporters argue that the rats had so much comfrey to eat they actually suffered from the effects of malnutrition and maintain that the alkaloids are not extracted in conventional herbal preparations (infusions and ointments). Health authorities have tended to disagree and comfrey is now banned in many parts of the world, including Australia and Canada. In the USA and Germany use of the herb is limited to topical applications on skin without open wounds. In the UK internal lay use is discouraged and most health food stores no longer offer comfrey tablets for sale, although the dried leaf for use in teas is generally readily available; creams, infused oils and ointments are freely available.

using comfrey

The herb is still easily found in the wild or can be grown in gardens (although it does have tenacious roots). The hot infused oil is easy to make and forms a useful base for massage oils for arthritis, sprains and similar traumatic injuries — add 2-5 drops of rosemary or lavender essential oil to 10ml/2tsp of comfrey,

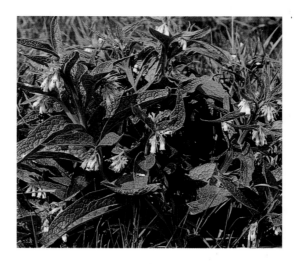

and rub into aching joints and limbs. Regular treatment can help repair the damage of old injuries which may be contributing to osteoarthritis. Comfrey is also extremely healing for any sort of bruising and the ointment can be particularly healing for nappy rash in small babies.

The dangers of pyrrolizidine alkaloids apart, the herb should not be used on fresh wounds before they are thoroughly cleaned since the rapid healing caused by the allantoin may trap dirt, so leading to abscesses.

cautions do not take internally for longer than 1-2 weeks, and preferably only in consultation with a qualified practitioner. Do not use on open wounds. Avoid in pregnancy.

dandelion
Taraxacum officinale

A perennial with a long tap root and a basal rosette of toothed leaves. Erect yellow composite flowers appear from spring to autumn followed by the characteristic puffball of hairy seeds.

comfrey

parts used
root, collected in autumn, or leaves, collected during early flowering.

commercial products
included in numerous ointments and rubs for bruises, sprains and strains; tincture, capsules and infused oil available from health food shops although internal use of the remedy is restricted in some countries.

how to use
tincture – up to 5ml/1tsp per dose, three times daily;
fresh herb – can be used in poultices for bruises and sprains;
ointments, infused oils and creams – use as need be.

dandelion

parts used

root generally gathered in spring, leaves gathered before flowering

commercial products

included in numerous proprietary remedies for digestive and urinary tract problems; capsules (250-520mg) and tincture (both root and leaf) available from health food shops; *Pu Gong Ying* is available from Chinese herbal shops.

how to use

tincture (leaf or root) - 5ml/1tsp per dose, three times daily;

capsules - up to 600mg per dose, three times daily;

infusion (leaf) - 25g/1oz to 500ml/1pt of water taken in three equal doses during the day;

decoction (root) - 25g/1oz to 750ml/1½pt of water taken in three equal doses during the day.

Use of dandelion in Western medicine is first mentioned in the *Ortus Sanitatis*, a guide to health written in 1485, making it a comparative newcomer to the repertoire. The name dandelion was apparently invented by a 15th-century surgeon known only as Master Wilhelm, who compared the shape of the leaves to a lion's tooth or *dens leonis*. Initially the herb was regarded as a variant of endive or chicory and recommended as a liver remedy. Its botanical name actually derives from the Arabic *tarakhaqún*, which means "wild chicory". The leaves are still eaten in salad (especially in France) and are extremely effective at increasing urination – hence the French name, *pissenlit,* and Old English pissabed or piddlybeds.

Master Wilhelm and his contemporaries regarded dandelion as a cooling herb, as do the

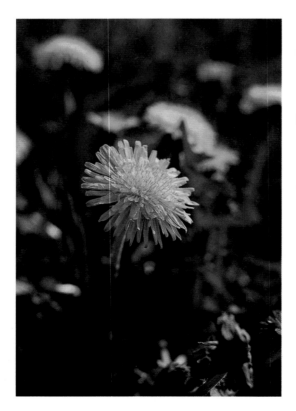

Chinese. They have used it in medicine since the seventh century and recommend it for both liver problems and skin eruptions, where it is considered to "cool the blood". Both the aerial parts of the European dandelion and an Oriental species (*T. mongolicum*) are known as *Pu Gong Ying* in China.

using dandelion

Dandelion is unusual in that it is extremely rich in potassium, which is generally lost in urination, so the plant helps to restore natural balance despite its diuretic action. Although the whole plant has a tonic action on the liver, the root is rather more stimulating and cleansing, and dandelion root tea makes a good laxative and liver stimulant for a sluggish digestion. It also makes a useful cleansing remedy in rheumatism, helping to clear toxins from the system.

Dandelion is commonly included in OTC slimming preparations because of its diuretic and laxative properties – although this is not an ideal way to attempt to lose weight, as it simply depletes body fluids.

Dandelion leaves are very nutritious (rich in vitamins A, B-complex, and C, plus iron, manganese, phosphorus, sulphur, calcium, silica and potassium), so are well worth adding to salads. Dandelion leaf tea can help with mild fluid retention and a decoction of the root makes a cleansing drink for the liver. Dandelion is unusual in that it is generally recommended to gather the roots in the spring rather than autumn, when most roots are lifted. This is because the starch content is lower then, so the active medicinal constituents are in

◄ Dandelion *Taraxacum officinale*

greater concentration. However, the French recommend the juice of the root, gathered in autumn, as a liver tonic.

Externally the white sap from dandelion stems can be used on warts, while a decoction of aerial parts can be used in an eye-bath for eye inflammations.

coltsfoot *Tussilago farfara*

A creeping perennial with round or heart-shaped leaves with a cobweb-like surface pattern. The flowers look rather like short, tufted dandelions on scaly stems and appear before the leaves in early spring.

Coltsfoot was once one of our most popular remedies for coughs and catarrh and its botanical name comes from the Latin for "cough dispeller". Its use has declined in recent years and, indeed, it has been banned in some countries due to the discovery of pyrrolizidine alkaloids in the leaves. These chemicals are known, in extremely high doses, to cause liver disease in rats (see page 205), although there is no firm evidence that coltsfoot can cause similar damage. Even so, it has fallen from favour and many herbalists advise its short-term use only.

The plant is unusual in that its flowers appear before the leaves, hence its old name *filius ante patrem*, meaning the son before the father. The flowers can be difficult to find, so try to identify your coltsfoot patch in summer, when you gather leaves, and return in spring for the flowers. It is a virulent weed and can be difficult to eradicate from gardens, so is best gathered from the wild.

➤ Coltsfoot *Tussilago farfara*

using coltsfoot

As well as helping to ease coughs and clear phlegm, coltsfoot is soothing and anti-catarrhal so is ideal for coughs caused by catarrh trickling down the throat. It is especially helpful for irritating and spasmodic coughs, including whooping cough, asthma and bronchitis and was an ingredient in herbal "tobacco" smoked for asthma. It also helps to relieve the muscle spasms associated with persistent coughing and reduces inflammation.

The yellow flowers can be dried or made into syrups; the leaves can be collected later in the year and similarly processed. Flowers and leaves (or the relevant syrups) are both used in the West and can be combined as desired. In traditional Chinese medicine only the flowers are used (also for coughs and catarrh) and are known as *Kuan Dong Hua*.

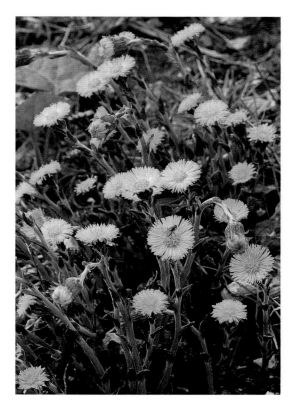

coltsfoot

parts used
flowers collected in spring, leaves collected in summer.

commercial products
sometimes included in proprietary cough mixtures and lozenges; tincture and juice available from health food shops; *Kuan Dong Hua* are sold in Chinese herbal shops.

how to use
tincture (flowers or leaves) – 5ml/1tsp per dose up to three times daily; *infusion* – 25g/1oz to 500ml/1pt of water, taken in three equal doses during the day or made into a syrup (see page 218) and taken in 10ml/2tsp doses every 2-3 hours.

stinging nettle
Urtica dioica

A perennial growing up to 2m/6 1/2ft tall, when well established, with upright stems covered in fine hairs and oval, serrated dark green leaves. Flowers appear in pendulous clusters in the leaf axils during summer and autumn; roots are bright yellow and often extensive.

Over-familiar in suburban gardens, hedgerows and on any ground that has ever been cultivated, stinging nettles were once used in a rather bizarre treatment known as urtication which involved beating paralysed limbs with the plant in an attempt to stimulate sensations. The same remedy was also recommended for rheumatic pains, while the Romans reputedly planted the small annual continental nettle (*U. pilulifera*) along British roads because they believed the country was so cold they would need to beat their bodies with nettles to keep warm.

Nettles sting because the hairs on their stems and leaves contain histamine, which is a potent skin irritant. Thanks to their ability to "rob the soil" and concentrate minerals and vitamins in their leaves they are a good nutrient and the plant makes a useful "spring tonic" as well as a good supplement in iron-deficient anaemia. Processing fresh young nettles in a juicer is a good way to make an energising tonic; they can also be cooked in soups to help clear out the stagnations of winter. It is best to gather the nettles when the plants are young, before flowering – and to wear gloves when picking and preparing them.

using stinging nettle

Nettles can be used externally in washes or infused oils for irritant skin rashes and the same oil can be used as the base for a massage rub for rheumatism. Internally, nettle tea is a popular folk remedy for rheumatism and can also help to relieve the acute painful stage of gout thanks to its ability to encourage urination and clear excess uric acid from the system. Nettles can also be helpful in urinary disorders while recent trials suggest that the root can be helpful for benign prostate enlargement. In pregnancy, nettle tea makes a useful additional source of calcium and iron and it also stimulates milk flow when breast-

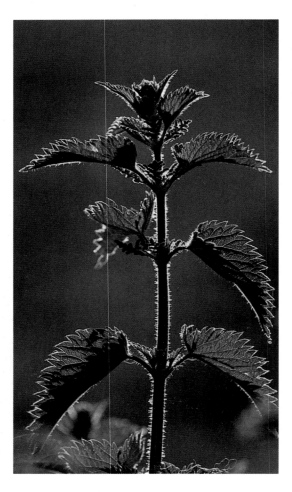

◄ Stinging nettle *Urtica dioica*

➤ Mullein *Verbascum thapsus*

feeding. Drinking nettle tea can be helpful for allergic skin rashes, especially those connected with salicylate sensitivity (see page 53). Furthermore, the plant will reduce blood sugar levels, so is a useful addition to dietary control of late-onset diabetes.

mullein *Verbascum thapsus*

A tall (up to 2m/6ft), erect biennial with soft, woolly, grey-green leaves which form a basal rosette in the first year; flowers are sessile, yellow and held in clusters on dense, erect 2½cm/1in wide spikes and appear from mid-summer to early autumn.

Mullein is a distinctive plant variously known as witch's candles, torches or candlewick from its old use as lamp wicks in the days before cotton. The stem was sometimes soaked in tallow to form a link light for use out of doors. The plant is also known as bunny's ears or donkey's ears from its large woolly leaves; these were once used as a preservative for wrapping delicate fruits such as figs and peaches.

The common name of mullein is variously said to derive from the Latin word *mollis*, meaning soft or, via Old English *moleyn*, from the Latin *malandrium*, meaning leprosy. The word *malandre* came to be applied to various diseases and lung disorders in cattle, and the herb – according to William Cole writing in 1657 – was regularly used by farmers to prevent coughs and lung diseases in their herds. It was once known as bullock's lungwort for this reason.

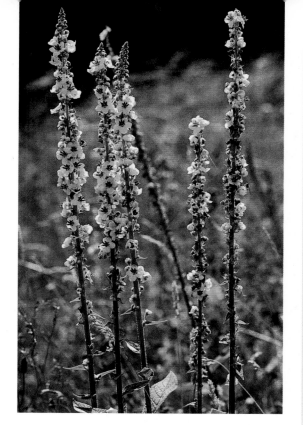

using mullein

Mullein is an excellent cough remedy which is soothing, reduces inflammations and encourages the production of phlegm. The dried leaves were once made into a smoking mixture to relieve bronchitis and other chronic coughs. Although flowers and leaves are often used together in commercial products, the flowers were once separated and made into syrups for catarrh. It is a mucilaginous plant which also makes a soothing wound remedy.

The infused oil made from the flowers (using the cold infusion method) is a traditional remedy for ear problems such as earache, discharges from the ear and eczema in the external ear and canal; 2-3 drops of the oil are often all that is needed to clear quite stubborn conditions. The same oil is used in Germany for piles, inflammations, bruises and frostbite.

mullein

parts used
leaves, flowers

commercial products
included in a few proprietary remedies for coughs; infused oil and tincture available from health food shops.

how to use
tincture – up to 5ml/1tsp per dose, three times daily;
infusion – 25g/1oz to 500ml/1pt of water, taken in three equal doses during the day.

helpful houseplants

We can also make use of the numerous exotic potted plants which are now available from nurseries and garden centres for home cultivation – both as medicinal remedies and generally to help improve the environment.

Plants have been grown in houses for centuries, sometimes for decoration but originally to serve more practical functions. The ancient Egyptians grew boswellia trees in tubs in palace courtyards as a source of frankincense, while the perfumed geraniums brought back to Europe from South Africa in the 17th century soon became popular for scenting rooms. Modern research has revealed an even more useful property for houseplants – many of them suck polluting chemicals from the atmosphere, breaking them down into harmless substances. Growing houseplants in town centre offices or inner city homes can really make the environment healthier for people who live and work there.

Philodendron spp., spider plants (*Chlorophytum elatum*), azaleas, Boston fern (*Nephrolepsis exaltata*) and weeping figs (*Ficus benjamina*) are all efficient at removing formaldehyde – a pollutant produced by some modern building materials as well as floor coverings, foam insulation and cleaning agents and also found in cigarette smoke and natural gas – from

the atmosphere, while the common ivy (*Hedera helix*) rapidly clears both formaldehyde and benzene contained in some car exhaust fumes, and the peace lily or white flag (*Spathiphyllum* spp.) soaks up trichloroethylene from dry cleaning fluid with enthusiasm. Bamboo palm (*Chamaedorea seifrizii*) will suck benzene, formaldehyde and trichloro-ethylene from the air helping to add moisture to centrally heated rooms at the same time. The dwarf date palm (*Phoenix roebelenii*) will clear the chemical pollutant xylene from the atmosphere.

Recent work has also focused on yuccas, which absorb urea from the atmosphere, welcoming it as a source of nitrogen and this makes the plant ideal for growing in lavatories to help reduce smells.

Also worth growing in pots indoors are:

aloe vera, which also absorbs atmospheric pollutants (see page 140), makes an immediately available remedy for minor burns, cuts and grazes if kept growing in a pot in the kitchen. The plant can be put outside in warm summers in temperate areas but prefers a more sub-tropical environment. It may look like a succulent but as a member of the lily family needs to be kept moist.

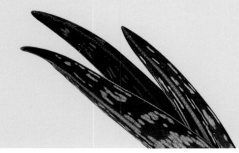

dendrobium nobile orchids, commonly grown as houseplants in Europe, help to clear pollutants such as acetone, formaldehyde and chloroform from the atmosphere, and the stems are used in Chinese medicine for feverish colds and dry coughs as well as to replenish kidney energies. The stems, known as *Shi Hu*, can also be eaten as a vegetable and were a favourite tonic remedy for the ancient Taoists used to combat ageing. They are sold dried in Chinese herbal shops.

passion flower (see page 154) can easily be grown outside in warm areas or against a south-facing wall; otherwise keep it as a conservatory or indoor climber and use the leaves in teas for insomnia.

the florist's chrysanthemum (*Dendranthema x grandiflorum*) is another Chinese medicinal plant. The flowers are known as *Ju Hua* and are used for liver and high blood pressure remedies. They are popular as a tea in China – sold Western-style in ready-made drinks and tea bags – but they do need to be steamed before use to reduce the bitter taste.

basil (see page 92) is another essential plant to keep in the house – not only for its culinary use but to promote a peaceful atmosphere and clarity of mind.

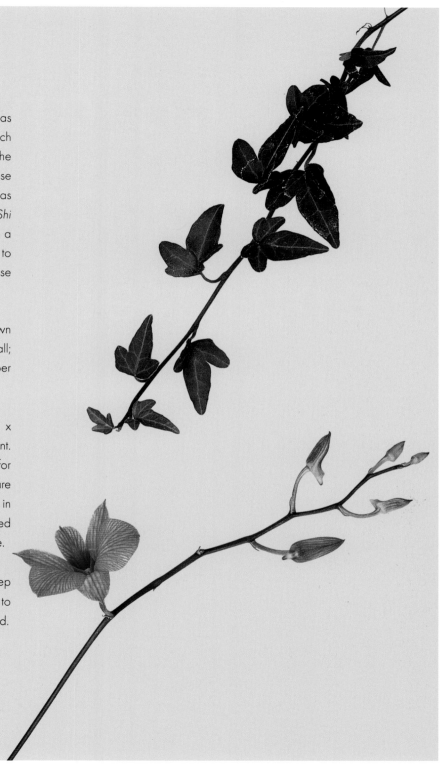

making and buying natural remedies

Herbal medicine has always been a "medicine of the people" – simple, easily found plant or vegetable remedies that could be brewed at home to treat a wide variety of ailments. For all too many of us today those remedies are no longer quite so easily found. Urban lifestyles make gathering wild plants a rare experience, while the pressures of modern life mean that few of us have spare time to make creams and tinctures.

Rediscovering some of the old household healing arts is not difficult. Simple remedies can be made quickly in the kitchen and even if access to the countryside is limited we can still grow healing plants in the garden or buy dried supplies from health food shops and by mail order. There is also something extremely satisfying about going into your garden to collect a few sprigs of lemon balm to make a relaxing tea when you feel stressed, or getting your own back on the rampant chickweed by putting it to good use as a healing ointment.

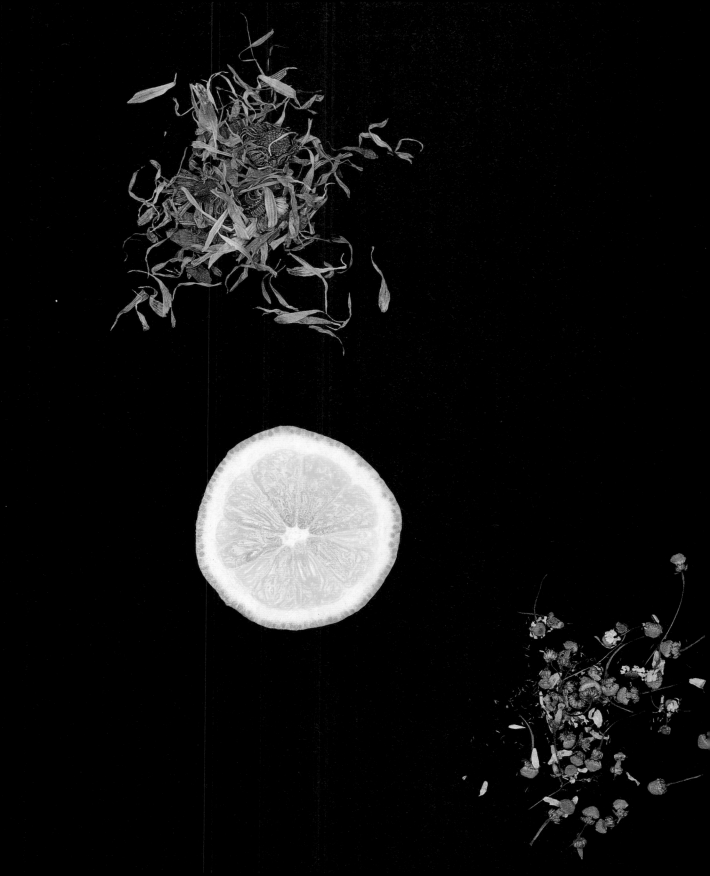

making remedies

Making herbal medicines at home is not only satisfying, it is also extremely low cost – and just because home-grown products are virtually free, it doesn't make them any less effective.

There are many ways to use herbs – both internally and externally. Some techniques are quick and easy, such as making teas; others require preparation: it can take at least two weeks to prepare a tincture, so this is not a method to use if you need medication in a hurry. Ointments and creams also take time and practice, although it is not difficult to make good-quality products with a little experience. Remember also that herbs vary in quality, character and moisture content throughout the year, so that at some times a good yield of juice is available or you may need to add less liquid to creams made from fresh herbs.

Having mastered the basic production skills, the next problem is deciding which herbs to use: they can, of course, be used individually – as simples – and will often prove very effective, however, herbs generally work best in combinations. Some herbalists will limit their mixtures to four or five herbs, others may include up to 20 in a single prescription. In traditional Chinese medicine, practitioners use classic formulae for particular syndromes. These prescriptions have often been unchanged for hundreds of years and all students of traditional Chinese medicine have to learn many hundreds of recipes by heart before qualifying.

For home use it is always best to keep combinations as simple as possible, limiting mixtures to two or three well-chosen herbs. A cough made worse by catarrh, for example, could be treated by coltsfoot flowers with elder flowers and hyssop, or a tension headache may respond to a combination of relaxing herbs, such as skullcap and vervain, with some which are more closely targeted at headaches – wood betony or lavender flowers, perhaps. It can also be useful to combine external and internal remedies. Rosemary oil, used topically, for example, can bring fast relief for arthritic pains while devil's claw taken internally may need four to six weeks to start controlling the problem.

infusions

An infusion is simply a tea made by steeping the herb in freshly boiled water for 10 minutes. The traditional proportion, suitable for most herbs, was always given as 1oz (28g – but normally converted as 25g or 30g) of dried herb to 1pt (about 500ml) of boiled water, which is sufficient for three doses, and the method can be used for most leafy herbs and flowers.

If you are using fresh herb, as opposed to dried, you will need three times as much to allow for the additional weight of water in fresh plant material (i.e. 75-90g/3oz to 500ml/1pt of water. It is best to make only enough infusion for one day's doses, although

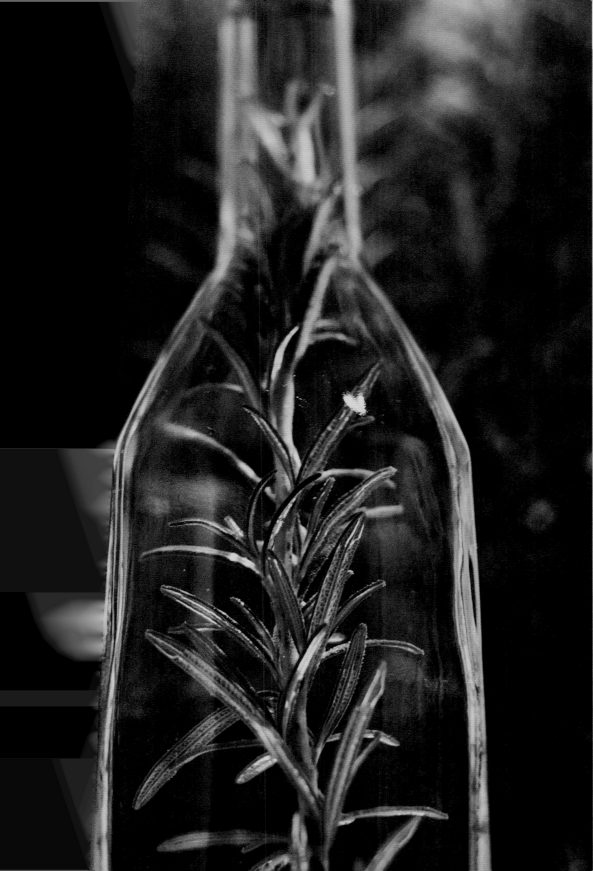

herbs for infusions
(continued from opposite)

linden
marigold
marsh woundwort
marshmallow
meadowsweet
motherwort
mugwort
mullein
olive
parsley
passion flower
peppermint
pilewort
plantain
purple loosestrife
raspberry
rosemary
sage
self-heal
shepherd's purse
skullcap
St John's wort
stinging nettle
strawberries
tea
thyme
toadflax
vervain
white deadnettle
witch hazel
wood avens
wood betony
yarrow

surplus can be stored in a refrigerator for up to 48 hours. Specific amounts for individual plants are included in Part 2 of this book (pages 70-209)

to make an infusion

• Put the required amount of herb into a ceramic or glass teapot or jug (with a lid).
• Add 500ml/1pt of water that is just off the boil to prevent loss of too many aromatic plant constituents in excessive steam.
• Leave the mixture to infuse for 10 minutes.
• Strain through a sieve – as with conventional tea leaves – into a clean jug.
• Drink a cup or wine-glass dose (about 150ml/6fl oz) three times a day. Sweeten with a little honey if required.
• The infusion can either be reheated before each dose or be drunk cold. Warm infusions are best for "cold" conditions, such as chills or arthritis.

Infusions are often best made from combinations of herbs and as combining a few grams of herbs for a day's dosages can be complicated, it is easiest to mix a larger batch for several days. One can mix equal amounts of herbs or use more of whichever one seems most appropriate for the current health problem: a cold remedy, for example, might include 10g/⅓oz of elder flowers, 10g/⅓oz of yarrow and 10g/⅓oz of peppermint for the daily dose. In this example one would combine, say, 50g/2oz each of elder flowers, yarrow and peppermint. Shake the dried herbs together thoroughly and store in a clean, dry jar. It is then easy to measure out 30g/1oz of the combination to make the day's dose of infusion as required.

decoctions

A decoction is like a tea, but it is made by simmering the plant material for 15-20 minutes and is ideal for tougher plant components such as bark, roots and berries, where it can be more difficult to extract the active ingredients. The traditional quantities, suitable for most herbs were always 1oz of herb to 1½pt of cold water – in metric parlance, about 25g to 750ml. Quantities needed for individual herbs are included in Part 2. It is best to make only enough for one day's doses at a time, although surplus can be stored in a refrigerator for up to 48 hours.

to make a decoction

• Put the required amount of herb into a stainless steel, glass, ceramic or enamel saucepan (not aluminium).
• Add 750ml/1½pt of water and bring to the boil, then reduce the heat to a gentle simmer.
• Continue to simmer until the mixture has been reduced by about a third which generally takes 15-20 minutes.
• Strain through a sieve – as with conventional tea leaves – into a clean jug.
• Drink a cup or wine-glass dose (about 150ml/6fl oz) three times a day. Sweeten with a little honey if required.
• The decoction can either be reheated before each dose or be drunk cold. Warm decoctions are best for "cold" conditions, such as chills or arthritis.

Decoctions can be reduced down to 100-250ml/3½-9fl oz with further heating and then this mix can be used in drop dosages (see page 221) either neat or in water. This can be a good

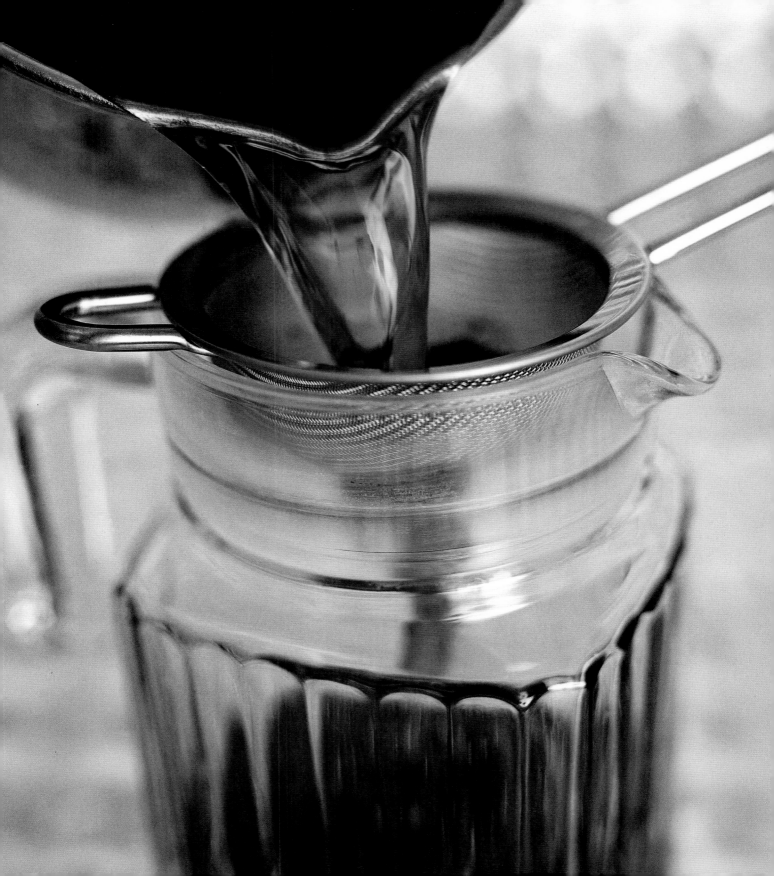

way to administer decoctions to children who are often reluctant to drink whole cups of herbal brews.

As with infusions (see above) different combinations of roots can be selected as required and it is best to mix these in larger quantities for later use as need be. A chesty cough associated with infection, for example, might be treated with a mixture of elecampane, liquorice, and echinacea; 12½g/½oz each of elecampane and echinacea roots and 5g/¹⁄₁₆oz of liquorice could be combined and simmered in 750ml/1½pt of water for 20 minutes before straining and taking in three equal doses. In China decoctions are generally preferred to infusions with as much as 100g/3½ oz or more of dried herbs heated in ½-1 litre/1-2pt of water for the day's dose. This thick mix is referred to as a *Teng* or soup and can often taste extremely unpleasant.

macerations

Although most roots can be made into decoctions (see above), some respond better to the process of cold maceration, which helps to preserve many active constituents which tend to be broken down by heating. As with decoctions and infusions, macerations are best prepared on a daily basis, although they can be stored in a refrigerator for up to 48 hours. This method is ideal for marshmallow and valerian roots.

to make a maceration
• Put the chopped root into a teapot or basin; use around 75g/3oz of fresh roots or 25g/1oz of dried.

• Cover with 500ml/1pt of cold water and leave overnight.
• Next day, strain the mixture through a sieve into a clean jug.
• Drink a cup or wine glass dose (about 150ml/6fl oz) of the cold mixture three times a day. Sweeten with a little honey if required.

combined infusions and decoctions

When using a number of herbs in a tea it is often necessary to use some as infusions and some as decoctions as with a tea of yellow dock root with burdock leaves for skin problems. The mixture may contain equal weights of roots and leaves or could have perhaps 20g/⅔oz of root and 10g/⅓oz of leaves for the day's doses.

to make a combination tea
• Put the required amount of herb into a stainless steel, glass, ceramic or enamel saucepan (not aluminium).
• Add 750ml/1½pt of water to the pan and bring to the boil, then reduce the heat to a gentle simmer.
• Continue to simmer until the mixture has been reduced by about a third which generally takes 15-20 minutes.
• Meanwhile, put the required amount of leafy plant material into a ceramic or glass teapot or jug (with lid).
• When the decoction mixture has reduced to about 500ml/1pt of water pour this onto the leaves and allow to infuse for 10 minutes.
• Strain through a sieve – as with conventional tea leaves – into a clean jug.

• Drink a cup or wine-glass dose (about 150ml/6fl oz) three times a day. Sweeten with a little honey if required.

• The combination can be reheated before each dose or drunk cold. Warm infusions are best for "cold" conditions, such as chills or arthritis.

syrups

Either sugar or honey can be used to preserve herbal infusions and decoctions and both are ideal for cough remedies as the sweetness is also soothing.

to make a syrup

• First make an infusion, decoction, or combination tea depending on the choice of herbs (see earlier methods).

• Strain the tea through a sieve – as with conventional tea leaves – into a measuring jug and check the amount.

• Then pour the liquid into a clean cast iron or stainless steel saucepan.

• For every 500ml/1pt of liquid add 500g/1lb of unrefined sugar or honey.

• Heat the mixture, stirring constantly to dissolve the sugar or honey and continue simmering gently and stirring to produce a light syrup.

• Remove from the heat and allow the mixture to cool.

• Store in clean glass bottles with a cork, not a screw top – the cork is important, as syrups often ferment and tight screw tops can easily cause exploding bottles.

• Take in 5-10ml/1-2tsp doses every 3-4 hours as required.

tinctures

A tincture is an alcoholic extraction of the active ingredients in a herb made by soaking the dried or fresh plant material in a mixture of alcohol and water.

Commercially produced tinctures are usually made from ethyl alcohol. In many countries this is subject to tax, and supply is strictly controlled; furthermore, several of the more pleasant-tasting tinctures are classified by customs officials as liqueurs so duty is often charged on extracts such as aniseed, caraway, cinnamon, lavender, lemon balm, orange peel and rosemary.

Although any alcohol can be used to make tinctures, not all alcohols are safe to drink, so great care needs to be taken with home production. Methyl alcohol (also known as methylated spirit) is extremely poisonous and, although some herbalists have used isopropyl alcohol (rubbing alcohol) for tincture-making, this too can be very toxic. Glycerol has the benefit of being very low cost, and is ideal for children and others who should avoid alcohol, however the resulting tinctures are slightly slimy to the taste.

For home use, probably the safest and most accessible source of alcohol is in the drinks cabinet – in the form of spirits and wines. Most tinctures are made from a mixture containing 25% alcohol in water (i.e. 25ml/1fl oz of pure alcohol with 75ml/3fl oz of water). This is slightly weaker in strength than most proof spirits – vodka, whisky, rum, gin etc. – so a suitable mixture can easily be made by diluting drinks bought over the counter. Of the commonly available spirits, vodka is generally considered the most appropriate as it has fewer

herbs listed in this book which can be used in cough syrups include

anise
coltsfoot
elecampane
hyssop
lemon
liquorice
marshmallow
onion
ribwort plantain
thyme

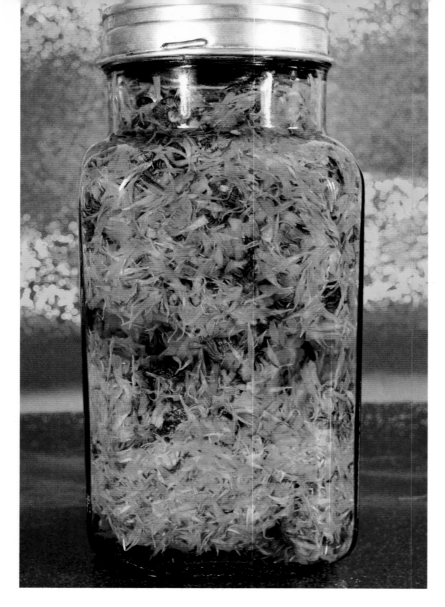

alcohol (such as vodka) to reduce the alcohol content and produce 1½ litres/3pt of a 25% mixture.

• Store the mixture in clean bottles, clearly labelled.

• Put 100g/4oz of dried herb into a large, wide-mouthed, glass jar such as an empty catering size mayonnaise pot or an old sweet jar. If using fresh herb then you will need 300g/12oz.

• Add 500ml/1pt of the diluted alcohol mixture to the jar, screw the lid tight and shake well.

• Leave the jar in a cool dark place for two weeks, shaking thoroughly every couple of days.

• After two weeks, strain the mixture through a wine press or jelly bag and store the resulting liquid in clean, dark glass bottles. The yield is generally 80-90% depending on how effective the wine press is. The herbal residue makes an ideal addition to the compost heap.

• Take the tincture in a little warm water three or four times daily; doses vary with herb but are generally 2½-5ml/½-1tsp. Fruit juice can be used instead of water to disguise unpleasant tastes if preferred.

Some herbs — mainly roots, barks or those which contain a lot of resins or essential oils — need to be extracted in 45-60% alcohol mixtures. This is more difficult to obtain for domestic use. Using the 37½% alcohol available from most commercial spirit will give a slightly weaker product compared with commercial tinctures, although if using home-grown herbs their freshness will more than make up for any loss of potency.

Tinctures will generally last for two years or more without deterioration — although Ayurvedic medicine actually argues that the tinctures increase in potency as they age.

other flavourings or herbal ingredients. Using rum is a good way to disguise the less palatable herbs. Standard tinctures are usually made in the weight:volume proportion 1:5 (i.e. 1kg of herb to 5 litres of alcohol/water or 1lb of herb to 5pts of alcohol/water).

to make a tincture

• First dilute your supply of alcohol. Add 500ml/1pt of water to 1 litre/2pt of 37½%

Unlike combinations of herbs used in teas, it is best to make tinctures of single herbs and then combine them as need be. A catarrhal cold, for example, might be treated with a combination of echinacea, elder flower and yarrow in the proportion 2:1:1. In this case pour 50ml/2fl oz of the echinacea tincture and 25ml/1fl oz of each of the elder flower and yarrow tinctures into a 100ml/4fl oz glass bottle. Shake well and use this in 5ml/1tsp doses, three times daily.

Recommended dosages for tinctures can vary enormously. Occasionally up to 20ml/⅔fl oz could be suggested, for example, as with some remedies for period pain. In other cases a number of drops is specified and many tinctures packaged for the over-the-counter market are sold in convenient dropper bottles.

Obviously drop sizes vary but a general rule of thumb is to count 20 drops as 1ml. Dropping pipettes and dropper bottles are often available from the chemists but if in doubt about the size of your chosen dropper, simply count the number of drops required to fill a teaspoon and then divide by five to give the drop/ml equivalent.

tonic wines

Tincture-like extracts can be made with wine, although they tend not to keep so well. Steeping the herb in wine was a traditional way of making medicines in the past and many early herbals mention this method. It is also a good way to make tonics. Tonic roots such as elecampane, ginseng, *Dang Gui, Huang Qi, He Shou Wu* or *ashwagandha* are ideal made into wines in this way.

to make a tonic wine
• Ideally use a clean vinegar vat (available from good cook shops) which is basically a large wide-mouthed jar with a tap near the bottom and a cork lid.
• Pack the herb or root loosely into the vat to around 5cm/2in from the top.
• Cover the herb completely with a good-quality red wine and leave the mixture for at least two weeks.
• Using the tap on the vinegar vat, draw off a sherry glass or small wine glass (around 75ml/3fl oz) of the wine each evening.
• Add more wine as need be to keep the herb totally covered otherwise the plant material will go mouldy and must be discarded. The vat can be used for up to 6 months before the herb will need to be renewed.

Traditional flower wines can also be made in this way. Simply gather healing petals as they appear through the year – start with coltsfoot, sweet violet (*Viola odorata*), primroses (*Primula vulgaris*) and cowslips (*Primula veris*), and add honeysuckle (*Lonicera japonica*), heartsease (*Viola tricolor*), St John's wort, roses (*Rosa* spp.), mullein, hollyhock, mallow and wood betony as the summer progresses. Put the fresh flowers into the vinegar vat and cover each layer of petals with wine. By the end of the year the vat will be filled and the liquid can be run off to make a revitalising drink for cold winter days.

juices

Processing a herb through a liquidiser is an easy way to make a juice of the entire plant,

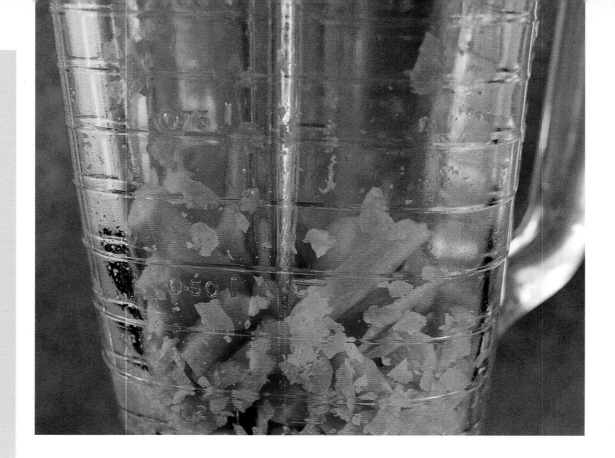

rather than trying to extract constituents by water or alcohol. The method is ideal for soft, leafy plants such as cleavers, lemon balm, St John's wort or fennel; if a juicer is available then it can also be used for fruits and vegetables.

to make a herb juice

- Loosely fill a small food processor or liquidiser with fresh herb.
- Process the mixture to produce a thick green slurry.
- Take in 10ml/2tsp doses, mixed with a little water if preferred, three times a day.
- The juice will last only for a few days in a refrigerator and soon deteriorates, so it is best to make small quantities (100ml/4fl oz or so) at a time.

Commercial herb juices are available from specialist suppliers and can often been found in health food shops or pharmacies; it is, of course, very easy to find carrot, tomato or beetroot juices in supermarkets.

ointments and creams

Creams are a mixture of oils or fats and water and are described as being miscible (meaning that they mix in with or can be absorbed by the skin), while ointments contain only oils or fats and form a separate layer over the skin. Ointments are suitable where the skin is already weak or soft or where some protection from additional moisture is needed (as in nappy rash).

Traditionally, ointments were made using animal fats.

to make an ointment

• Melt 250g/10oz of lard or Vaseline in a saucepan over a very low heat.
• Add 50g/2oz of dried herb and stir well.
• Continue heating gently until the herb is slightly crisp – this generally takes about 2 hours.
• Warm a metal measuring jug in the oven (160°C/320°F/gas mark 4) for 5-10 minutes and have ready five sterilised 50g/2oz glass ointment pots.
• Strain the mixture through a fine nylon sieve or jelly bag into the warm jug, which will prevent it solidifying too quickly, and then pour immediately into the ointment pots. Once the ointment has set, store in a cool dry place and use as required. Ointments will usually last for at least a year if the pots have been well sterilised.

Creams can easily be made using emulsifying ointment (available from most pharmacists). This is a mixture of oils (usually hydrocarbons or paraffins) which can be blended with a certain proportion of water to make a cream.

to make a cream from emulsifying ointment

• Use a large double saucepan or else a stainless steel bowl placed on top of a large saucepan. Fill the lower pan with water.
• Put 300g/10oz emulsifying ointment into the top saucepan and heat the double pan.
• When the emulsifying ointment has melted add 135ml/4½fl oz of glycerol and 165ml/5½fl oz of water. The cold liquid will cause the

ointment to resolidify so continue heating until the mixture is fully liquid once more.
• Add 60g/2oz dried herb to the mixture and heat for at least three hours.
• Check on the water level of the lower pan regularly and add additional boiling water as need be to prevent the pan from boiling dry.
• After three hours, pour the hot mixture through a wine press or jelly bag (placed over a basin and suspended from the legs of an upturned stool as in jam making). This needs to be done fairly quickly as the cream will start to solidify once the heat is removed.
• Collect the still melted cream in a basin and stir gently until it cools. It should remain smooth throughout, if the mix begins to go lumpy or separate out it will need to be remelted in a fresh double saucepan again. Adding a little more emulsifying ointment at this stage can help.
• Once the cream is completely cold store in small dark glass jars for use as need be. The cream will usually keep for at least a year if stored in a cool dry place although the shelf-life can be extended by adding five drops of benzoin (sold alongside aromatherapy oils or in pharmacies) to the mixture as a preservative.

to make a cream from beeswax and lanolin

• Use a large double saucepan or else a stainless steel bowl placed on top of a large saucepan. Fill the lower pan with water.
• Put 25g/1oz of white beeswax and 25g/1oz of anhydrous lanolin (available from a chemist) into the top saucepan and heat the double pan.
• When the beeswax and lanolin have melted add 100ml/4fl oz of sunflower oil (or similar), 75ml/3fl oz of water, 25ml/1fl oz of glycerol.

The cold liquids will cause the fats to resolidify so continue heating until the mixture is fully liquid once more.

• Add 50g/2oz of dried herb to the mixture and heat for at least three hours.

• Check on the water level of the lower pan regularly and add additional boiling water as need be to prevent the pan from boiling dry.

• After three hours, pour the hot mixture through a wine press or jelly bag (placed over a basin and suspended from the legs of an upturned stool as in jam making). This needs to be done fairly quickly as the cream will start to solidify once the heat is removed.

• Collect the still melted cream in a basin and stir gently until it cools.

• Once the cream is completely cold store in small dark glass jars for use as need be. The cream will usually keep for at least a year if stored in a cool dry place although the shelf-life can be extended by adding five drops of benzoin (sold alongside aromatherapy oils or in pharmacies) to the mixture as a preservative.

When making herbal creams and ointments the proportions of herb to fat/water mixture are important so the metric/imperial measures given here may seem inconsistent but maintain the proportions in different measuring systems.

infused oils

Infused oils can be used in making ointments or as a base for massage oils and are an excellent and simple way of creating external herbal remedies. There are two techniques: hot infusion or cold infusion.

to make a hot infusion

• Use a large double saucepan or else a stainless steel bowl placed on top of a large saucepan. Fill the lower pan with water.

• Put 100g/4oz of dried (300g/12oz of fresh) herb and 500ml/1pt of sunflower oil (or similar) into the top saucepan or bowl and heat.

• Remember to refill the lower saucepan with boiling water from time to time to prevent it from boiling dry.

• After about three hours strain the oil through a fine sieve, muslin jelly bag or wine press into a jug.

• When cool, pour the infused oil into clean glass bottles and store away from direct sunlight.

to make a cold infusion

Because the oils are not heated in this method, one can use good-quality seed oils that are rich in essential fatty acids (EFAs) — such as *gamma*-linolenic or *cis*-linoleic — which have significant therapeutic properties. Oils high in EFAs include walnut, safflower and pumpkin.

to make a cold infused oil

• Use a medium-sized jar with a wide mouth, such a 1kg/2lb storage jar or large size mayonnaise jar.

• Pack the jar quite tightly with either dried or fresh herb material, about 2½cm/1in from the top.

• Completely cover the herb with oil, such as walnut or safflower oil.

• Leave the jar on a sunny windowsill or in the greenhouse for at least three weeks.

• Then, strain the mixture through a wine press, fine sieve or jelly bag.

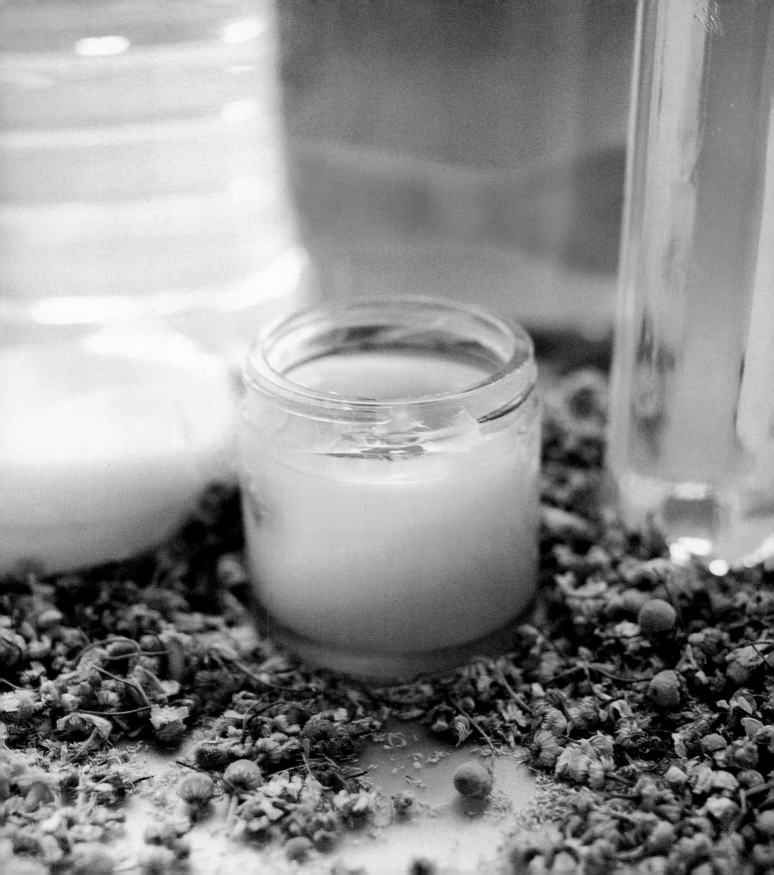

strains and sprains – use 5-10 drops each of rosemary, eucalyptus, juniper and lavender oil in 50ml/2fl oz of infused comfrey or St John's wort oil.

arthritis and rheumatism – use 5-10 drops each of rosemary, lavender, sage and marjoram in 50ml/2fl oz of infused bladderwrack or infused rosemary oil.

migraine and headaches – use 5 drops each of lavender, marjoram and lemon balm oil in 25ml/1fl oz of sweet almond or wheat germ oil.

general relaxing oil – use 5 drops each of basil, sandalwood, lemon balm and lavender in 25ml/1fl oz of St John's wort or sweet almond oil.

chest rubs are ideal for treating many respiratory and throat problems, including coughs, bronchitis, whooping cough, laryngitis and asthma. Use 5-10 drops of thyme, hyssop and eucalyptus oil in sweet almond or wheat germ oil and massage into the chest two or three times a day.

• Ideally, the whole process should be repeated once more using fresh herb and the once-infused oil and again leaving it in a sunny place for a further two or three weeks.

• Finally strain the twice-infused mixture through a wine press, fine sieve or jelly bag and store in a cool, dry place in clean dark glass bottles.

These infused oils – which will generally last for at least a year, often longer – can also be used in ointments or creams with beeswax and anhydrous lanolin (which you can order through your pharmacist).

For suggested herbs for infused oils, see panel on page 224

to make an infused oil ointment

• Use a large double saucepan or else a stainless steel bowl placed on top of a large saucepan. Fill the lower pan with water.

• Melt 25g/1oz of beeswax and 25g/1oz of anhydrous lanolin in the top bowl of the double saucepan and heat for a few minutes until the fats are well melted.

• Add 100ml/4fl oz of the infused oil. If the fats have been solidified by adding the cooler liquid, stir the mixture and heat for a few minutes longer.

• Pour the liquid into clean glass jars while still warm and allow to cool.

to make an infused oil cream

• Use a large double saucepan or else a stainless steel bowl placed on top of a large saucepan. Fill the lower pan with water.

• Melt 25g/1oz beeswax and 25g/1oz anhydrous lanolin in the top bowl of the double saucepan and heat for a few minutes until the fats are well melted.

• Add 100ml/4fl oz infused oil, stir, and heat for a few minutes longer if the fats have been solidified by adding the cooler liquid.

• Remove the bowl from the heat and slowly add 50ml/2fl oz of a herbal tincture, stirring constantly. Continue stirring until the mixture is completely cool and the cream smooth.

• Once the cream is completely cold store in small dark glass jars for use as need be. The cream will usually keep for at least a year if stored in a cool, dry place.

Various combination creams using different oil and herb/tincture mixtures are easy to make using this method. For suggested herbs, see panel on page 224.

massage oils

The sort of massage oils used in aromatherapy are very easy to make at home by adding a few drops of essential oil to some sort of oil base. Suitable bases include sweet almond oil, wheat germ oil, avocado oil or any of the infused herb oils made from walnut or sunflower oil described above.

Essential oils are made commercially, usually by steam-distilling various parts of the plant. This is not a technique for home use. In general do not use more than 10% of essential oil (½ml/10 drops of essential oil in 5ml/1tsp of carrier oil), as many essential oils can irritate sensitive skins. Always buy good-quality essential oils as many cheap ones are chemically adulterated. The higher the price and the more reputable the brand name, the more likely the oil is to be good quality.

MENTHE
MINT

S ESSENTIELLES
TIAL OILS

Essen

LE CORPS
BODY CARE

CHAMOMILE
BLUE

ESSENTIAL OIL 2.5ml
THIS IS A HIGHLY CONCENTRATED PURE
PLANT ESSENCE. ALWAYS DILUTE
BEFORE USE. DO NOT TAKE INTERNALLY
WITHOUT PROFESSIONAL ADVICE
KEEP OUT OF REACH OF CHILDREN

25116.10

herbs mentioned in this book suitable for making steam inhalants include

chamomile
thyme
eucalyptus
hyssop
peppermint

the following essential oils are readily available from health shops; adding them to the bath can be helpful

aches and pains – rosemary, lavender, eucalyptus, juniper, marjoram

anxiety and stress – benzoin, chamomile, cypress, rose geranium, jasmine, lavender, marjoram, lemon balm, rose, sandalwood

catarrh – peppermint, eucalyptus, lavender

coughs and colds – hyssop, thyme, benzoin, anise, sandalwood, eucalyptus

fatigue – basil, lemon balm, rosemary, sage, peppermint

headaches – lavender, rose, marjoram

period pain – chamomile, cypress, marjoram, lemon balm, rosemary, sandalwood

Use small dark glass bottles and pour the carrier oil in first and then add drops of essential oil as required. When you are ready to use, pour about 2½ml/½tsp of oil on to the palm of your hand, rub the hands lightly together to spread the oil and then massage the affected area.

See panel on page 226 for some of the most relaxing massage combinations.

steam inhalants

Inhaling aromatic oils is a good way to clear the respiratory system of mucus in conditions such as catarrh, sinusitis, bronchitis or asthma. Either infusions or well-diluted essential oils can be used. It is important to stay in a warm room for 30 minutes after treatment to allow the airways time to return to normal.

to make a steam inhalation
• Put a large handful of the fresh herb or 25g/1oz of dried herb into a large (2 litre/ 4pt) basin.
• Pour on around 500ml/1pt of boiling water.
• Lean over the basin and cover your head completely with a towel.
• Inhale the steam for 10 minutes or as long as you feel comfortable.
• Stay in a warm room for at least 30 minutes after the treatment and repeat once or twice a day.
• Up to ½ml/10 drops of an essential oil can be used instead of the dried herb if preferred.

For helpful herbs to use as inhalants, see the panel on the left.

foot baths

Soaking your feet in a hot bath can bring relief to aching feet, ease sprains and stimulate the circulation for those prone to chilblains; it also helps combat the common cold. Suitable essential oils (see under Baths, below) or hot infusions can be used, or you can opt for a traditional mustard bath, using 1tbsp of powdered mustard to a basin of hot water.

Alternating hot and cold treatments can help reduce bruising and provide emergency relief for badly sprained ankles. Soak the affected area in a basin of very hot water containing a large quantity of rosemary sprigs or 1ml/20 drops of rosemary essential oil for 3-5 minutes; then plunge into a water and ice mixture for 2-3 minutes. Repeat the process for as long as you can bear it.

baths

Adding essential oils or an infusion to bath water is an excellent way to ease aching limbs, clear a stuffy nose or relax after a stressful day. Use 2-5 drops of essential oil neat in the bath water and stir well to disperse the oil. Alternatively add 500ml/1pt of a freshly made and strained infusion. Suitable oils for adding to baths are listed in the panel (left).

pessaries and suppositories

Pessaries are waxy pellets containing medication which can be inserted in the vagina and will melt at body temperature, delivering the remedy to the site of infection or irritation.

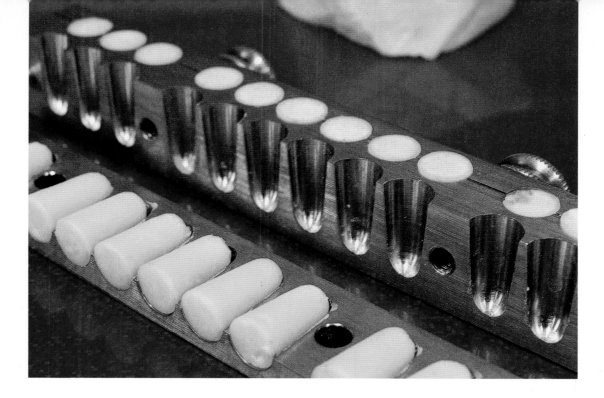

Suppositories are similar, but intended for anal insertion. They are often used where treatments are needed in the lower bowel and the medicines would otherwise be broken down during the digestive process.

Both can be made at home in the same way, although the process can be time consuming without a pessary mould (sometimes available from chemists). An ideal base is cocoa butter which melts at body temperature. Substitute moulds can be made by shaping cooking foil into small thimble-like holders about 1cm/½in in diameter and 2cm/⅘in long.

to make pessaries and suppositories

• Pessary moulds are available which will hold up to 24 pessaries.
• First lubricate the mould. Mix 10g/⅖oz of soft soap, 50ml/2fl oz of glycerol and 40ml/1⅓fl oz of methylated spirit. Shake this together and leave for a couple of days for the soft soap to dissolve thoroughly.
• Pour enough lubricant into the mould to just fill it, leave for a few seconds, then pour away. The lubricant can be reused several times.
• Use a double saucepan or else a stainless steel or ceramic bowl placed on top of a saucepan. Fill the lower pan with water.
• To make 24 pessaries/suppositories, melt 20g/¾oz of cocoa butter in the top pan of the double saucepan. Remove from the heat.
• Add 1½ml/30 drops of essential oil to the melted cocoa butter, stir and pour into the mould. Leave to set.
• Remove the pessaries/suppositories from the mould and store in a jar between layers of greaseproof paper.

Some suitable oils for pessaries to treat vaginal infections, such as thrush, can be found in the panel on page 231.

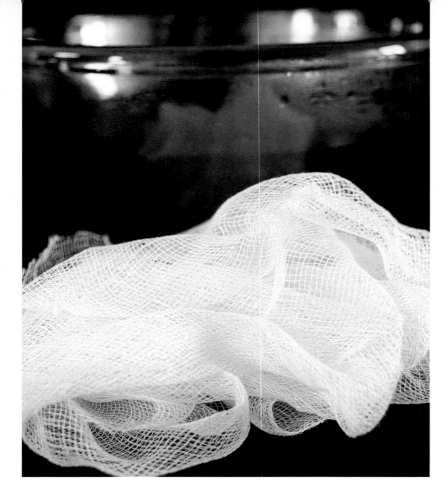

headaches, when a pad soaked in cold lavender infusion can be helpful.

poultices

Poultices have a very similar action to compresses, but involve applying the whole herb to an affected area directly rather than using a liquid extract. Poultices are usually applied hot for swellings, sprains or to draw pus and splinters. As with hot compresses, renew the hot poultice as it cools or place a hot-water bottle on top to keep it hot.

to make a poultice
• Cut a piece of of surgical gauze, muslin, lint or cotton about three times the size of the area to be treated.
• Fold fresh or dried herbs in the fabric to make a small pack and then place the parcel flat on a small pie dish or similar container. Pour boiling water on to it and soak for 3-5 minutes.
• Pour off the water and place the poultice directly onto the affected area. Replace with a fresh poultice after 1-2 hours.
• Cold poultices can be made by softening fresh herb material by either bruising with a vegetable mallet or mixing in a food processor for a few seconds. Spread this onto the gauze and chill in a freezer for 5 minutes. Then use in the same way as a hot poultice, replacing with a fresh chilled pack after 1-2 hours.
• If using dried herbs or powder, mix with equal amounts of runny honey and vegetable oil to make a soft paste.

For suitable herbs to use in poultices, see panel opposite.

compresses

Compresses are often used to accelerate healing of wounds or muscle injuries. They are basically cloth pads soaked in herbal extracts and usually applied hot to painful limbs, swellings or strains.

To prepare a compress, use a clean piece of cotton, cotton wool ball, linen or surgical gauze soaked in a hot, strained infusion, decoction or tincture (20ml/1fl oz of tincture to 500ml/1¼pt of hot water) and apply to the affected area. When the compress cools repeat using fresh, hot mixture.

Occasionally a cold compress may be more suitable than a hot one – as with some types of

buying over-the-counter remedies

Some types of herbal extracts can be rather more complicated to make at home and it is best to buy them ready-made from herbal suppliers and health food shops. Fluid extracts, powders and capsules as well as essential oils are all in this category and can be found in good health food shops.

fluid extracts

More concentrated alcohol/water extracts are available commercially as "fluid extracts". The herb to liquid ratio is around 1:1 and these are rather complex for home production. Fluid extracts are generally made by heating the basic tincture mixture in a percolator to reduce the volume to around a half. This liquid is collected and reserved and then a fresh quantity of herb and alcohol/water is added and the cycle of maceration and percolating repeated twice more.

Because the alcohol will have evaporated during the process, fluid extracts do not last as long as tinctures and often need to have extra alcohol added for long-term storage.

Fluid extracts are, by definition, five times stronger than the average 1:5 tincture, so need be used only in very small quantities. If the dose of a tincture is 5ml/1tsp, then 1ml/20 drops of a fluid extract will deliver the same amount of herb.

Professional herbalists often use fluid extracts when large amounts of a herb are needed such as meadowsweet used in arthritis.

powders and capsules

Although it is possible to grind herbs in a domestic coffee grinder, they usually become very hot in the process and this can cause chemical changes within the plant: grinding hard roots can also damage the coffee grinder! It is best to use powders produced using commercial mills, which do not cause quite so much heating, and many powdered herbs are now available from specialist suppliers.

Two-part gelatine capsules (generally size 00, which holds around 200-250mg of powder) are available from pharmacists or specialist health food shops, but filling them by hand is a laborious process and it is often easier simply to take an equivalent amount of the powder stirred into a little water instead.

To fill capsules put some herb powder in a saucer or flat dish and then separate the two halves of the capsule. Slide them together through the powder, scooping it into the capsule. Capsule-filling machines are used by many herbalists. These mechanically separate 100 capsules at a time, holding the two halves in plastic frames. Powder is spread over the lower frame, filling the capsules, and then the top frame replaced to reassemble them.

Many common herbs are now available ready prepared in capsules from health food shops and pharmacies. These may be packaged as single herbs or in combinations and can also use differently-sized capsules so it is important to check recommended dosages.

essential oils suitable for making pessaries include

thyme
marigold
tea tree

herbs mentioned in this book suitable for making poultices include

comfrey
chamomile
slippery elm
marshmallow
chickweed
St John's wort

patent remedies

Well over 1,000 different herbal remedies can now be found in health food stores and pharmacies. Many of these are based on traditional remedies devised by herbalists 50 or 100 years ago, while others use more recently discovered herbs or Oriental plants that have little history of traditional use in the West.

Production and distribution of herbal medicines is, quite rightly, strictly regulated in most countries. Despite the popular view that herbs are natural and therefore "safe", many plants are extremely potent and misuse can have serious side-effects. Controlling legislation varies significantly around the world. In some European countries, such as Germany, the market is highly regulated and herbal products are manufactured to the same standards and licensing rules as pharmaceutical drugs. Elsewhere, such as New Zealand, product licences are virtually unknown.

There have been moves in recent years to standardise the rules governing herbal products throughout Europe and the European Scientific Cooperative on Phytotherapy (ESCOP) has been working on a series of herbal monographs detailing usage, which are likely to be adopted as standard within the European Union. These monographs define the claims that can be made for particular herbal products. At present labelling and licensing rules, which limit the therapeutic claims that can be made for products, vary between countries. Garlic, for example, tends to be licensed in Britain as a remedy for catarrh and colds, whereas in Germany it is usually licensed as a preventative tonic for heart and circulatory problems since it lowers cholesterol levels.

Currently, in the UK, licences issued by the Medicines Control Agency (MCA), are only ever given for remedies used to treat minor self-limiting ailments so the printed claim is only a part of the picture. OTC products are not allowed to make claims for treating chronic problems, such as arthritis or high blood pressure, so remedies that can tackle these ailments either have to be sold as suitable for something else or relegated to the unlicensed category. Echinacea tablets, for example, have been licensed as a remedy for minor skin problems while evening primrose oil is licensed only for eczema and breast discomfort associated with pre-menstrual syndrome. Products granted licences by the MCA have the product licence details (a code number starting PL) printed on the packages and can make carefully worded claims which generally start: "A herbal remedy traditionally used for the symptomatic relief of…". Such products usually also need to include an instruction to "consult your doctor if symptoms persist" on the label.

Unlicensed products – generally classified as food supplements – can include single crude herbs sold in tablets and tinctures as well as some proprietary combinations. These products cannot even make the limited claims of licensed products, so selecting an appropriate remedy can be difficult as very little information about use will be found on the label. The antidepressant effects of St John's wort, for example, can only be hinted at in descriptions of the "sunshine herb".

The European Herbal Practitioners' Association (EHPA), among others, is currently trying to change the official view of herbal medicines so that traditional products could more easily be licensed and regulated without

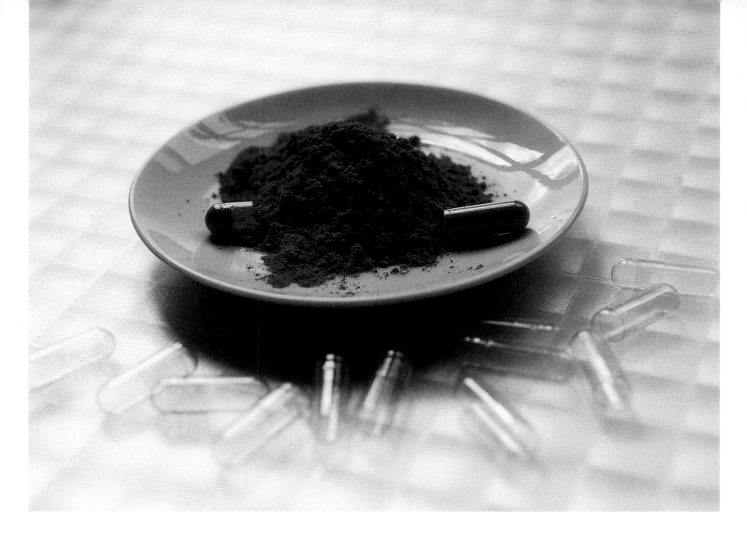

having to undergo the sort of clinical trials and tests demanded for new pharmaceutical drugs. It is also hoping to extend the range of approved remedies available to newer herbs from non-European traditions.

Existing European product licensing rules are generally based on traditional and well-documented uses for a particular herb. This emphasis on tradition means that there are virtually no licensed products based on the more recently introduced herbs such as devil's claw. Newcomers from the Amazonian jungle or the Far East, such as Peruvian cat's claw or *noni*, are similarly neglected by the legislators.

Currently there are no licensed Ayurvedic and Chinese herbal preparations in the UK and in some countries – including Australia – there are already bans on the importation of certain Chinese herbs. Indeed, the quality of imported Oriental herbs can be questionable and although these are improving, errors in labelling and packaging do occur.

The OTC market remains something of a minefield for the unwary. Always try to check actions in a herbal before buying to ensure that the product is going to be suitable and be highly suspicious of products listing exotic ingredients or those with dubious botanical names.

growing and storing herbs

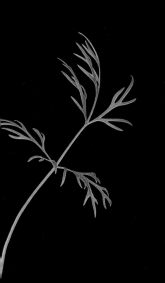

While gathering wildflowers from hedgerows is available to only fortunate country dwellers, every garden or window box – no matter how small – has the potential to supply basic medicinal needs. Herbs are no more difficult to cultivate than any other herbaceous plants or shrubs, while garden herbs provide a constant array of healing aromas to enjoy. Herbs can prove attractive, too: variegated varieties generally have only slightly less therapeutic properties than basic species and are usually less vigorous, so may be preferable if space is limited. For the less common medicinal herbs, home cultivation can also ensure a constant supply.

While fresh leaves from some garden herbs, such as rosemary and sage, can be gathered throughout the year, most plants are highly seasonal and so need to be collected, dried and stored for winter use. This is not as demanding of time or space as it may seem as the quite small quantities – just enough to fill an average jam-jar or two – will generally be enough to meet the family's needs. Try to grow and store a cross-section of remedies to cope with common ailments such as colds, headaches, muscular aches, nervous tension or digestive upsets.

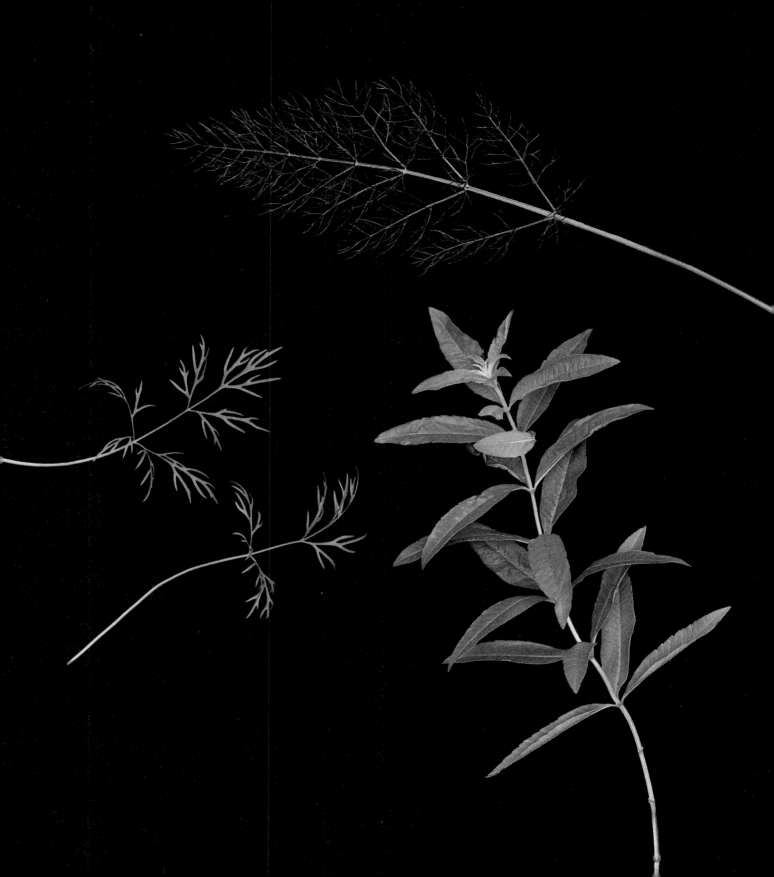

growing herbs

Home-grown and freshly dried herbs tend to be far more potent than commercial specimens which may have been stored for many months before sale – and not always kept in ideal conditions.

When growing herbs for home use, it is obviously very important to avoid chemical pesticides. Ideally use organic growing methods and avoid artificial fertilisers.

buying plants

As always when buying nursery-grown plants, look for strong, healthy specimens with plenty of new growth and space in the pot for expansion. Straggly, yellowing herbs will not improve when planted out in the garden – they will simply be a disappointment.

Although it is especially satisfying to watch your herbs grow from seeds, some species are slow growing or difficult to propagate, so are worth buying as plants to help establish the herb garden – especially for plants such as comfrey or elecampane which will very soon grow to an impressive size. If you want the more decorative varieties of herbs then a visit to a good specialist nursery is essential: worth looking for are variegated lemon balm, variegated mugwort, red ribwort plantain, variegated comfrey, and the various pink-, white- and blue-flowered versions of hyssop, lavender and rosemary.

Most specialist herb nurseries expect a peak in sales in mid- to late spring and will gear production to these times. Later in the season plants are likely to become pot bound with a mass of tangled roots emerging at the bottom and sometimes numerous annual weeds sharing the pot. Good nurseries will regularly pot up their products to larger containers as the season progresses, but then the price usually rises accordingly.

When buying plants always examine them closely for any pests: red spider mite, aphids and whitefly can congregate on the underside of leaves or on new growth and will prove unwelcome additions to a healthy garden. You can check on roots and potting practices by upturning the pot and tapping gently so that plant and compost slide out of the container. Healthy root growth should be evident and the compost should hold its shape. Loose soil suggests that the plant has only recently been potted up and there has been little time to establish the root system.

Always check that plants are correctly labelled: garden centres and even specialist nurseries do not always get names quite right and plant tags can be misplaced. Try to have a little idea of what the plant should look like before buying or ask nursery staff to check if you are unsure.

Herbs mentioned in this book which are worth buying as established plants include: agrimony, comfrey, fennel, hyssop, lavender, lemon balm, marshmallow, marjoram, meadowsweet, motherwort, mugwort, passion flower, peppermint, rosemary, purple sage, skullcap, thyme, wood betony and yarrow.

growing from seed

It is never worth buying annual herbs in pots – as with garden flowers, they are far better grown from seed, ideally planted directly in the garden where they will spend the summer. The patient can cultivate their own perennial medicinal herbs from seed, too, although generally taking cuttings or dividing established plants is quicker, more efficient and avoids any hybridisation. Seeds for common herbs are often sold alongside vegetable seeds in garden centres, although many medicinal herbs (including toadflax and wood betony) are more likely to be found in the wild flower sections.

Many herbs will self-seed enthusiastically, which can be both a useful source of new plants and a nuisance demanding ruthless weeding out. Particular culprits can include angelica, fennel, feverfew, lemon balm and skullcap.

Annual medicinal herbs to sow regularly include anise, basil, borage, Californian poppy, coriander, German chamomile, dill, and marigold. Sow annual seeds where they are intended to grow once the soil is warm enough. It is worth allowing some of the plants to go to seed to provide a ready-made crop for successive years – earmarking a plot in the vegetable garden where they can grow undisturbed is a good way of ensuring supplies.

Perennial and biennial herbs which are easy to grow from seed include angelica, catmint, coltsfoot, elecampane, fennel, feverfew, hyssop, mullein, parsley, green sage, wood betony, wild thyme, hops, St John's wort, ribwort plantain and skullcap. Sow biennial or perennial seeds in a seed tray or 7½cm/3in cm pot containing well-watered, good-quality compost. Cover larger seeds with a fine layer of compost roughly equal in depth to the size of the seed, but leave small seeds uncovered. Cover the tray with glass or place the pot in a plastic bag and store in a warm place (up to about 20°C/68°F). Alternatively, use a heated propagator.

As soon as the seedlings are large enough to handle prick them out into a second seed tray, eventually potting on into 7½-10cm/3-4in pots before hardening off and planting out. Most seeds should be sown in spring, although perennials are often best sown in late summer or early autumn. Pot these on, over-winter in a greenhouse or cold frame and plant them out the following spring.

growing from cuttings

Woody perennial herbs are best propagated by cuttings rather than grown from seed. Select cuttings from the side shoots of bushy herbs such as sage and rosemary, using semi-ripe sprigs, in late summer or early autumn, or choose the new softwood growth in spring and early summer when roots need to develop quickly if the cutting is to survive. Semi-ripe cuttings are usually more successful for medicinal herbs such as elder, hyssop, lavender, marjoram, rosemary, purple sage and thyme.

Simply break or cut off suitable shoots, keeping a heel of the main stem attached if possible. Dip the base of the cutting into hormone-rooting powder and set half a dozen cuttings in good-quality compost in a 10cm/4in pot. Water well. After a few weeks roots should appear at the base of the pot.

Pot on the rooted cuttings into individual 7½-10cm/3-4in pots ready for hardening off and planting out.

root division

Herbs can also be propagated by root division. Use a small fork to lever clumps of ramsons, for example, apart or divide large roots with a sharp spade in the early spring when growth has just started. Replant immediately after division and water thoroughly. Roman chamomile, peppermint and elecampane can be propagated by taking the small offsets and runners they develop and replanting.

keeping them under control

Herbs can grow rapidly and need vigorous pruning to keep in check. For medicinal herb cultivation, regular cropping usually limits the need to do too much pruning. If you cut herbaceous herbs back to 10-15cm/4-6in when collecting aerial parts for drying that is usually all that is needed. Where specific parts of a plant are used (e.g. lavender flowers), then normal gardening rules for pruning apply.

Prune shrubby herbs, such as rosemary, sage and lavender, after flowering in late summer, cutting back to leave around 10-20cm/4-8in of the new growth.

a healthy window box

Herbs will grow happily for one or two seasons in containers or window boxes, although fresh planting each spring will ensure healthier plants and a better balance in sizes. Remember, too, that herbs thrive in poor soil, so rich potting compost can encourage excess growth. Use a loam-based compost or add one part of grit to five parts of peat-based compost to improve the soil texture and drainage.

Suitable plants for a medicinal herbal window box include: variegated lemon balm, Roman chamomile, wood betony, creeping thyme (*Thymus serpyllum*), a small sage plant, nasturtiums (*Tropaeolum majus*), and variegated ground ivy (*Glechoma hederacea*) – a useful anti-catarrhal for colds and running noses that is often sold in garden centres for hanging baskets or tubs.

harvesting herbs

The time when herbs are gathered can significantly affect the constituent chemicals and thus the therapeutic properties. In the past complex rituals were followed so that herbs were gathered when they were at their most potent; old herbals often give detailed instructions as to when to gather plants – at what time of day, phase of the moon or in which sign of the zodiac.

Today, many of these traditions appear bizarre and groundless, but often they did in fact pinpoint the time of year when the herb was at its peak. Vervain, for example, was gathered when the dog star, Sirius, could be seen in the heavens (during the so-called "dog days" from early July to August), which – in the northern hemisphere – is generally a time when the plant is coming into flower and is probably at its best. Sage was reputedly best "in May" and it is generally at its peak just before flowering time, which usually starts in early June.

Harvesting traditions such as these survive most obviously today in Tibetan medicine, in which herbs are often collected at times that are astrologically significant for the individual patient. The practitioner will study the history of the disease, the precise time of onset and so on, and will then choose the correct time to collect the remedy in this particular case.

For Western herb gatherers, however, more prosaic considerations include collecting the herbs on a dry day, which makes them easier to preserve, and when the plants are at the peak of maturity so that the concentration of active ingredients is highest.

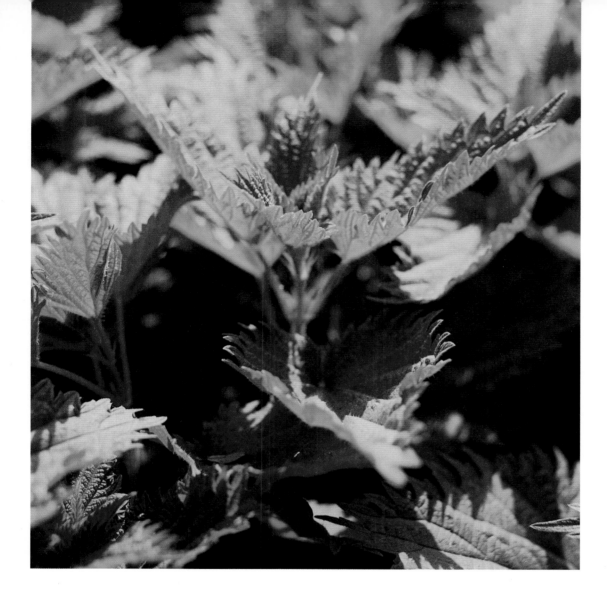

flowers

These should be collected when fully open and handled carefully as they are easily damaged. Small flowers such as lavender can be dried on their stems but if the stem is fleshy – like mullein – the flowers must be removed and dried individually. It is best to keep the flowers whole if possible and separate the petals once they are dry. An easy way to dry individual flowers is to spread them on trays and place in an airing cupboard for a couple of days.

leaves

Large leaves (such as burdock) can be gathered individually, but smaller ones (such as lemon balm) are best left on the stem. Leaves of deciduous herbs should generally be gathered just before flowering; evergreen ones like rosemary can be collected throughout the year. Sometimes young leaves are picked early in the season for cooking or spring tonics – such as stinging nettles or dandelions for use in soups and salads. A second crop of the more mature leaves can then be taken closer to flowering time. Coltsfoot and butterbur leaves appear after the flowers and should be gathered then.

aerial parts

If you are using all the aerial parts (leaves, stem, flowers and seed-head) then the best time to collect is in the midst of flowering, giving a mixture of all of them. Skullcap, for example, should be collected when at least half or more of the flowers have formed the characteristic cap-shaped seed pod.

seeds

These should be collected when ripe. For plants with large seed-heads such as fennel, it is best to gather them when around two-thirds of the seeds on a particular head are ripe and before too many have been dispersed by the wind or taken by birds.

fruit

Berries and other fruits should be gathered when just ripe, before the fruit becomes too soft or pulpy to dry effectively.

roots

Roots are generally gathered in the autumn when the aerial parts of the plant have died down and before the ground becomes too hard to make digging difficult. An exception is dandelion, whose roots should be gathered in spring when the carbohydrate content of the root is at its lowest and the concentration of medicinal constituents is thus greater.

bark

This is generally best collected in the autumn, when the sap is falling, to minimise damage to the plant. Never remove all the bark – or a band of bark completely surrounding a tree – unless you really do want to sacrifice the plant to herbal medicine.

saps and resin

These can be collected from trees by making a deep incision in the bark in autumn when the sap is falling. In most cases a cup attached to the tree will be an adequate receptacle, but sometimes a large bucket may be needed: a substantial amount of birch sap, for example, can be collected overnight at certain times of year. Aloe gel can be obtained by splitting the leaf open and scraping the thick gelatinous sap into a bowl using the blunt side of a knife. Latex from plants such as wild lettuce and greater celandine can be extracted by squeezing the leaf stems over a bowl. Many saps can be corrosive, so protective gloves should be worn. Saps can generally be stored for a few days in a refrigerator or can be preserved by boiling to form a reduced paste.

bulbs and corms

These should be gathered after the aerial parts have died down. Collect garlic corms quickly as they tend to move downwards in the soil once the leaves have wilted and can be difficult to find.

drying herbs

Herbs need to be dried as quickly as possible and away from bright sunlight to preserve the aromatic ingredients and prevent oxidation of other chemicals. A good circulation of air is also needed, so tie stems in small bunches. A dry

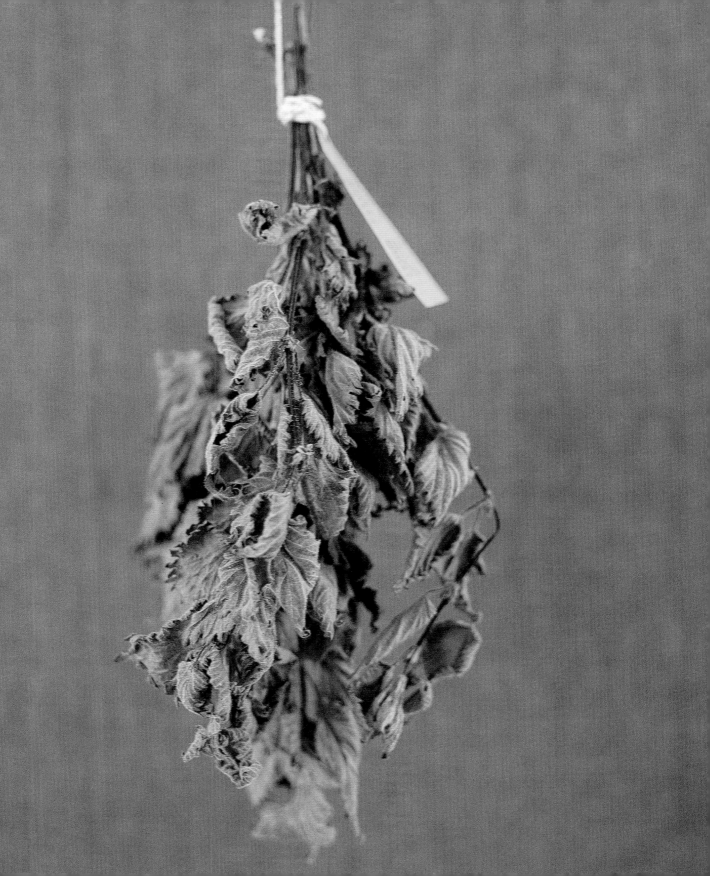

garden shed with a low-powered fan heater running is ideal, although an airing cupboard with door left ajar or a spare bedroom are also suitable. Avoid drying herbs in garages as they can become contaminated with petrol fumes. In warm conditions with a good circulation of air it is possible to dry herbs completely within five or six days, sometimes even less. The longer the plant takes to dry the more likely it is to discolour and lose its flavour. Ideally the temperature in the drying room should be between 20-32°C/70-90°F and should never go above 38°C/100°F.

With experience, it is possible to know precisely when the herbs are dry enough to bottle. They should be crumbled gently and stored in clean dry jars or pots with air-tight lids. If the herbs are stored when still slightly damp they will go mouldy. Jars should ideally be of coloured glass or pottery or kept out of direct sunlight which speeds deterioration. Do not store herbs in metal or plastic containers.

Some people use a microwave oven for drying herbs but research work has shown that such radiation can cause changes to the complex chemicals in herbs with entirely new substances, of unknown toxicity or efficacy, being produced in the process. It is therefore best to avoid this technique for medicinal herbs.

Some herbs freeze well – especially fennel, dill, parsley and basil. They can be chopped and frozen in ice cube trays or wrapped in plastic film in small bunches. This is ideal for culinary use but the sort of quantities needed for medicinal applications generally makes freezing impractical.

Remember to label dried herbs with the variety, source and date. If dried and stored properly, most will keep for 12-18 months without significant deterioration. However, there are exceptions: valerian and hops both change their chemical composition over time, so the action of the herb can vary with age.

flowers

Collect the flowers on a dry day when the morning dew has evaporated and remove obvious dirt, grit, insects, etc. Then spread the flower heads on newspaper or trays and place in the airing cupboard or in a warm spare room to dry. Lavender flowers are best treated like seeds and dried in bunches covered with a loosely tied paper bag. Small flowers can be left intact but marigold petals are best pulled from the flower heads when dried and the central part of the flower discarded. Store in dark glass/pottery containers or in cupboards.

leaves/aerial parts

Collect on a dry day and tie in small bunches of about five to eight stems which can be hung in a garden shed, spare room or other dry, airy, warm place. When the leaves are brittle, but not so dry that they turn to powder when touched, the herb is ready. Always dry leafy herbs while still on the stem. Once dried, the leaves can easily be rubbed from the stem and the larger pieces discarded. If you are using the entire aerial parts of a plant, then flowers, stem, seed-heads and leaves can be crumbled together before storing.

seeds

Collect entire seed-heads, with about 15-25cm/6-10in of stalk, when the seeds are almost ripe and hang them in small bunches loosely covered with paper bags, away from direct sunlight. The seeds will fall off when they are ripe and will be collected in the bag during the following couple of weeks.

berries

These should be picked when just ripe and spread on trays in an airing cupboard. Fleshy fruits should be turned regularly to ensure even drying and that any berries with signs of mould are discarded.

roots

Wash roots thoroughly to remove soil and dirt. It is best to chop large roots into small pieces when still fresh as they can be difficult to cut when dry. Spread the pieces on trays and dry for two to three hours in a cooling oven (i.e. an oven with no direct heat). Repeat this process for large roots, then transfer to an airing cupboard or quiet sunny room to complete drying undisturbed. Roots need to be stored in dry, air-tight containers away from sunlight. Some tend to reabsorb moisture from the air and should be discarded if they become soft.

bark

Dust or wipe bark to remove moss or insects – avoid soaking in water too much. Then break into manageable pieces (1-3cm/1-1¼in square) and spread on trays in an airing cupboard or warm, dry, airy room.

buying dried herbs

For those with limited growing space, there is now – fortunately – a good choice of suppliers of dried herb both in shops and by mail order (see page 251). Always buy in small quantities (250-500g/8oz-1lb) to avoid unnecessary home storage and where possible examine material before buying to check on quality. Choose herbs which have a good colour and aroma and are not faded or musty-smelling.

Avoid shops which display herbs in clear glass jars on sunny shelves – the quality will probably be disappointing. Poor storage can lead to rapid deterioration with mouse droppings, mould and insects among unwanted pollutants.

Ideally buy organic herbs or those labelled as "wild crafted", which means they have been collected in the wild rather than grown as a commercial – and often heavily sprayed – cash crop. Although, in the interests of conservation, it is best to avoid wild-crafted supplies of rare species such as golden seal or some types of echinacea. Poor harvesting can lead to many unwanted additions – dried grass, for example, is often found with herbs which have been gathered from meadow areas. With practice, one soon learns to recognise the characteristics of many dried herbs so it becomes easier to check on the accuracy of labels. Skullcap, for example, has characteristic seed pods, agrimony has small burrs and many herbs can be identified from their aroma.

Mistakes can and do happen, however. A classic error was confusion over wood sage (*Teucrium scorodonia*) and skullcap which for many years led to a description of wood sage being included in herbals under skullcap. Another well-documented error concerned the supplier who sold sea mayweed (*Matricaria maritima*) as feverfew – the plants are similar in appearance but the mayweed lacks feverfew's therapeutic constituents, so would be useless for treating migraine.

a medicinal herb garden

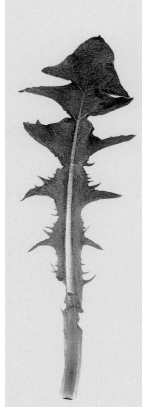

Many common garden flowers are actually potent medicinal plants, so the label "herb garden" can cover a multitude of specimens. Lily of the valley (*Convallaria majalis*), for example, is used by professional herbalists to treat heart problems, while in Chinese medicine decorative shrubs also have their uses: buddleia (*Buddleja davidii*) provides a remedy for cataracts and forsythia (*Forsythia suspensa*) is a favourite to clear deep-seated infections. Many of the wildflower healers listed in Part 2 of the book – such as shepherd's purse, dandelion and cleavers – can also usually be found lurking in weedy corners. Although many commonly grown culinary herbs, such as sage, thyme and parsley, are also useful medicinally, some of the more valuable therapeutic plants are unlikely to be grown in a basic herb garden, so it is well worth sowing some native wild flowers such as St John's wort, agrimony and wood betony.

Many of the plants discussed in detail in Part 2 are ideal to grow at home. Others that deserve a place in the medicinal herb garden include:

lady's mantle (*Alchemilla xanthoclora*) – the aerial parts are useful as a menstrual regulator and styptic. The dew which collects in lady's mantle leaves was once thought to contain magical properties.

heartsease or **wild pansy** (*Viola tricolor*) – ideal for a variety of skin conditions and inflammations, including nappy rash, heartsease is also used internally for coughs and chest problems. Use the aerial parts.

melilot or **king's clover** (*Melilotus officinalis*) is an excellent remedy for varicose veins and eczema. The plant is tall with bright yellow flowers. Collect while flowering and use in creams and washes.

southernwood (*Artemisia abrotanum*) is a highly aromatic shrubby perennial with delicate green/grey foliage. The plant can be rubbed on the skin to repel insects and is a traditional remedy to encourage hair growth – an infused oil massaged into the scalp can help thinning hair.

calamint (*Calamintha officinalis*) is a mint-scented perennial which will spread rapidly and can fill odd corners of the garden. It can be used to make a pleasant-tasting tea for indigestion and stomach upsets while Culpeper recommended it for all "afflictions of the brain" and the plant was once popular for nervous excitability and hysteria.

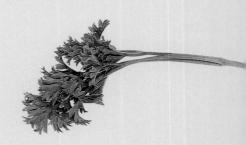

goat's rue (*Galega officinalis*) makes a splendid clump at the back of a herbaceous border with attractive pink/white flowers during much of the summer. It was traditionally used to stimulate milk flow in breast-feeding but will also help to reduce blood sugar levels and is useful to control late onset diabetes.

bergamot (*Monarda didyma*) is not to be confused with the bitter orange peel oil of the same name. It is a colourful plant flowering in mid-summer with showy red or purple blooms and was brewed as oswego tea by native Americans. It was also taken for digestive upsets, nausea and diarrhoea. The leaves can be used in cooking to provide a gentle minty flavouring and are also antiseptic so can be a useful addition to teas to combat colds and infections.

nasturtiums (*Tropaeolum majus*) are a colourful addition to any garden. The flowers are edible and can be added to salads while the leaves are bitter, antiseptic and increase urination so can helpful for urinary infections, wounds, or to stimulate the digestion.

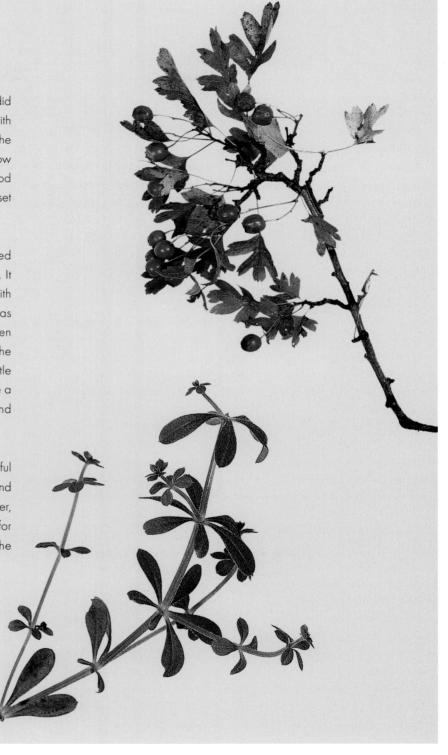

glossary

adrenal cortex part of the adrenal gland located above the kidneys, which produces several steroidal hormones.

agni the digestive fire of Ayurvedic medicine (see below).

alkaloid active plant constituent containing nitrogen and which usually has a significant effect on bodily function.

allergen any substance which triggers an allergic response.

allopathy prevalent system of Western medicine which treats illness by prescribing substances to provoke an opposite condition from the disease – thus a fever is treated with temperature suppressants or an ache with painkillers.

alterative a substance which improves the function of various organs – notably those involved with the breakdown and excretion of waste products – to bring about a gradual change of state.

amino acids the building blocks of proteins.

amoebacidal kills amoeba.

analgesic relieves pain.

anaesthetic causes local or general loss of sensation.

anaphrodisiac reduces sexual desire and excitement.

anodyne allays pain.

antacid corrects the effects of stomach acid and relieves indigestion.

antibiotic destroys or inhibits the growth of micro-organisms such as bacteria and fungi.

anti-bacterial destroys or inhibits the growth of bacteria.

anti-fungal destroys or inhibits the growth of fungi.

anti-inflammatory reduces inflammation.

anti-microbial destroys or inhibits the growth of micro-organisms such as bacteria.

anti-oxidant prevents or slows the natural deterioration of cells that occurs as they age due to oxidation.

anti-rheumatic relieves the symptoms of rheumatism.

antiseptic controls or prevents infection.

antispasmodic reduces muscle spasm and tension.

anti-tussive inhibits the cough reflex, helping to stop coughing.

aperient a very mild laxative.

aphrodisiac promotes sexual excitement.

aril fleshy or hairy outgrowth of certain seeds.

arteriosclerosis build up of fatty deposits in the blood vessels leading to narrowing and hardening, and associated with heart disease and strokes.

astringent used to describe a herb which will precipitate proteins from the surface of cells or membranes causing tissues to contract and tighten; forms a protective coating and stops bleeding and discharges.

Ayurvedic system of medicine which originated in southern India around 5000BC based on a model of body humours (see below) and the inner life force *prana* (see below)

Bach Flower Remedies extracts of flowers collected as dew and preserved in brandy, discovered by Dr Edward Bach in the 1930s and widely used to treat emotional upsets and disturbances (see p. 48 for details of Dr Bach's 38 healers).

bactericidal kills bacteria.

beta-carotene an orange-yellow plant pigment which is converted in the body into vitamin A.

biennial a plant which lives for two years.

bile thick, bitter fluid secreted by the liver and stored in the gall bladder, which aids the digestion of fats.

bitter stimulates secretion of digestive juices.

blood clotting the process by which the proteins in blood are changed from a liquid to a solid by an enzyme, in order to check bleeding.

blood sugar levels of glucose in the blood.

bronchial relating to the air passages of the lungs.

bulk laxative increases the volume of faeces producing larger, softer stools.

capillary permeability the exchange of carbon dioxide, oxygen, salts and water between the blood in capillaries and tissues.

carcinogenic causes cancer.

carminative expels gas from the stomach and intestines to relieve flatulence, digestive colic and gastric discomfort.

cathartic a strong, purging laxative.

cerebral circulation blood supply to the brain.

cholagogue stimulates bile flow from the gall bladder and bile ducts into the duodenum.

choleric one of the Galenic (see below) temperaments associated with yellow bile, heat and dryness.

cholesterol fat-like material present in the blood and most tissues which is an important constituent of cell membranes, steroidal hormones and bile salts. Excess cholesterol has been blamed for the build-up of fatty deposits in the blood vessels seen in arteriosclerosis.

choleretic increases the secretion of bile by the liver.

circulatory stimulant increases blood flow.

cleansing herb a herb that improves the excretion of waste products from the body.

colitis inflammation of the colon (lower bowel)

cooling used to describe herbs that are often bitter or relaxing and will help to reduce internal heat and hyperactivity.

coumarin active plant constituent which affects blood clotting.

decongestant relieves congestion, usually nasal.

demulcent softens and soothes damaged or inflamed surfaces, such as the gastric mucous membranes.

depressant reduces nervous or functional activity.

diaphoretic increases sweating.

diuretic encourages urine flow.

Doctrine of Signatures a mediaeval theory which argued that plants contained clues to their medicinal properties in their appearance: yellow flowered herbs, for example, were believed to be helpful for jaundice while pilewort with its nodular roots was clearly ideal for treating haemorrhoids. Some of these interpretations were in fact quite valid (pilewort *is* good for haemorrhoids and yellow-flowered dandelion makes a good liver herb) although others, now largely forgotten, were less accurate. Similar beliefs are found in most cultures worldwide.

emetic causes vomiting.

emollient softens and soothes the skin.

essential fatty acids these are classified by chemical structure and the two groups most commonly found in supplements are known as omega-six and omega-three acids. The omega-six group includes arachidonic acid and *gamma*-linolenic acid (GLA) while the omega-three category includes linoleic acid, *alpha*-linolenic acid and two commonly found in fish oil – eicosapentanoeic acid (EPA) and docasahexaenic acid (DHA). In recent years these acids have been found to be of significant nutritional importance and lack of them is believed to contribute to a very wide range of common Western ills – including arthritis, skin diseases, menstrual and menopausal problems and heart disease. A number of acids can be metabolised in the body from linoleic acid but only when in its chemical *cis*-linoleic form. Commercially produced vegetable oils often convert this form into *trans*-linoleic acid in processing and this is less beneficial. *Gamma*-linolenic acid is found in evening primrose oil, borage oil and blackcurrant oil and these oils also contain substantial amounts of *cis*-linoleic acid. *Alpha*-linoleic acid is found in significant amounts in linseed, hemp seed, and pumpkin seed oils with less in walnut and soy bean oils. Not all essential fatty acids are beneficial – erucic acid is believed to damage heart tissue, for example, and is found in high proportion in certain varieties of rape seed (and in trace amounts in some borage seed extracts). The essential fatty acids are important in the production of prostaglandins (see below). More than 50 of these have been identified and they have wide-ranging and important functions in the body. The PGE_1 series is particularly beneficial and these are often at low-levels in people who are prone to allergies, depressives, alcoholics, and diabetics. In the usual metabolic pathway *cis*-linoleic is converted to *gamma*-linolenic acid which in turn is made into *dihomogamma*-linolenic acid in the body, which is then used to make PGE_1.

essential oil volatile chemicals extracted from plants by such techniques as steam distillation; highly active and aromatic.

expectorant enhances the secretion or sputum from the respiratory tract so that it is easier to cough up.

febrifuge reduces fever.

flavonoids active plant constituents which improve the circulation and may also have diuretic, anti-inflammatory and anti-spasmodic effects.

Galenic traditional Western medicine practised throughout Europe until the 18th century and largely based on ancient Greek principles dating back to Hippocrates. The theory took its name from Galen, a Roman physician, and regards human health and temperament as controlled by four bodily humours: phlegm, yellow bile, black bile and blood giving rise to the temperaments: Phlegmatic, Choleric, Melancholic, and Sanguine (see below).

gamma-**linolenic acid (GLA)** see Essential fatty acids.

haemostatic stops bleeding.

hormone a chemical substance produced in the body which can affect the way tissues behave. Hormones can control sexual function as well as emotional and physical activity.

humours substances associated with bodily states or temperaments in both Galenic (see above) and Ayurvedic medicine. The Galenic humours were blood, yellow bile, black bile and phlegm. Ayurvedic humours are *vata*, *pitta,* and *kapha*.

hyperacidity excessive digestive acid causing a burning sensation.

hyperglycaemic increases blood sugar levels.

hypertensive raises blood pressure.

hypoglycaemic reduces blood sugar levels.

hypotensive lowers blood pressure.

kapha phlegm, an Ayurvedic humour associated with earth and water elements.

labyrinth the inner ear.

laxative encourages bowel motions.

lipids fat-like chemicals (such as

cholesterol) which are present in most tissues and are important structural materials for the body.

lubricant reduces friction.

melancholic one of the Galenic (see above) temperaments associated with black bile, cold and dryness.

Meniére's disease a disorder of the iner ear which leads to nausea, vertigo, tinnitus and deafness. The cause is largely unknown.

menthol a volatile oil with a peppermint aroma extracted from various mints (including peppermint), which is carminative, locally anaesthetic, decongestant and antiseptic. Used in a number of herbal products for colds and indigestion.

mucilage complex sugar molecules found in plants that are soft and slippery and provide protection for the mucous membranes and inflamed surfaces.

nervine herb that affects the nervous system and which may be stimulating or sedating.

peripheral circulation blood supply to the limbs, skin and muscles (including heart muscles).

peristalsis the waves of involuntary contractions in the digestive tract which move food and waste products through the system.

phlegm catarrhal-like secretion or sputum. In both Galenic (see above) and Oriental medicine phlegm is a more complex entity related in internal balance and sometimes associated with spleen deficiency.

phlegmatic one of the Galenic (see above) temperaments associated with phlegm, cold and dampness.

photosensitivity desensitive to light.

physiomedicalism system of medicine developed in 19th-century North America which focused on disease as a result of cold conditions.

pineal gland a pea-shaped mass of tissue found in the brain, believed to have some function in sexual development and known to secrete melatonin.

pitta bile, an Ayurvedic humour associated with the fire element.

pituitary gland – a major gland in the endocrine system controlling production of of many vital hormones. Located at the base of the skull.

prana the inner life force of Ayurvedic medicine (see above) associated with breath.

prostaglandins hormone-like substances that have a wide range of functions in the body. They can act as chemical messengers and some also cause uterine contractions. Various series of prostaglandins are known usually as PGE_1, PGE_2, etc.

pungent having an acrid smell and bitter flavour.

purgative drastic laxative.

pyrrolizidine alkaloids chemicals found in a number of plants (including comfrey, borage and coltsfoot) which in excess can be associated with liver damage although many regard the research evidence for this as inconclusive.

Qi (ch'i) the body's vital energy as defined in Chinese medicine.

relaxant relaxes tense and overactive nerves and tissues.

rubefacient a substance which stimulates blood flow to the skin causing local reddening.

sanguine one of the Galenic (see above) temperaments associated with blood, heat and dampness. It was regarded in the Middle Ages as the ideal temperament.

saponins active plant constituents similar to soap and producing a lather with water. They can irritate the mucous membranes of the digestive tract which, by reflex, has an expectorant action. Some saponins are chemically similar to steroidal hormones.

sedative reduces anxiety and tension.

simple a herb used as a remedy on its own.

soporific induces drowsiness and sleep.

stimulant increases activity.

styptic stops external bleeding.

systemic affecting the whole body.

tannin active plant constituents which are astringent and combine with proteins. The term is derived from plants used in tanning leather.

thyroid gland in the neck which controls metabolism and growth; it requires iodine for normal function.

tincture liquid herbal extract made by soaking plant material in a mixture of alcohol and water.

tisane an infusion.

tonic restoring, nourishing and supporting for the entire body.

tonify a tonic action: strengthening and restoring for the system.

topical local administration of a herbal remedy.

vata wind, an Ayurvedic humour associated with air and aether elements.

venous return the blood flow back to the lungs and heart from the body's extremities.

volatile oils complex, often aromatic, substances with a low boiling point which rapidly evaporate in the air. The smells associated with different herbs and extracts are often due to such oils.

vulnerary wound herb.

warming a remedy which increases body temperature and encourages digestive function and circulation. Warming herbs are often spicy and pungent to taste.

yang in Chinese theory, aspect of being equated with male energy dry, hot, light, ascending.

yin In Chinese theory, aspect of being equated with female energy – damp, cold, dark, descending.

consulting a herbalist

While over-the-counter herbal remedies can be helpful for a range of ailments, more serious problems need professional help. Approaches to herbal medicine vary considerably around the world. In the UK, primary health care is dominated by conventionally trained general practitioners whose attitudes to alternative or complementary therapies range from the sympathetic to openly hostile: a few GPs may be trained in herbal or homeopathic medicine or, if not, may be willing to refer patients to suitable practitioners but many more dismiss herbal medicine as "quackery". In France herbal practitioners or *"phytotherapists"* are almost always trained doctors who have studied plant medicine at post-graduate level while in Germany, alternative practitioners qualify as *"Heilpraktiker"* and have comparable status to orthodox GPs.

In China, traditional herbal medicine is available in special hospitals as an alternative to Western medicine, while in Japan herbal remedies are available on the equivalent of the National Health Service. In some countries – including some states of the USA – it is illegal for anyone to prescribe herbal remedies or set themselves up as a herbal practitioner, although self-medication with herbs is permitted. In other countries just about anyone – well trained or not – can set up in business as a medical herbalist and dispense all manner of inappropriate "cures".

Britain's unique tradition

Britain is probably unique within Europe in having a well-established and reputable system for training herbal practitioners, who have not necessarily obtained any other medical qualifications. The National Institute of Medical Herbalists was founded in 1864 and until recently members qualified by examination after four or five years of specialist study. Now several UK universities offer first degrees in herbal medicine and graduates can apply for membership of the institute after a further period of clinical experience guided by established practitioners. Members of the National Institute use the initials MNIMH or FNIMH after their names which gives the patient some guarantee that they are consulting a suitably trained practitioner.

The UK's other main professional herbal body is The General Council and Register of Herbalists whose members use the initials MH. It has a rather different philosophical approach from that usually adopted by the NIMH practitioners with its members tending more towards homoeopathy: herbal tinctures are likely to be prescribed in drop doses rather than the teaspoonful generally favoured by NIMH members. A third, more recently formed organisation is the Register of Traditional Chinese Medicine whose members largely use a combination of acupuncture and Chinese herbs, while an association of Ayurvedic pracitioners has also recently been formed to help standardise training in this area, too.

visiting a practitioner

Consulting a professional herbalist is not all that different from visiting a GP – or rather, visiting a GP as one would have done 40 or 50 years ago. Indeed, many herbalists liken their approach to that of the old-fashioned family physician – using a lot of patient listening and probing questions to uncover all the relevant symptoms, along with time-honoured diagnostic techniques: feeling pulses, looking at tongues, testing urine and with clinical examinations dependent on palpation, auscultation and percussion rather than laboratory tests. A first consultation will generally take at least an hour and subsequent ones 20 minutes or so. A wide range of ailments is commonly treated: both the sort of problems one may normally take to a GP – infections, aches and pains, menstrual disorders, high blood pressure, urinary dysfunction, digestive problems etc. – and those chronic conditions for which herbalism is often seen as a "last resort", such as rheumatoid arthritis, ME, emphysema and so on.

As well as reviewing the current illness, the herbalist will ask about medical history – previous health problems that may be contributing to the current imbalance, family tendencies and allergies, diet, lifestyle, stresses and worries.

Examinations may include taking blood pressure and pulses, palpating the abdomen to identify the cause of pain or discomfort, listening to chest wheezes (auscultation) or checking the degree of movement in an arthritic knee or shoulder. Simple clinical tests undertaken on site could include urine analysis or measuring haemoglobin levels using a tiny drop of blood. Existing orthodox medication also needs to be checked.

complementary treatments

Herbalists would certainly not recommend dropping vital drugs, but any incompatibility of these with herbal remedies obviously needs to be considered when prescribing plant medicines. Similarly, many patients turn to herbs because they are anxious to phase-out their drugs, for whatever reason, and a safe programme of replacing them with gentler herbal remedies needs to be devised – preferably with the support and co-operation of the patient's GP. Herbal remedies, for example, can be very helpful for sufferers trying to break an addiction to tranquillisers or sleeping pills – or as alternatives for those suffering the side-effects from non-steroidal anti-inflammatory drugs used for arthritis.

At the end of the consultation, the patient does not simply leave with a prescription for the local pharmacist to dispense. In Britain, few pharmacies are willing to stock the hundreds of tinctures, creams, oils, powders, capsules or dried herbs that the medical herbalist needs to keep in stock, so medical herbalists are permitted by law to make and dispense their own remedies. This was, until recently, the situation in Ireland as well, although, in 2000, changes were made to the law there and many herbal remedies are now available on prescription only.

As well as a combination of herbs, specially selected to help the unique health problems of each individual, the patient may leave the consultation room with a list of dietary suggestions, foods to avoid or details of those to eat more of. There may also be recommended relaxation routines to follow or Bach Flower Remedies to help emotional factors affecting physical well-being. Or perhaps the patient will be sent away with a small growing plant to bring a little love and beauty into their life. Whatever the remedy, healing is a two-way process and the patient must take responsibility for their own health and actively participate in any cure. Those who expect a "magic pill" to solve their problems with little of their own effort, may be happier with orthodox therapies.

Generally herbalists like to see patients fairly soon after the first consultation to check on progress – perhaps after two or three weeks – with regular meetings every four to six weeks for six months or more in chronic cases. Herbal medication is likely to be altered slightly after each consultation to reflect changes in the condition.

all sorts of therapy

Just as all patients are different, so too are all herbalists and finding a practitioner with whom you feel empathy and can trust, can be just as important in treatment as taking the right herbs. Some herbalists follow a semi-orthodox path prescribing remedies to ease symptoms just as modern drugs do, others will focus on holistic treatments urging major lifestyle changes. Some will use only Western herbs, others a combination of Chinese or Ayurvedic remedies. Some will talk mainly of pathological conditions, others will suggest Qi stagnation, allergies or define just about anything in terms of emotional stress. Some will depend on the consulting couch and the results of clinical tests for diagnosis – others will swing a pendulum or try applied kinesiology (a manipulative theraphy based on muscle testing techniques). If possible, choose your practitioner by personal recommendation from like-minded friends to ensure a good relationship with someone who understands your problem and whom you can also understand.

further reading

Bartram, T. (1995) *Encyclopaedia of Herbal Medicine*, Grace Publishers, Christchurch.

Benfield, H., and Korngold, E. (1991) *Betwen Heaven and Earth: A guide to Chinese medicine*, Ballantine Books, New York.

Bown, D. (1995) *Encyclopaedia of Herbs and their Uses*, Dorling Kindersley, London.

Brooke, E. (1992) *A Woman's Book of Herbs,* The Women's Press, London.

Chancellor, P. M. (1971) *Handbook of the Bach Flower Remedies*, C W Daniels, Saffron Walden.

Conway, P. (2001) *Tree Medicine,* Piatkus, London.

Davis, P. (1995) *Aromatherapy: An A-Z,* 2nd Edition, C W Daniels, Saffron Walden.

Erasmus, U. (1986) *Fats and Oils,* Alive Books, Canada.

Foster, S., and Yue, C. (1992) *Herbal Emissaries,* Healing Arts Press, Rochester, VT.

Frawley, D., and Lad, V. (1986) *The Yoga of Herbs,* Lotus Press, Santa Fe.

Frawley, D. (1989) *Ayurvedic Healing: A Comprehensive Guide,* Passage Press, Salt Lake City, Utah.

Griggs, B. (1981) *Green Pharmacy,* Jill Norman & Hobhouse, London.

Gursche, S. (1993) *Healing with Herbal Juices,* Alive Books, Canada.

Harrison, J. (1984) *Love Your Disease,* Angus & Robertson, Sydney.

Hobbs, C. (1995) *Medicinal Mushrooms,* Botanica Press, Santa Cruz.

Maury, M, (1974) "How to cure yourself with wine" in Montignac, M.

(1991) *Dine Out and Lose Weight,* Editions Artulan, Paris.

McIntyre, A. (1988) *Herbs for Pregnancy and Childbirth,* Sheldon Press, London.

Mills, S. Y. (1991) *Out of the Earth,* Viking, London.

Newell, C. A., Anderson, L. A., and Phillipson, J. D. (1996) *Herbal Medicines,* The Pharmaceutical Press, London.

Ody, P. (2000) *The Complete Guide: Medicinal Herbal,* Dorling Kindersley, London.

Ody, P. (2000) *Practical Chinese Medicine,* Godsfeld Press, London.

Ody, P., Lyon, A., and Vilinac, D. (2001) *The Chinese Herbal Cookbook,* Kyle Cathie, London.

Ody, P. (2001) *The Holistic Herbal Directory,* Chartwell Books, New Jersey.

Rogers, C. (1995) *The Women's Guide to Herbal Medicine,* Hamish Hamilton, London.

Strelow, W., and Hertzka, G. (1988) *Hildegard of Bingen's Medicine,* Bear & Co., Sante Fe.

Vogel, V. J. (1970) *American Indian Medicine,* University of Oklahoma Press.

Weiss, R. F. (1988) *Herbal Medicine,* Beaconsfield Publishers, Beaconsfield.

Wren, R. C. (1988) *Potter's New Cyclopaedia of Botanical Drugs and Preparations,* C W Daniels, Saffron Walden.

useful addresses

associations and professional bodies

British Herbal Medicine Association, Sun House, Church Street, Stroud, Gloucestershire GL5 1JL.

College of Ayurveda, 20 Annes Grove, Great Lifod, Milton Keynes MK14 5DR.

The General Council and Register of Consultant Herbalists, Marlborough House, Swanpool, Falmouth, Cornwall TR11 4HW.

The Herb Society, Deddington Hill Farm, Warmington, Banbury, Oxon OX17 1XB.

National Institute of Medical Herbalists, 56 Longbrook Street, Exeter, Devon EX4 6AH.

The Natural Medicines Group, PO Box 5, Ilkeston, Derbyshire DE7 8LX.

The Register of Chinese Herbal Medicine, 19 Trinity Road, London N2 8JJ.

mail order herb suppliers

G. Baldwin & Co, 171-174 Walworth Road, London SE17 1RW.

East West Herbs Ltd, Langston Priory Mews, Kingham, Oxon OX7 6UW.

Greenways (Ayurvedic herbs), The Old Clinic, 10 St John's Square, Glastonbury, Somerset BA6 9LJ.

Hambledon Herbs, Court Farm, Milverton, Somerset TA4 1NF.

Neal's Yard Remedies, 26-34 Ingate Place, London SW8 3NS.

nurseries and specialist suppliers

Cheshire Herbs, Fourfields, Forest Road, Little Budworth, Tarporeley, Cheshire CW6 9ES.

Iden Croft Herbs, Frittenden Road, Staplehurst, Kent TN12 0DN.

The Cottage Herbery, Mill House, Boraston, Tenbury Wells, Worcs. WR15 8LZ.

The Herb Garden, Hall View Cottage, Hardstoft, Pilsley, Chesterfield, Derbyshire.

National Herb Centre, Banbury Road, Warmington, Banbury, Oxon OX17 1DF.

Poyntzfield Herb Nursery, Black Isle, By Dingwall, Ross & Cromarty IV7 8LX.

index

Picture Acknowledgements

LH: Laura Hodgson   GPL: Garden Picture Library   Holt: Holt International

1, 2–3, 5, 7 LH; 14 Friedrich Strauss/GPL; 15 LH; 22 Lamontagne/GPL; 23 Jerry Pavia/GPL; 28 David Cavagnaro/GPL; 29 Nigel Cattlin/Holt; 34 Nigel Cattlin/Holt; 35 Inga Spence/Holt; 38 Duncan Spence/Holt; 41 (left) Rosie Mayer/Holt; 41 (right) Nigel Cattlin/Holt; 43 Nigel Cattlin/Holt; 47 (left) Tim Spence/GPL; 47 (right) Howard Rice/GPL; 52 (above) Rowan McOnegal; 52 (below) Erika Craddock/GPL; 57 Nigel Cattlin/Holt; 61 (above) Nigel Cattlin/Holt; 61 (below) A I Lord/GPL; 63 (left) Neil Holmes/GPL; 63 (right) Mark Bolton/GPL; 67 Primrose Peacock/Holt; 68–9, 70–1, 72–3 LH; 74 Jacqui Hurst/GPL; 75 Tim Spence/GPL; 76 Brigitte Thomas/GPL; 77 Peter Wilson/Holt; 78 Howard Rice/GPL; 79 Inga Spence/Holt; 81, 83 Nigel Cattlin/Holt; 84 Sunniva Harte/GPL; 85 Christi Carter/GPL; 87 A I Lord/GPL; 88–9 David Burton/Holt; 90 Willem Harinck/Holt; 91 Nigel Cattlin/Holt; 92 Juliette Wade/GPL; 93 Christi Carter/GPL; 95 Alan & Linda Detrick/Holt; 96 Friedrich Strauss/GPL; 97 John Miller/GPL; 98 Michel Viard/GPL; 99 John Glover/GPL; 101 Bob Gibbons/Holt; 102–3 LH; 104 Mayer/Le Scanff/GPL; 105 Primrose Peacock/Holt; 107 Nigel Cattlin/Holt; 108 John Glover/GPL; 109 Nigel Cattlin/Holt; 110 Howard Rice/GPL; 112–3 Nigel Cattlin/Holt; 114 (main picture) Lamontagne/GPL; 114 (inset) David Cavagnaro/GPL; 116 Emma Peios/GPL; 117 P Karunakaran/Holt; 118 Willem Harinck/Holt; 120 Nigel Cattlin/Holt; 121 Inga Spence/Holt; 122 Nigel Cattlin/Holt; 123 Mayer/Le Scanff/GPL; 125 (main picture) Ron Sutherland/GPL; 125 (inset) Linda Burgess/GPL; 126 Lamontagne/GPL; 127 (main picture) Mayer/Le Scanff/GPL; 127 (inset) Mark Bolton/GPL; 128 Christopher Gallagher/GPL; 130 Friedrich Strauss/GPL; 131 Inga Spence/Holt; 132 (both pictures) Nigel Cattlin/Holt; 133, 134 Inga Spence/Holt; 137 (main picture) Nigel Cattlin/Holt; 137 (inset) Inga Spence/Holt; 138–9 LH; 140 A I Lord/GPL; 144 Alan & Linda Detrick/Holt; 147 Mark Bolton/GPL; 151 Chris Burrows/GPL; 154 Nigel Cattlin/Holt; 159 Janet Sorrell/GPL; 161 J S Sira/GPL; 163 Primrose Peacock/Holt; 164–5 LH; 166 Howard Rice/GPL; 167 Nigel Cattlin/Holt; 168 Rowan McOnegal; 169 Nigel Cattlin/Holt; 170, 171, 172 Bob Gibbons/Holt; 173, 174, 175, 176 Nigel Cattlin/Holt; 177 (left) Mayer/Le Scanff/GPL; 177 (right) Bob Gibbons/Holt; 178 Juliette Wade/GPL; 179 Sunniva Harte/GPL; 180 Deni Bown; 181 Inga Spence/Holt; 182 Nigel Cattlin/Holt; 183 (left) Rowan McOnegal; 183 (right) Deni Bown; 184–5 Rowan McOnegal; 186 John Glover/GPL; 187 Bob Gibbons/Holt; 188 Peter Wilson/Holt; 189 (left) Nigel Cattlin/Holt; 189 (right) Sunniva Harte/GPL; 190 Geoff Dann/GPL; 191 Nigel Cattlin/Holt; 192 Bob Gibbons/Holt; 193 Nigel Cattlin/Holt; 194 Rowan McOnegal; 195 Duncan Smith/Holt; 196 Juliette Wade/GPL; 197 Bob Gibbons/Holt; 198 Nigel Cattlin/Holt; 199 (left) Christopher Gallagher/GPL; 199 (right) Nigel Cattlin/Holt; 200 (left) Janet Sorrell/GPL; 200 (right) Howard Rice/GPL; 201 Rowan McOnegal; 202 Howard Rice/GPL; 203 Heather Angel; 204; 205 Nigel Cattlin/Holt; 206 LH; 207 Nigel Cattlin/Holt; 208 Wayne Hutchinson/Holt; 209 Phil McLean/Holt; 210–11, 213, 215, 217, 220, 222, 225, 227, 229, 230, 233, 235, 239, 241, 244–5 LH